Applied Cranial-Cerebral Anatomy

Applied Cranial-Cerebral Anatomy

Brain Architecture and Anatomically Oriented Microneurosurgery

Guilherme C. Ribas
Hospital Israelita Albert Einstein

CAMBRIDGE
UNIVERSITY PRESS

CAMBRIDGE
UNIVERSITY PRESS

Shaftesbury Road, Cambridge CB2 8EA, United Kingdom

One Liberty Plaza, 20th Floor, New York, NY 10006, USA

477 Williamstown Road, Port Melbourne, VIC 3207, Australia

314–321, 3rd Floor, Plot 3, Splendor Forum, Jasola District Centre, New Delhi – 110025, India

103 Penang Road, #05–06/07, Visioncrest Commercial, Singapore 238467

Cambridge University Press is part of Cambridge University Press & Assessment, a department of the University of Cambridge.

We share the University's mission to contribute to society through the pursuit of education, learning and research at the highest international levels of excellence.

www.cambridge.org
Information on this title: www.cambridge.org/9781107156784

DOI: 10.1017/9781316661567

First published 2018

A catalogue record for this publication is available from the British Library

Library of Congress Cataloging-in-Publication data
Names: Ribas, Guilherme, author.
Title: Applied cranial-cerebral anatomy : towards an understanding of human brain architecture and of an anatomically oriented microneurosurgery / Guilherme Ribas.
Description: Cambridge, United Kingdom ; New York, NY : Cambridge University Press, 2018. | Includes bibliographical references and index.
Identifiers : LCCN 2017043871 | ISBN 9781107156784 (hardback)
Subjects: | MESH: Brain – anatomy & histology | Skull – anatomy & histology | Brain – surgery
Classification: LCC QP360 | NLM WL 300 | DDC 612.8/2–dc23
LC record available at https://lccn.loc.gov/2017043871

ISBN 978-1-107-15678-4 Hardback

To my now quiet but eternal Tina . . .

Contents

Foreword

Neurosurgery is like bank robbery: you need to get in, get the money, and get out without being caught. The "success" of the "job" depends on a large number of considerations, starting with the question of whether the job is worth doing and what exactly it entails. There can hardly be a perfect robbery without perfect knowledge of the streets, corridors, basements, the building and neighborhood drainage and electricity infrastructure, security systems, etc. Sometimes, one may also need to study local geology, and architectural and construction history. Similarly, each stage, and ultimately the success of a "neurosurgical job," depends heavily on the understanding of anatomy, ontogenetic and phylogenetic history, and function of the brain, the skull, and the surrounding soft tissues. This book gives one a unique opportunity to gain and deepen such understanding.

Applied Cranial-Cerebral Anatomy is unique because of its author's unique credentials. Professor Guilherme C. Ribas has over three decades of experience in performing operations on the brain. He spent over three decades studying brain anatomy, initially as a fellow in the now legendary laboratory of Dr. Albert Rhoton (1932–2016) in Gainesville, Florida, and more recently, as a professor of anatomy at the University of São Paulo. For over two decades, he has been teaching and lecturing brain and applied brain anatomy in Brazil and around the world.

In 2005, together with Professor Ribas, we founded the Cambridge Lectures in Neurosurgical Anatomy. During the many Cambridge and lately also Southeast Asia editions of the Lectures, we marveled at the 3D photographs of his and his fellows' exquisite dissections. But no less we appreciated his didactic approaches to explaining the concepts behind the anatomical architecture of the brain. Together with many course delegates, we had suggested to Professor Ribas that he writes his lectures up as a book. We are thrilled to see it happen.

One of the most exciting features of this book is named in its subtitle, "the brain architecture." The brain's shape, its folds, fissures, gyri sulci, ventricles, and the relative relationships of substructures are not random; there is an order to it. The shapes have evolved throughout the millennia of phylogenesis and 40 weeks of intrauterine life (with only some minor changes thereafter). Knowledge of the order and architecture is relevant not only to medical students and neuroscientists, but to neurologists, psychiatrists, neuropsychologists, neuroradiologists, and neurosurgeons. The understanding of the choroidal fissure, for example, will help a neuroradiologist understand how an epidermoid tumor grows from the tectal cistern to the lateral ventricle with little or no impact on the function of the surrounding, highly eloquent brain. It will help the oncologist to explain the migration of cells in "multifocal gliomas" and plan radiotherapy more safely. It will make it easier for the neurosurgeon to understand the location of a lesion in relation to surrounding brain structures and to plan an optimal approach through the natural spaces to minimize the risk of brain injury. Deeper knowledge of white matter pathways and cortical and subcortical structures will help a speech and language specialist to better understand the neurological deficits and rehabilitation potential of patients with strokes and other focal lesions.

Much of the advanced imaging and navigation technology is too expensive and simply not affordable to the majority of patients with neurosurgical conditions worldwide. Yet, the knowledge of craniometric points as well as intrinsic brain anatomy detailed in this book can circumvent a great deal of the perceived handicap resulting from the lack of access to such technology. By the same token, having the latest gadgets does not replace the need of anatomical knowledge as "the fool with a tool is still a fool, only a more dangerous one."

As surprising as it may seem, neurosurgery can be performed with relatively little anatomical knowledge, just as it is possible to break into a bank by ramming a digger through the bank's wall. This, however, does not guarantee that any money can be taken or that one can get away with it. Gaining understanding of neuroanatomy is not easy and, let's be honest, never complete. It is, however, our duty as neurosurgeons and other clinicians to make our work more "accurate, gentle, and safe" (Dr. Albert Rhoton). This book goes a long way to help us on the never-ending quest for excellence. It is not a one-off reading, but a text to which we will be returning to find new insights that will emerge on the background of our newly acquired clinical experience.

Ramez Kirollos, MD, FRCS
Thomas Santarius, MD, PhD, FRCS
Cambridge

Preface

Neuroanatomy can and should be studied throughout all its different dimensions (morphological, histological, functional, biochemical, genetic, radiological), but for their proper understanding, and particularly for the medical practice thereof, comprehension of brain architecture is fundamental.

The notion of brain architecture comprises appraisal of the sizes and shapes of the neural structures, their relationships with each other, their relationships with the intracranial natural spaces which are the cerebrospinal fluid spaces, with their related vessels and cranial nerves, and the relationships of the cerebral surfaces with the skull.

With this in mind, the aim of this book is to provide a tridimensional understanding particularly of the cerebral hemispheres, and of the relationships of the cerebral surfaces with the skull outer surfaces. Although more directed to neurosurgeons and neuroradiologists, it might also be of interest to neurologists and to anyone in the field of neuroscience.

The book is divided into three main chapters. Chapter 1 is about historical remarks more pertinent to the knowledge of the cerebral surface and to the methods of establishing cranial-cerebral relationships for neurosurgery. Chapter 2 describes the cerebral anatomy as seen more from an architectural perspective, and with more emphasis on the sulci and gyri of the cerebral surface. Chapter 3 describes the cranial-cerebral relationships through the concept of sulcal and cerebral key points and as applied to the practice of modern microneurosurgery. Repetitions of concepts, of descriptions, and also of a few illustrations throughout the text, are intentional.

This book has its origins in my passion for anatomy, and is mostly based on my anatomical research initiated during a brief stay at Dr. Rothon's lab in Gainesville, Florida, and continued at the University of São Paulo Medical School. It incorporates my two theses completed and presented at the University of São Paulo Medical School and their related articles that were subsequently published, the related knowledge described by other authors, and, above all, answers to some questions that were borne out of actual clinical doubts and dilemmas I had throughout my decades-long neurosurgical career.

The privilege of giving numerous regular lectures about these subjects has helped me to shape concepts and polish the way they should be presented, and my audiences provided the main motivation to gather this knowledge together as a book.

The recent tenth anniversary of the Cambridge Lectures in Neurosurgical Anatomy, with its unabating popularity, definitely makes this a special moment to have this book published by the prestigious Cambridge University Press.

Acknowledgments

I would like to acknowledge Evandro de Oliveira, teacher and friend, who introduced me to and guided me through the universe of microneurosurgical anatomy; John A. Jane Jr., teacher and mentor, for his constant motivation and support; Albert Rhoton Jr., for the opportunity of a brief fellowship which had a major impact on my career; Aldo Junqueira Rodrigues Jr., chairman and friend, who gave me the unique opportunity to develop my anatomical research at the University of São Paulo Medical School; Richard Gonzalo Párraga Choque, for his devotion and superb dissections which much enrich this book (Figures 2.22 C and D; 2.24 A, B, C, and D; 2.25; 2.27 A and B; 2.28 A and B; 2.31; 3.13 A, B, C, and D; 3.14 A and B; 3.15 A and C; 3.16 A, B, C, D, E, and F; 3.17 A and B; 3.24 C, D, E, F, G, and H; 3.33 A, B, C, and D); Eduardo Santamaria Carvalhal Ribas, son and colleague, for his dedicated collaboration and updates; André Felix Gentil, colleague and associate, for his support and dynamic help; Thomas Santarius, colleague and friend from Cambridge, whose counseling and help were decisive for the accomplishment of this project; Camila Querido Tanizaka and Carmen Dulce Querido Marotta Tanizaka, for their tireless work on this book; José Falcetti, for the illustrations; the organizers of regular yearly courses who invited me to give lectures which motivated this book; the residents of the Department of Neurosurgery at the University of Virginia, Charlottesville, USA, for their enthusiasm and eagerness to learn during our regular visits and lectures since 1995; Evandro de Oliveira, organizer of the course "Anatomy of Sulci, Gyri and Ventricles, and Dissection of White Matter Fibers," in the Hospital Beneficência Portuguesa de São Paulo, in São Paulo, Brazil, from 2003 to 2014; Carlos Alegria and all his personnel, organizers of the course "Sulci, Gyri and Dissecting Fibers," in Braga, Portugal, since 2003; Thomas Santarius, Ramez Kirollos, and all their personnel, organizers of the Cambridge Lectures in Neurosurgical Anatomy, in Cambridge, UK, since 2005; Rod J. Oskouian and all SSF (Seattle Science Foundation) personnel, organizers of the Annual SNI (Seattle Neuroscience Institute) Brain Anatomy with Neurosurgical Applications Course, in Seattle, USA, since 2011; and George Samandouras, Mitchel Berger, and all their personnel, organizers of the Advanced Techniques in Neurosurgical Oncology Course, in London, UK, since 2012.

Chapter 1 Historical Remarks

Interesting that just as with brain evolution, brain anatomical knowledge also took place from the bottom up, with the cerebral sulci and gyri being the last structures to be understood!
G. C. Ribas, 2017

1.1 The Cerebral Surface

Knowledge of brain anatomy in general and of its surface in particular is very recent. This is despite human interest in the brain being very old, with the making of cranial trepanations probably being the oldest systematized surgical procedure in our history (Sachs, 1952) and having been done successfully (on the basis of new bone growth after these procedures) in European Neolithic cultures about 10 000 years ago, and more frequently in South America by the pre-Inca and Inca cultures in Peru with findings that date until 2000 years ago (Finger, 1994; Graña *et al.*, 1954; Lyons and Petrucelli, 1978; Sachs, 1952).

The Egyptians were the first to provide systematic medical records with the writing of the Edwin Smith surgical papyrus (seventeenth century BC) based on the teachings of Imhotep (ca. twenty-seventh century BC), father of Egyptian medicine. The text deals particularly with traumatic lesions; but its hieroglyphics mention for the first time in history the equivalents for the words "brain" and "corrugations of the brain," and also mention a note about a patient with an opened skull wound who became "speechless" during its palpation (Breasted, 1930 apud Catani and Schotten, 2012; Catani and Schotten, 2012). The Egyptians believed that the heart, and not the brain, was responsible for intellectual, emotional, motor, and sensation

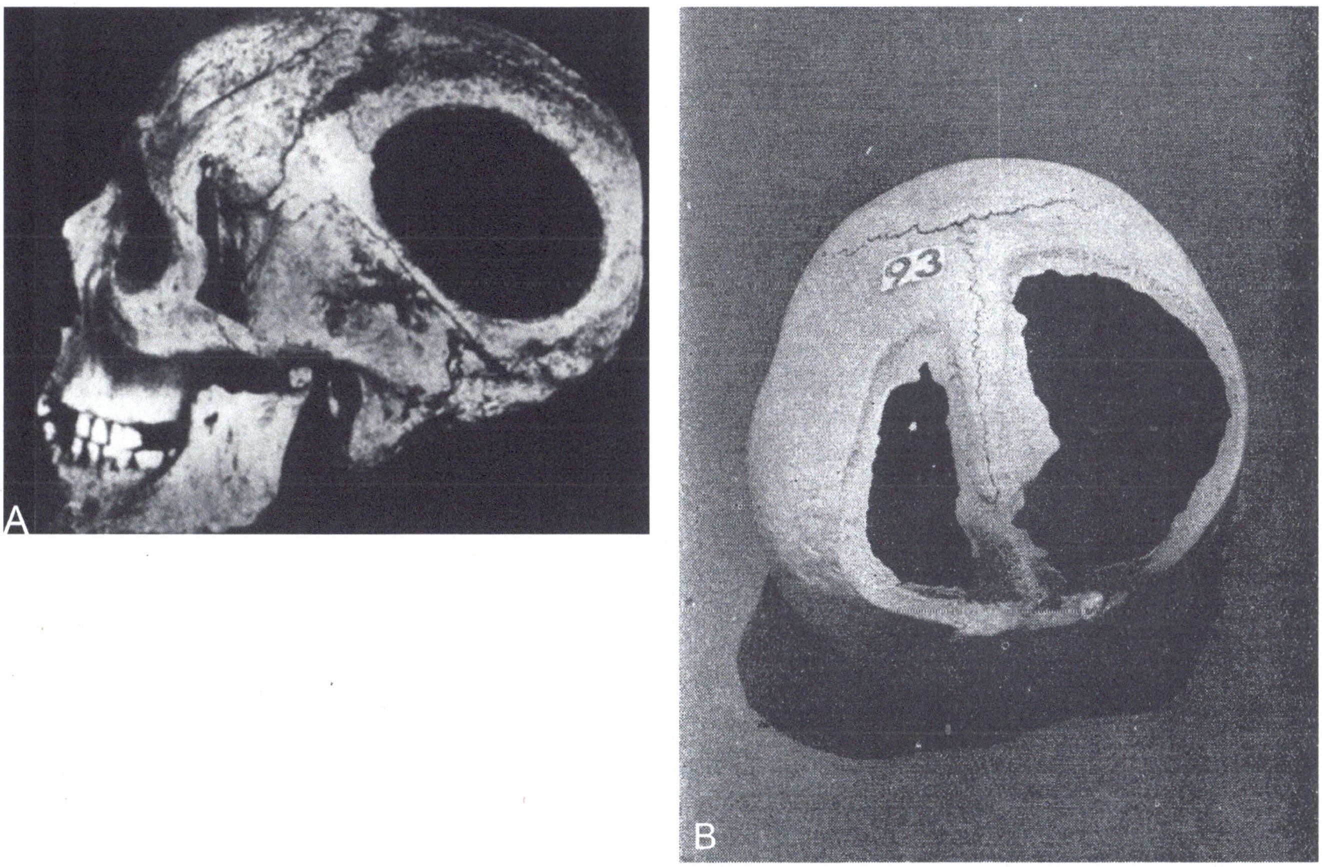

Figure 1.1 (A) Trephine skull opening from the Neolithic Period (Neolithic skull, Nogent-les-Vierges, Oise, France. Musée de l'Homme, Paris) (Sachs, 1952), and (B) trephine skull openings from the pre-Colombian Peruvian civilization, apparently with the aim of preserving bone over the superior longitudinal sinus (Graña *et al.*, 1954).

functions, and the brain was treated by them with indifference as also shown in the subsequent and much longer Ebers papyrus (Finger, 1994). Nevertheless, it is interesting to point out that, during their New Kingdom era, it was common to remove the brains of cadavers to be mummified through the nostrils and the base of the skull with the help of a small chisel and an iron hook (Finger, 1994), pioneering a trans-sphenoidal surgical route.

During antiquity, no significant contributions to neuroanatomy were made until the development of the Greek culture. Alcmaeon from Crotona (ca. fifth century BC) performed some of the earliest recorded dissections, described the optic nerves, identified that the sense organs were connected to the brain through nerves, and was the first to propose that the brain was the central organ of sensation and thought, which was also suggested by Anaxagoras (500–428 BC) at about the same time. Alcmaeon's cephalocentric concept is known to have deeply influenced later philosophers and anatomists such as Pythagoras, Plato, Herophilus, Erasistratus, and Galen (Catani and Schotten, 2012; Debernardi *et al.*, 2010).

Hippocrates (460–370 BC), the father of medicine, emphasized that the brain was responsible for mental activity and convulsions, although some important Greek philosophers of that time, like Aristotle (384–322 BC), the Stoics, and the Epicureans, still believed that the heart was the seat of intellectual, perceptual, and related functions (Finger, 1994).

Previously forbidden in Greek culture, human dissections began to be performed around 300 BC in Alexandria, Egypt, then a Greek city which was particularly culturally developed. There, Herophilus (ca. 335–280 BC), follower of Hippocrates and considered the father of anatomy, studied the brain, its ventricles, and the cerebellum, discriminated the motor from the sensitive nerves, and described the torcula of the cranial venous sinuses that bears his name (torcular Herophili). Erasistratus (ca. 310–250 BC), studying the comparative anatomy of the brain surface, already suspected a relationship between intellect and gyri complexity (Finger, 1994) and compared the arrangement of brain convolutions to the jejunum (Clarke and O'Malley, 1996).

With the decline of the Greek Empire, the Roman medicine that followed was largely a continuation of Greek ideas, particularly because many Greek physicians settled in Rome. Aurelius Cornelius Celsus (25 BC–AD 50), though not formally trained, practiced medicine and wrote the first Roman work *De Medicina*; however, it was Galen (AD 130–200) who left the best known anatomical contributions from this period (Finger, 1994; Singer, 1952; Sarton, 1954).

Galen was born in the Greek city of Pergamon, trained in Alexandria, and later settled in Rome where he was a surgeon for gladiators and performed dissections mainly on animals. Among all his anatomical contributions, in neuroanatomy, Galen numbered the cranial nerves and described the autonomic nervous system, but since most of his dissections and experiments were performed on cattle and on many other kinds of animal, he incorrectly considered that many of these findings were also pertinent to human anatomy (Sarton, 1954; Finger, 1994).

He followed Hippocrates in also rejecting Aristotle's ideas that the brain simply served to cool the passions of the heart and in believing that the brain was also responsible for imagination, cognition, and memory (for Hippocrates, the basic components of intellect), but he did not believe that the convolutions of the brain were associated with intelligence as previously proposed by Erasistratus.

Galen believed that a natural spirit was produced in the liver, converted in the heart to a higher form, named the vital spirit, and was then carried to the brain through the carotid and rete mirabile ("wonderful net"). This is a vascular plexus located at the base of the brain as observed by him in the dissections of some animals, particularly of oxen (Clarke and Dewhurst, 1975; Finger, 1994; Singer, 1952). It was then transformed into animal spirits within the brain ventricles as already proposed previously by Herophilus of Alexandria almost five centuries before (Dobson, 1925 apud Catani and Schotten, 2012).

The Church fathers of the fourth and fifth centuries adopted Galen's ideas associating the higher human functions mostly with the brain ventricles. One of the earliest advocates of the so-called ventricular theory of brain functions was Nemesius, Bishop of Emesa, a city in current Syria, and others that followed him in this period related the ventricular cavities with different functions (Clarke and Dewhurst, 1975; Finger, 1994), generating conceptions that lasted for many centuries.

The approximately 1000 years of the Middle Ages, roughly from the fourth to the fourteenth century, as is well known, were poor regarding scientific developments in general. Although having had the contributions of Avicenna (AD 980–1037) in the Arabic world who is credited with the first representation of the brain around the year AD 1000 by some authors (Tamraz and Comair, 2000), and the contributions of the first European human dissections by Mondino dei Luzzi (ca. 1270–1326) (Finger, 1994; Lyons and Petrucelli, 1978; Tamraz and Comair, 2000), anatomical studies were very limited, in particular because human cadaveric dissections were forbidden at that time.

The relative liberation of this practice that occurred during the Renaissance finally led to the progressive development of all anatomical knowledge, and the most preeminent figure in this field was undoubtedly Andreas Vesalius (1514–1564), professor of anatomy and surgery at Padua University, Italy.

Vesalius was a native of Brussels who studied anatomy in Paris with Jacobinus Sylvius (1478–1555), and his seminal work *De Humani Corporis Fabrica* (*On the Working of the Human Body*) (Saunders and O'Malley, 1950) was completed in Padua and Venice in 1542. It was published in Basel in 1543 (Finger, 1994; Singer, 1952) with the artwork probably done by Jan Stephan van Calcar (ca. 1499–1546) and/or by other students of the great painter Titian (ca. 1487–1586). The *Fabrica* was based on extensive human dissections, and Vesalius was particularly led to indicate Galen's anatomical errors, having counted some 200 of them. In 1544, Vesalius left Italy to become court physician to Charles V (1500–1558), which ended his career as an anatomist (Finger, 1994).

Vesalius left many contributions to neuroanatomy, with descriptions of the meninges, cerebral hemispheres distinguishing the white and gray matter, corpus callosum and septum pellucidum, ventricles, fornix, colliculi, and pineal gland, cerebellar hemispheres and vermis, infundibulum and pituitary body (Lyons and Petrucelli, 1978; Saunders and O'Malley, 1950; Singer, 1952; Tamraz and Comair, 2000). With regard to the cerebral gyri, Vesalius still illustrated them chaotically and understood their shape and folding to be responsible for anchoring the vessels that penetrate the brain through the sulci (Vesalius, 1543 apud Catani and Schotten, 2012).

Although having denied the existence of the rete mirabile in humans, Vesalius did not reject entirely the ideas defended by Galen and the ventricular localization theory itself, and this major interest in the ventricular cavities may explain the relative neglect of the brain gyri by all the anatomists throughout more than 20 centuries.

Other contemporaneous authors of this period were the great artist and also anatomist Leonardo da Vinci (1472–1519), who besides his well-known studies of the brain ventricles also made beautiful but incorrect illustrations of the cerebral surface (Cianchi and Breschi, 1997; Clayton, 1992), and Julius Casserius (ca. 1545–1616). His work represented the brain convolutions, which at that time were still understood to resemble the small bowel as described previously by Herophilus and by Erasistratus 18 centuries before (Singer, 1952).

Constanzo Varolio (1543–1575) started slicing the brain and described the pons in 1573 (Varolio, 1573 apud Clarke and O'Malley, 1996), and in 1587, Giulio Cesare Aranzi (1530–1589) described the hippocampus within the lateral ventricular cavity (Varolio, 1573 apud Clarke and O'Malley, 1996).

In 1663, Franciscus de le Boë (1614–1672), also known as Dr. Sylvius, described the lateral cerebral sulcus (Sylvius, 1663 apud Catani and Schotten, 2012), which came to be named the Sylvian fissure by Caspar Bartholin (Bartholin, 1641 apud Catani and Schotten, 2012; Catani and Schotten, 2012) in 1641. For some authors, the Sylvian fissure was primarily described by Girolamo Fabrici d'Aquapendente (ca. 1553–1619) (Collice *et al.*, 2008), who followed Andreas Vesalius (1514–1564) and Gabriel Fallopius (1523–1562) at the University of Padua (Finger, 1994).

In 1664, Thomas Willis (1621–1675) published his highly regarded *Cerebri Anatome*, which featured illustrations by the renowned architect Christopher Wren (1632–1723). In addition to describing the group of arteries surrounding the base of the brain now known as the circle of Willis, he introduced a variety of terms, including neurology, hemisphere, corpus striatum, peduncle, and pyramid, and related the cerebral gyri to memory, but still not representing the brain gyri and sulci properly. Interestingly, Willis related the striatum with movement and sensation, and the corpus callosum with imagination (Finger, 1994).

Raymond Vieussens (1644–1716) published the famous *Neurographia Universalis* in 1690 (Vieussens, 1690), describing in detail the centrum semiovale and other cerebral structures,

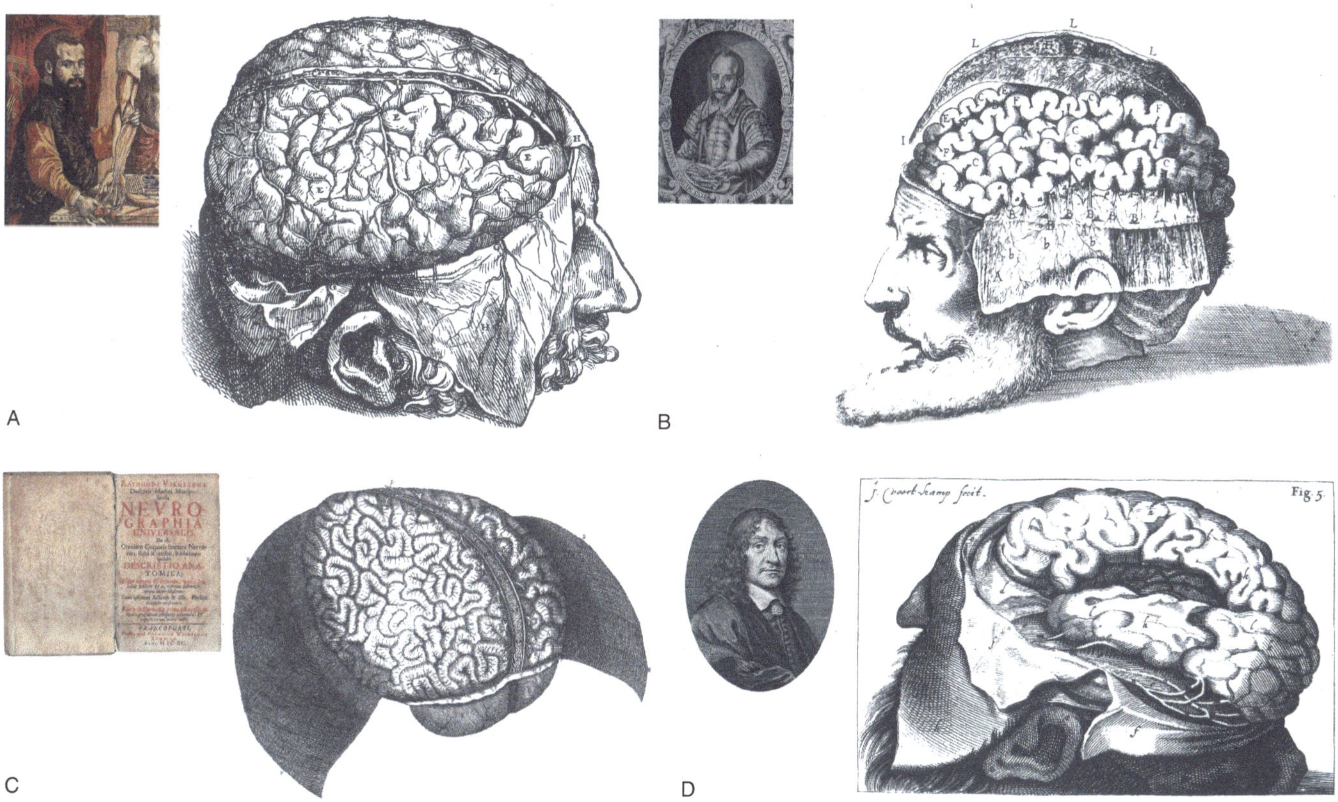

Figure 1.2 Illustrations of the cerebral surface from the Renaissance: (A) by Andreas Vesalius (1514–1564), (B) by Giulio Casserio (ca. 1545–1616), (C) by Raymond Vieussen (1641–1716), and (D) by Franciscus de le Boë, known as Dr. Sylvius (1614–1672) already depicting the lateral fissure that bears his name. (Illustrations from Clarke and Dewhurst (1975) and from Saunders and O'Malley (1950).)

but still illustrating the brain surface similarly to the small bowel (Finger, 1994; Tamraz and Comair, 2000). Godefroid Bidloo clearly displayed the central sulcus in his atlas and textbook published in 1685 (Tamraz and Comair, 2000), and subsequently Félix Vicq d'Azyr (1748–1794), famous for describing the mammillothalamic tract, also described the precentral and postcentral convolutions separated by the central sulcus, and coined the term uncus (Tamraz and Comair, 2000). In 1809, Johann Christian Reil (1759–1813) provided a comprehensive description of the insula (Lockard, 1977), which had already been identified by Bartholin in 1641 (Finger, 1994; Tamraz and Comair, 2000). In 1827, Herbert Mayo, student of the renowned anatomist and surgeon Charles Bell (1774–1842), published illustrations of the corona radiata and internal capsule, as well as other important tracts (Türe *et al.*, 2000). In 1829, the Italian anatomist Luigi Rolando (1773–1831) published his text *Della Struttura degli Emisferi Cerebrali* (Rolando, 1829 apud Türe *et al.*, 2000), becoming the first author to accurately portray the central sulcus, which is still also referred to as the fissure of Rolando (Finger, 1994; Tamraz and Comair, 2000).

In the early nineteenth century, Frans Joseph Gall (1758–1828) related the different brain convolutions to different mental faculties and "propensity," adopting the concept of organology where each brain convolution corresponded to a specific organ. For Gall, each gyrus would cause an impression on the skull, generating an external protrusion that would express each individual character (Clarke and Dewhurst, 1975; Gall and Spurzheim, 1810–1819 apud Catani and Schotten, 2012). Although not justified at all, Gall's concepts, altogether known as phrenology, encouraged the investigation of cortical localizations and hence the clinico-anatomical correlation method (Catani and Schotten, 2012).

Achille Loius Foville (1799–1891) was the first author in the history of neuroanatomy to illustrate perfectly the sulci and gyri of the brain surface, in his atlas of brain anatomy edited in 1844, but did not describe their organization within the text (Brogna *et al.*, 2012).

It was the German physiologist Friedrich Arnold (1803–1890) who first used the terms frontal, parietal, and occipital to describe the cranial bones. In a text published in 1851 (Broca, 1876b), Arnold recognized only the Sylvian fissure and the parieto-occipital sulcus (then known as the internal perpendicular fissure) (Déjérine, 1895) as anatomically constant sulci, and he described the temporal region as an anterior extension of the occipital region.

It is notable that, despite the intense interest that humankind has always had in relation to the brain, it was only in the middle of the nineteenth century that the general anatomical organization of the cerebral sulci and gyri was perceived and described by the French anatomist Louis Pierre Gratiolet (1815–1865) who succeeded his professor Francois Leuret (1797–1851) (Leuret and Gratiolet, 1857–1959 apud Türe *et al.*, 2000; Gratiolet, 1854 apud Pearce, 2006; Pearce, 2006). In addition to his well-known description of optic radiation, Gratiolet together with Leuret also distinguished between primary and secondary sulci based on their phylogenetic appearance, adopted the terms initially proposed by Arnold to divide each cerebral hemisphere into lobes, and coined the elegant term "plis de passage" to describe the connections between adjacent gyri. Gratiolet was the first anatomist to understand and describe the fact that, despite individual variations, the cerebral sulci and gyri are organized in accordance with a general arrangement (Gratiolet, 1854 apud Pearce, 2006; Pearce, 2006).

In relation to his original concept of brain lobes, it is interesting to point out that regarding the precentral and postcentral gyri, Gratiolet initially considered the former one, then called the "first anterior ascending gyrus" (Déjérine, 1895), as belonging to the parietal lobe (Gratiolet, 1854 apud Pearce, 2006), and only a few years later decided to consider it part of the frontal

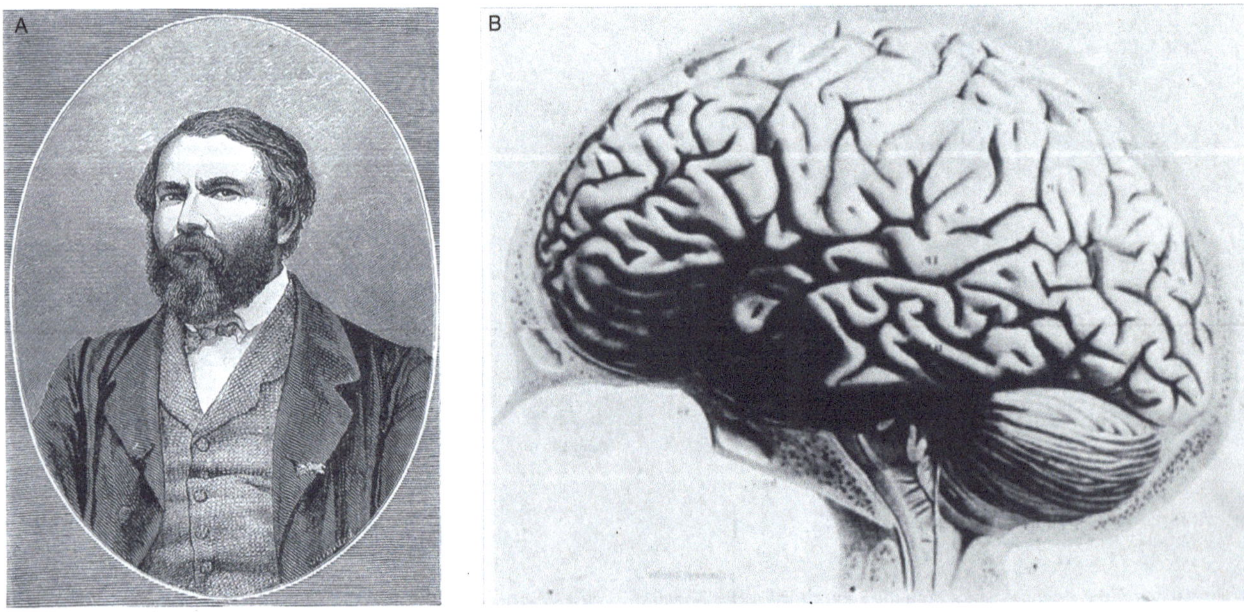

Figure 1.3 The cerebral surface as depicted by (A) Louis Pierre Gratiolet (1815–1865), who described (B) the basic organization of the cerebral gyri. (Illustrations from Clarke and Dewhurst (1975).)

lobe, leaving the latter, then called the "second anterior ascending gyrus" (Déjérine, 1895), part of the parietal lobe (Leuret and Gratiolet, 1857–1959 apud Türe *et al.*, 2000).

In 1869, Johann Alexander Ecker (1816–1887) also accurately described all of the cerebral sulci and gyri, introducing the designations orbital, precentral, parieto-occipital, and transverse occipital to describe these various sulci (Tamraz and Comair, 2000).

William Turner (1832–1916), who also studied the brain sulci in detail, with his name becoming an eponym of the intraparietal sulcus (Lockard, 1977), emphasized in 1866 that the central sulcus should be considered the posterior limit of the frontal lobe (Broca, 1876b; Tamraz and Comair, 2000; Turner, 1866 apud Catani and Schotten, 2012; Yasargil, 1994). On the other hand, regarding particularly a proposed concept of a central lobe of the brain, it is interesting to mention that, in 1868, the German anatomist T. L. W. Bischoff referred to the pre- and postcentral gyri, respectively, as "anterior and posterior central convolutions of the brain" (Broca, 1876b), as did Edward H. Taylor in 1900 (Taylor and Haughton, 1900 apud Uematsu *et al.*, 1992), already clearly suggesting to group these two gyri together and separate from the adjacent gyri.

The knowledge of the correlations between the nervous structures and their respective neurophysiological functions, in turn, only came to be developed from the second half of the nineteenth century, and the pioneers of the location of cerebral cortical functions were undoubtedly Pierre Paul Broca (1824–1880) in France, and John Hughlings Jackson (1835–1911) in England (Finger, 1994; Lockard, 1977; Schiller, 1992).

An anthropologist, anatomist, neurologist, and surgeon, Broca evidently relied initially on anatomical knowledge available at the time, and was particularly motivated and influenced by the aforementioned descriptions by Gratiolet (Broca, 1876b; Türe *et al.*, 2000). He introduced the concept of brain location (Lockard, 1977).

Following the previous observations of Bouillaud in 1825 (Schiller, 1992; Bouillaud, 1825 apud Catani and Schotten, 2012), and of Auburtin in 1861 (Schiller, 1992; Auburtin, 1861 apud Catani and Schotten, 2012) who described a transient aphasia secondary to the compression of an opened left fronto-opercular wound in a patient who had sustained a gunshot suicidal lesion, in 1861, Broca also outlined the cortical motor speech area based on the clinical-anatomical study of two patients who died after left fronto-opercular strokes (Broca, 1861 apud Finger, 1994), locating it in the "posterior portion of the third frontal gyrus, adjacent to the Sylvius fissure." It is interesting to note that only after two years did Broca note that this type of involvement was particularly related to the left side of the brain, and that he came to deal more clearly with this issue in 1865 (Finger, 1994).

Around the same time, in England, Hughlings Jackson suggested the existence of a somatotopical cortical motor area based on clinical observations of epileptic patients. In Germany in 1870, Gustav Fritsch and Edward Hitzig confirmed experimentally Jackson's conceptions in dogs, demonstrating that both motor and sensory functions are related to the cerebral cortex. In 1886 in England, David Ferrier mapped in detail the sensorimotor cortex of the monkey, as did other authors such as Sidney Grunbaum (1861–1921) and Charles Sherrington (1857–1952) in apes.

In 1874, the human cortical area responsible for language understanding was described by Carl Wernicke (1848–1904) as located within the left temporoparietal region (Wernicke, 1874 apud Catani and Schotten, 2012; Finger, 1994), and in 1892, Joseph Jules Déjérine (1849–1917) described the cortical area responsible for reading as located in the left angular gyrus based on clinical-anatomical findings (Déjérine, 1892 apud Catani and Schotten, 2012).

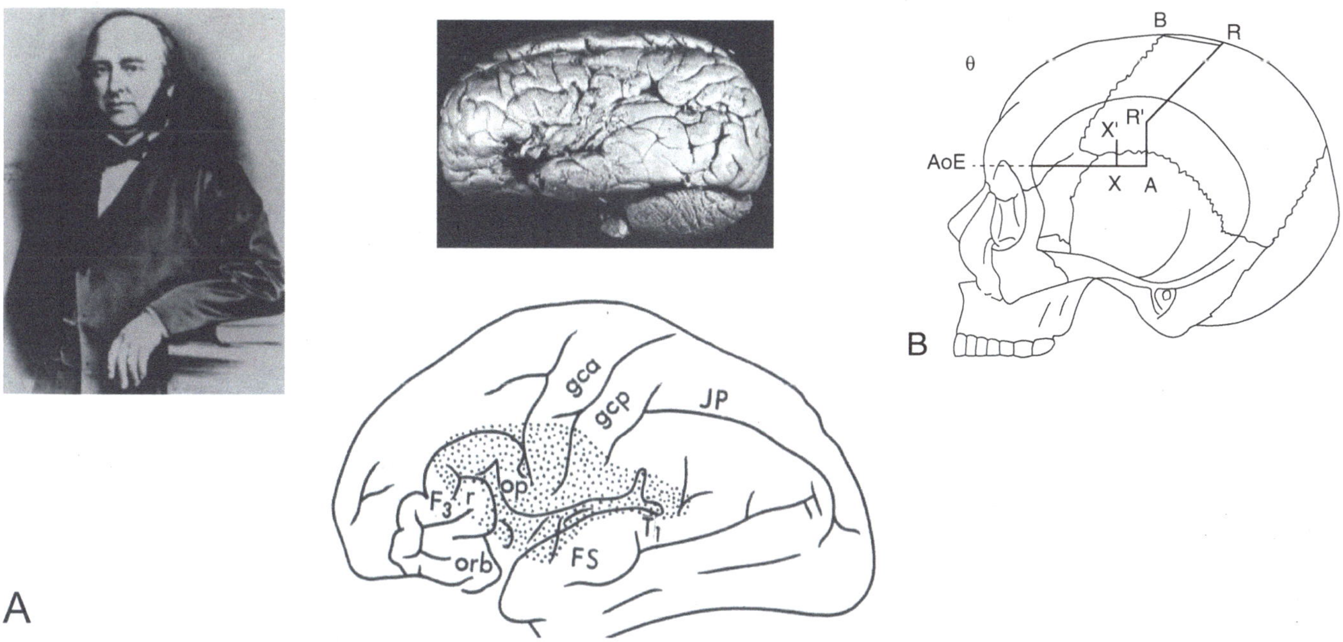

Figure 1.4 (A) Pierre Paul Broca (1824–1880), with the sketch of his description of the language motor cortical area in 1861, together with a picture of the brain of his patient Mr. Leborgne; (B) Broca's sketch of the cranial-cerebral relationships of the speech area, based on the Broca-Championnière Method, for the drainage of brain abscess causing a motor aphasia, in 1876 (from Stone (1991)).

Victor Horsley (1857–1916), considered the father of neurosurgery, was one of the pioneers of human trans-operatory cortical stimulation and, in 1885, observed that "the main motor cortical representation is anterior to the central sulcus" (Finger, 1994; Lyons and Petrucelli, 1978). After him, Harvey Cushing (1869–1939), who briefly trained with Horsley and became the most prominent surgeon in the establishment of neurosurgery as a specialty in the United States, repeated these procedures with patients under local anesthesia and was also able to reproduce such auras and seizures in epileptic patients (Finger, 1994; Lyons and Petrucelli, 1978).

The first human cortical map was developed by Fedor Krause (1857–1937) in 1911, but it was Wilder Penfield (1891–1976) who described in detail the motor, sensitive, and other functional cortical areas based on his trans-operatory studies of cortical stimulation of epileptic patients operated on by him under local anesthesia in the Montreal Neurological Institute (Penfield and Boldrey apud Brodal, 1981).

1.2 Cerebral Cortical Cytoarchitecture

The advent of the microscope invented by Marcello Malpighi (1628–1694) and Antony Van Leeuwenhoek (1632–1723) (Finger, 1994) allowed the study of the brain cortex, and in 1840, Jules Baillarger (1809–1890) described the six cortical layers and the two white lines or bands pertinent to layers IV and V of the cerebral cortex which are known as the Baillarger striae (Baillarger, 1840 apud Clarke and O'Malley, 1996; Lockard, 1977), and which correspond to the line of Gennari within the calcarine cortex previously described by Francesco Gennari (1750–1796) in 1782 (Lockard, 1977).

Preceded by Camillo Golgi (1843–1926) who developed the silver stain, Santiago Ramón y Cajal (1862–1934) utilized the same techniques and, concomitantly with Charles Sherington (1857–1952) who established the concept of the synapse, delineated the basics of the cortical cell connections. While Golgi proposed the syncytium theory with the notion that a network connected all neurons, Ramón y Cajal described the neuron theory with the proper concept that each neuron acts as a single cell (Squire *et al.*, 2003; Finger, 1994).

Following these pioneers of neurohistology, Alfred Walker Campbell (1868–1937), Korbinian Brodmann (1868–1981), and Constantin von Economo (1876–1931) studied and described the whole cerebral cortical cytoarchitecture and further brain sulci and gyri details.

Although less detailed than the von Economo map (von Economo, 2009), Brodmann's cytoarchitectonic map (Brodmann, 1909 apud Penfield and Baldwin, 1952) became much more popular. Oscar Vogt (1870–1959) and Cecile Vogt (1875–1962) partially based their myeloarchitectonic studies (Vogt, C. and Vogt, O., 1926 apud Catani and Schotten, 2012) on Brodmann's areas (Catani and Schotten, 2012).

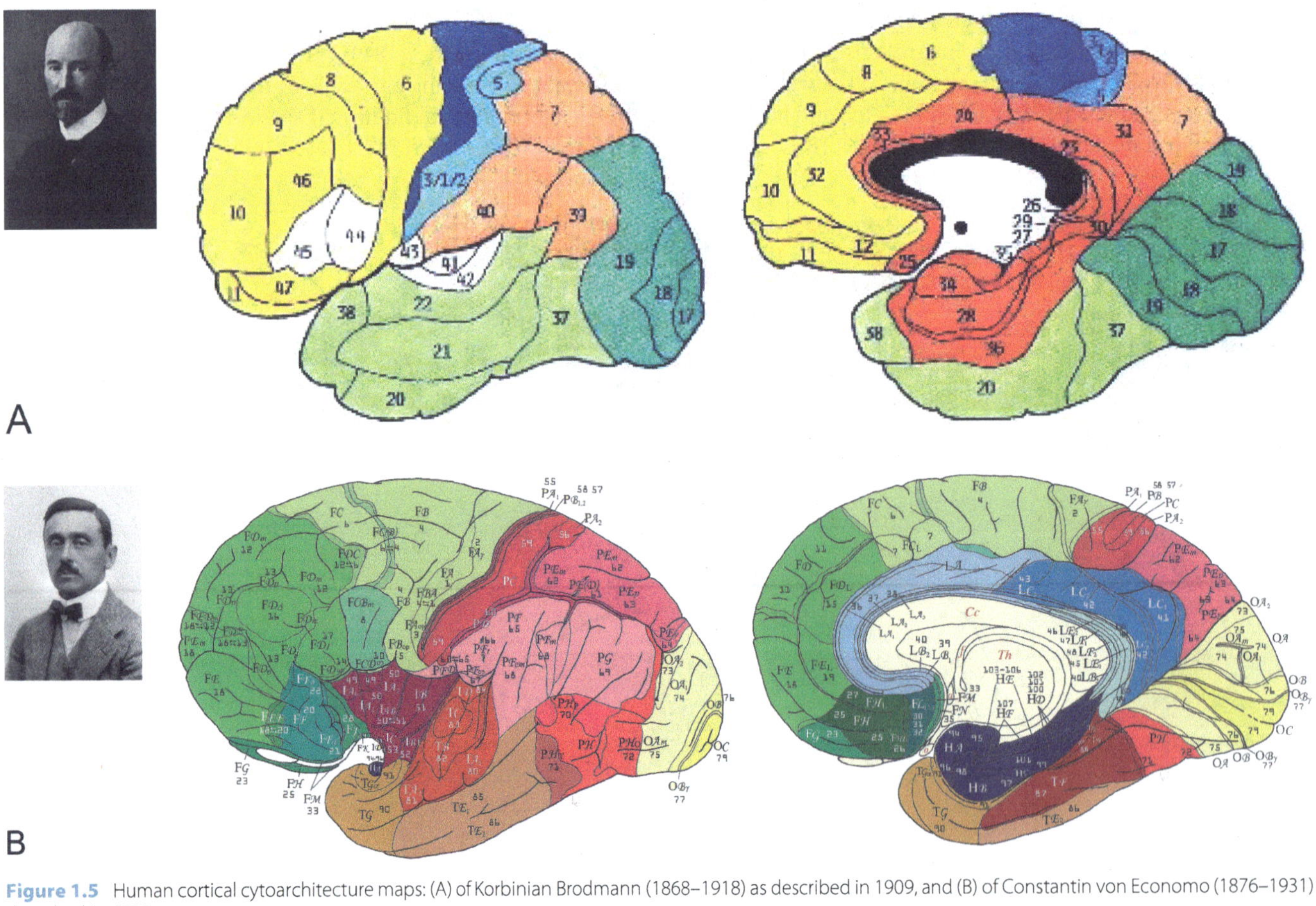

Figure 1.5 Human cortical cytoarchitecture maps: (A) of Korbinian Brodmann (1868–1918) as described in 1909, and (B) of Constantin von Economo (1876–1931) as described in 1925.

1.3 White Matter Fibers

Another major contribution of the microscope was to provide a clear differentiation between the gray and white matter, which had already been observed by Malpighi himself, and which encouraged further studies of the white matter bulk that until then was understood as having only a mechanical support function (Catani and Schotten, 2012).

Nicolaus Steno (1638–1686) was the first to suggest its study through fiber dissections (Steno, 1669 apud Clarke and O'Malley, 1996), which became possible with the aid of new methods to harden the soft brain tissue. Raymond Vieussens (1641–1716) boiled the brain in oil and was able to demonstrate the brain continuity of the corona radiata fibers with the internal capsule and within the brainstem, and to differentiate ascending and descending fibers from callosal fibers (Vieussens, 1690; Catani and Schotten, 2012); however, it was Félix Vicq d'Azyr (1748–1794) who further differentiated the inter-hemispheric from the intra-hemispheric association fibers (Vicq d'Azyr, 1786 apud Clarke and O'Malley, 1996; Catani and Schotten, 2012), which later supported Theodor Meynert's (1833–1891) classical classification of projection, commissural, and association fibers (Meynert, 1867–1868 apud Catani and Schotten, 2012; Meynert, 1885 apud Catani and Schotten, 2012; Meynert, 1872 apud Türe *et al.*, 2000). Meynert was a very important anatomist, neurologist and psychiatrist who had among his students Carl Wernicke, Sergei Korsakoff, August-Henri Forel, Paul Flechsig, and Sigmund Freud (Catani and Schotten, 2012). Among other contributions, he also described the fasciculus retroflexus and the substantia innominata with the basal nucleus that currently bears his name (Lockard, 1977).

The visual fibers were initially demonstrated by Bartholomeo Panizza (1785–1867), and the optic radiation was later completely described from the lateral geniculate body to the occipital cortex by Louis Pierre Gratiolet (1815–1865) (Párraga *et al.*, 2012).

Other important contributions in this field were made by Johann Christian Reil (1759–1813) who soaked the brain in alcohol and described the cingulum, the ansa peduncularis, the tapetum fibers underneath the optic radiation and also the substantia innominata (Reil, 1812 apud Catani and Schotten, 2012; Lockard, 1977), and by Karl Burdach (1776–1847) who, among many tracts, described the arcuate fasciculus and occipital-temporal connections (Burdach, 1819–1822–1826 apud Catani and Schotten, 2012) which were later identified as the inferior fronto-occipital fasciculus by Curran in 1909 (Curran, 1909 apud Catani and Schotten, 2012).

Regarding particularly the basal forebrain region previously known as the "Substantia Innominata (unnamed substance) of Reichert" and that currently corresponds to the ventral-striato-pallidal region, it received its original name of "Ungenannte Maksubstans" given by Johann Christian Reil in 1809, had its name later apparently erroneously attributed to the neuroanatomist Karl Bogislau Reichert due to its mention within his atlas of 1859, and was finally better described and popularized by Theodor Meynert (Heimer *et al.*, 1997; Lockard, 1977; Meynert, 1867–1868 apud Catani and Schotten, 2012; Meynert, 1885 apud Catani and Schotten, 2012).

More recently, the method of freezing the brain before its dissection proposed by Josef Klinger in 1935 (Klinger, 1935 apud Türe *et al.*, 2000; Ludwig and Klinger, 1956) reactivated the practice of fiber dissections, currently widely used for studying brain anatomy. The process of freezing the brain after its fixation causes the formalin to crystallize, which separates the fibers, easing their dissection.

1.4 Cranial-Cerebral Relationships

Knowledge of the locations of the main functions of the cortical surface led to anatomical-clinical correlations, but the absence of imaging technology that could demonstrate the precise location of potentially surgical intracranial lesions in relation to the cranial surface generated studies in the second half of the nineteenth century correlating the location of cortical areas and their recently discovered functions with repair points on the cranial surface.

Broca was also the pioneer of these studies, having reported to the Anatomical Society of Paris in 1861 the results of his first study on cranial-cerebral topographical correlations. The study was performed on 11 cadavers of adult males and was published in the same year (Broca, 1861 apud Finger, 1994). In his study, Broca introduced wooden pins through strategically located cranial perforations and then examined in detail their positions in the respective brains removed at their autopsies. In this first work, we note the observations that "the occipital cleft coincides with or is directly before the lambdoid suture," and that "the upper end of the Rolandic sulcus is between 40 and 52 millimeters behind the Bregma," contradicting and correcting Gratiolet's earlier findings which placed it under the Bregma (quoted from Broca (1876b)).

In 1876, Broca published the work "Sur la topographie crânio-cérébrale" (on cranial-cerebral topography) (Broca, 1876b), which constituted a true monograph on the subject where he described his findings and compared them with those of other authors of the time. In this text, Broca already distinguishes the sulci from the fissures, classifies the sulci as primary or secondary according to their major or minor anatomical findings, and recognizes as fissures only the fissure of Rolando that corresponds to the central sulcus, the lateral fissure of Sylvius, and the external occipital fissure which corresponds to the emergence of the occipital sulcus in the convexity. Besides the topographical correlations of these fissures, Broca also studied the cerebral correlations of the craniometric points he had previously described in anthropological studies (Broca, 1875; Gusmão *et al.*, 2000).

The methods of cranial-cerebral topographic correlations that were studied and proposed during the transition period between the nineteenth and twentieth centuries were mainly

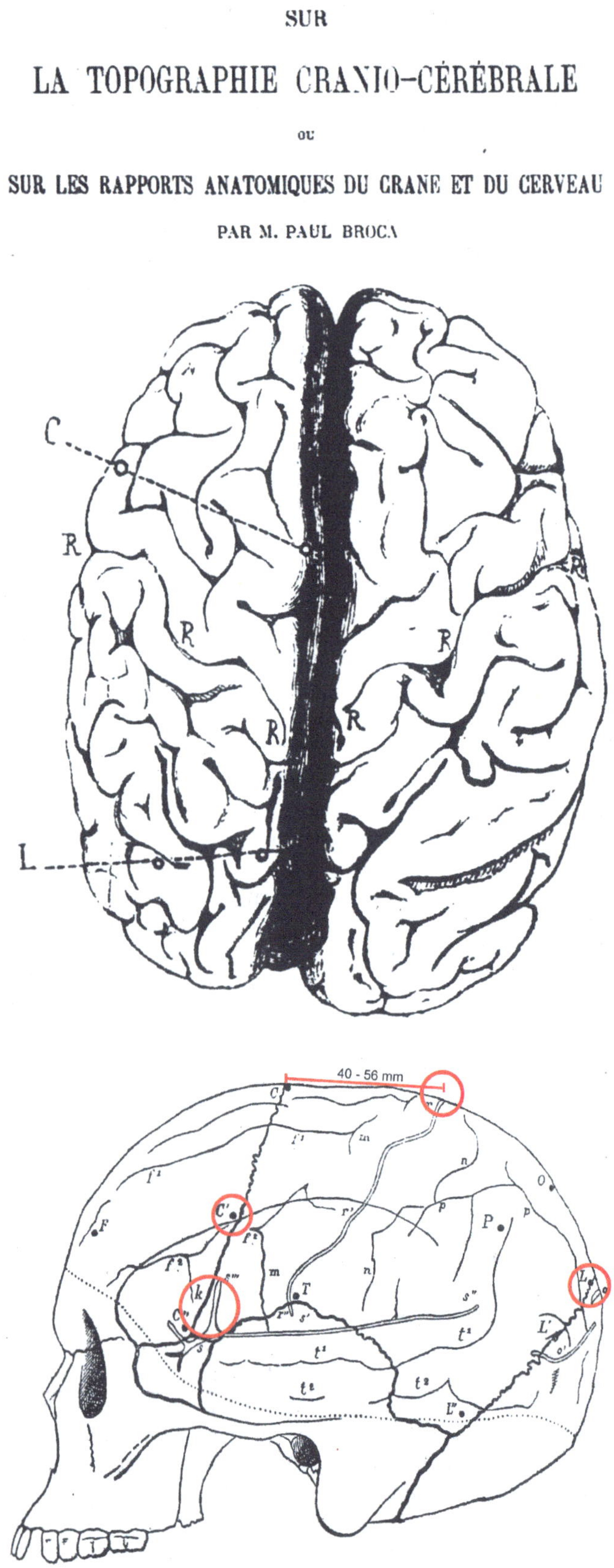

Figure 1.6 Illustrations from Broca's monograph "Sur la topographie crânio-cérébrale" of 1876, which pioneered the study of cranial-cerebral relationships (Broca (1876b)).

based on the establishment of measurements along lines drawn from easily identified cranial points.

Among those methods stand out those proposed by Championnière, Poirier, Le Fort and Chipault (Testut and Jacob, 1932) in the 1990s also in France; of Turner (Turner, 1873 apud Greenblatt, 1997) in 1873, Horsley (Horsley apud Ebeling *et al.*, 1987) in 1892, Thane and Godlee (Krause, 1912) in 1896, and Taylor and Haughton (Taylor and Haughton, 1900 apud Uematsu *et al.*, 1992) in 1900, in England; of McClellan (McClellan, 1896) in 1896 in the United States; and of Bischoff (Bischoff, 1868 apud Broca, 1876b) in 1868, of Krönlein (Krause, 1912) in 1898, and Kocher in 1907 (apud Krause, 1912; Krause, 1912) in Germany. It is interesting to mention that Emil Thiodor Kocher (1841–1917) and Rudolf Ulrich Krönlein (1847–1910) were both eminent Swiss surgeons, with Kocher being awarded the Nobel Prize in Medicine and Physiology in 1909 in the light of his studies in physiology and surgery of the thyroid gland, and with Krönlein being particularly known for his work on abdominal wall hernias (Anderson, 1999).

In relation to the actual surgical application of these cranial-cerebral relationships, Broca was a pioneer again in 1876 with the report of the surgical treatment of a patient with a cerebral abscess in the language area, drained by "a trepanation done 1.5 centimeters posterior to the coronal suture and 2 centimeters above the Sylvius fissure." With this operation, Broca established modern neurosurgery by making these procedures more scientifically oriented and hence less exploratory (Broca, 1876a apud Stone, 1991; Gusmão *et al.*, 2000).

In 1884, Rickman Godlee performed the first glioma surgery based on neurological findings (seizure and hemiparesis) in the patient and directed by the knowledge of cranial-cerebral relationships described by B. D. Thane and himself, in the Hospital for Epilepsy and Paralysis, in London, in the presence of Hughlings Jackson, David Ferrier, Victor Horsley, and Joseph Lister (Kaye and Laws, 2001).

With regard to the relationships of the cranial sutures with the brain sulci and gyri, it is interesting to note that the more classic textbooks present illustrations pertinent to these relationships, but barely mention them in their texts. Among these treatises and atlases that contain beautiful illustrations of the relationships between the cranial sutures and the brain surface, standouts are the *Treatise on Topographic Anatomy* by Testut and Jacob (1932) with its first edition dating back to the beginning of the twentieth century, the textbook *Surgery of the Brain and Spinal Cord* by Krause (1912), and the more recent *Atlas of Topographical and Applied Human Anatomy* by Pernkoff (1980), with its first edition dating back to 1968.

Neurosurgical texts published more recently rarely mention cranial-cerebral relationships, and when they do, the mentions are brief and only pertinent to the classic nineteenth century descriptions (Rhoton, 1999; Seeger, 1978; Hansebout, 1982).

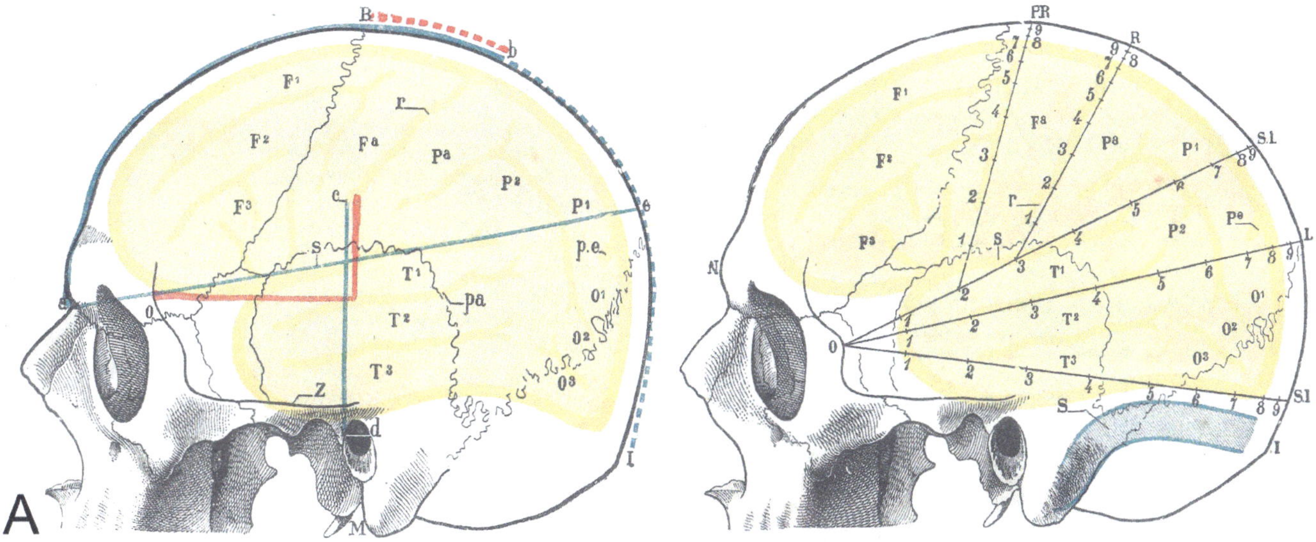

A

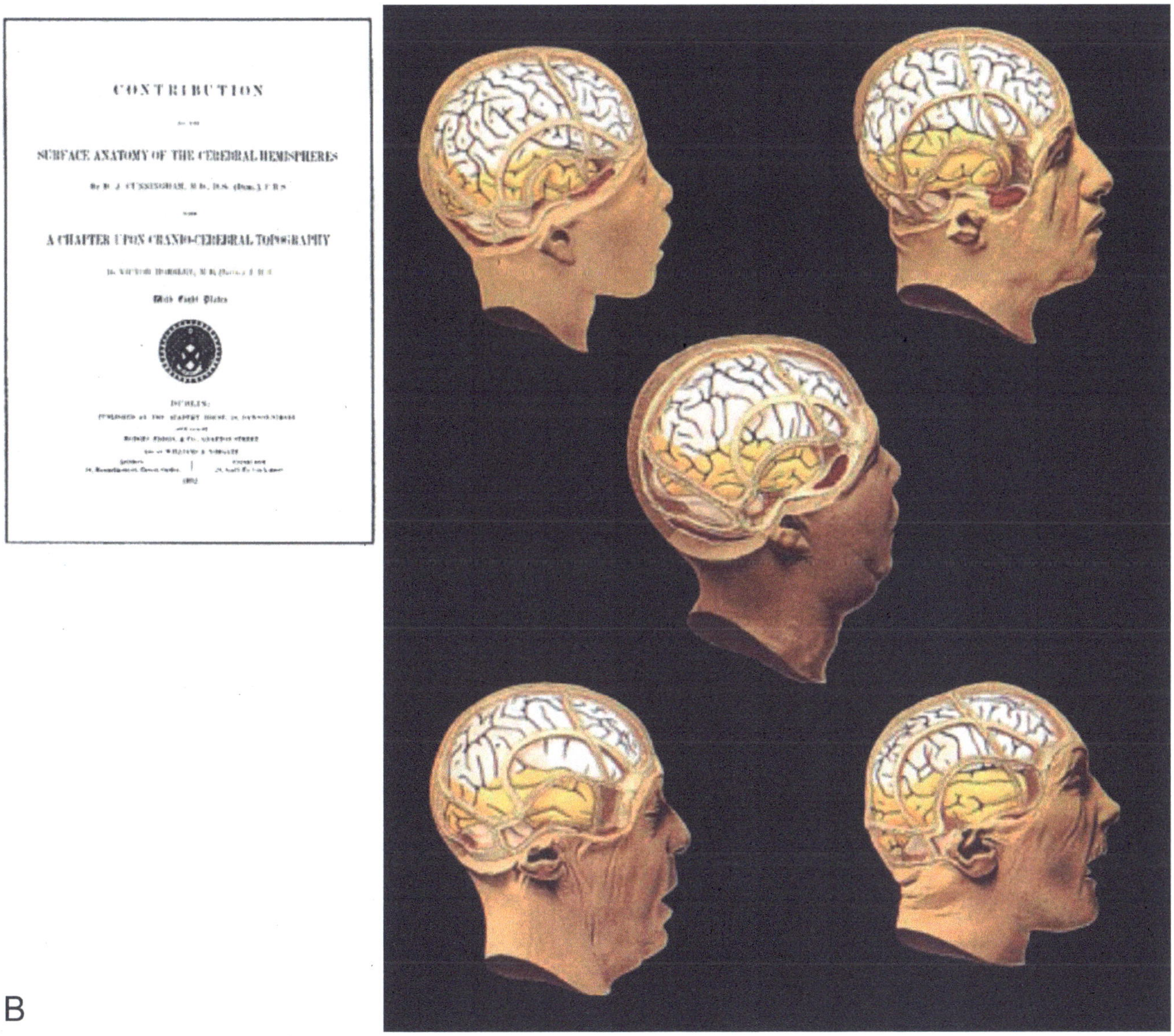

B

Figure 1.7 Other pioneering methods to establish the cranial-cerebral relationships:
(A) of Poirier-Chapionnière (1980), and of Chipault (1984) (see Testut and Jacob (1932)), in France;
(B) of Horsley (1892), in England;
(C) of Taylor and Haughton (1900), and of Thane and Godlee, 1896 (In Krause (1912)), in England;
(D) of Ferrier (1876), in England;
(E) of Krönlein (1898), and of Kocher (1907), in Germany;
(F) of McClellan (1896), in the United States.

SOME RECENT RESEARCHES ON THE TOPOGRAPHY OF THE CONVOLUTIONS AND FISSURES OF THE BRAIN.

By EDWARD H. TAYLOR, M.D., B.Ch., F.R.C.S.I.;
Surgeon to Sir Patrick Dun's Hospital;
University Examiner in Anatomy, Trinity College;

AND

WILLIAM S. HAUGHTON, M.B., B.Ch.;
Surgeon to Steeven's Hospital;
University Demonstrator of Röntgen Photography

[Read in the Section of Anatomy and Physiology, June 1, 1900.]

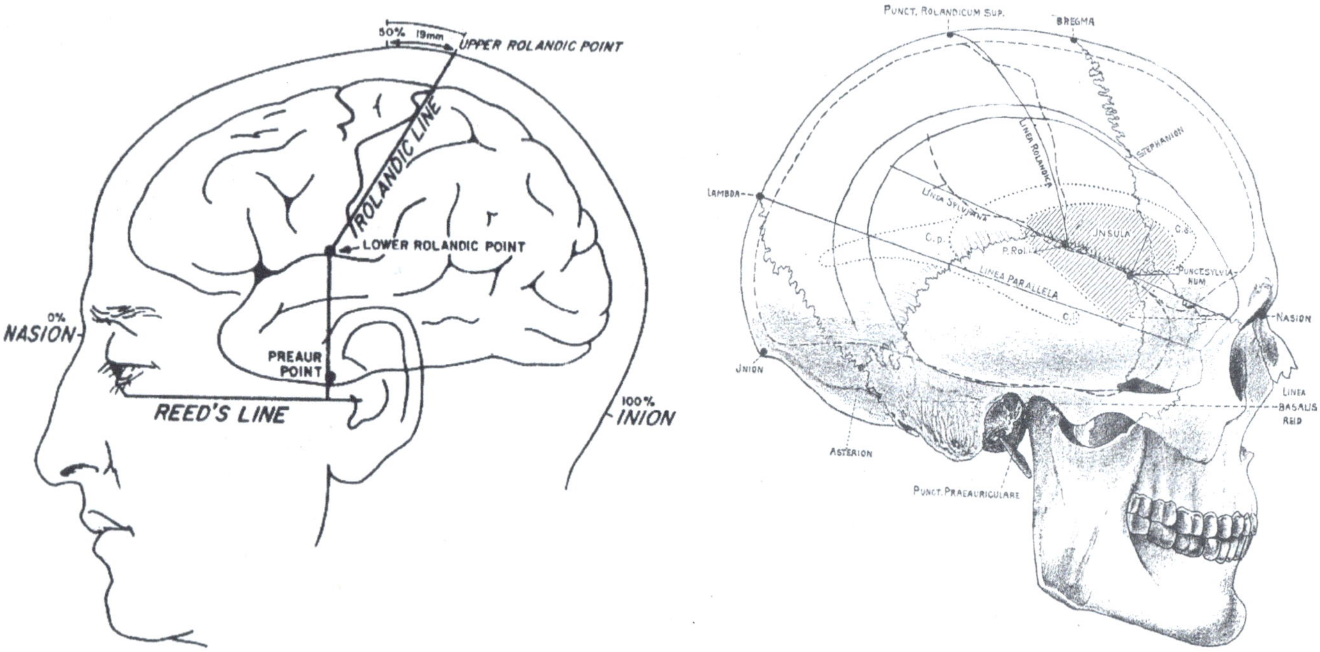

C

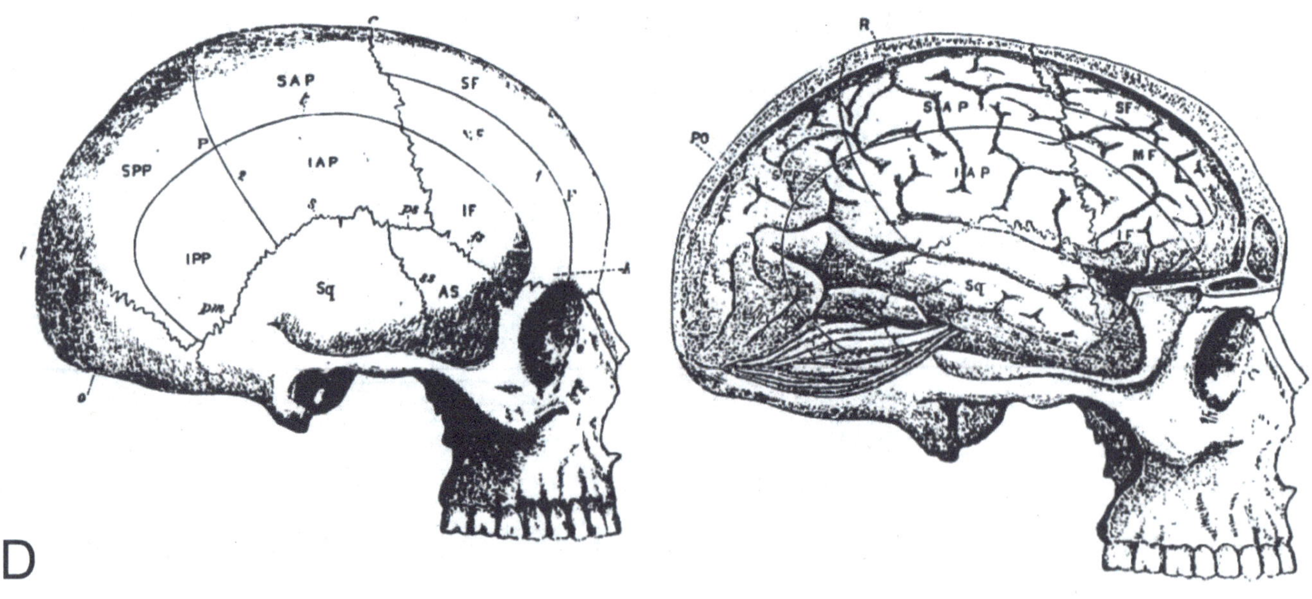

D

Figure 1.7 (cont.)

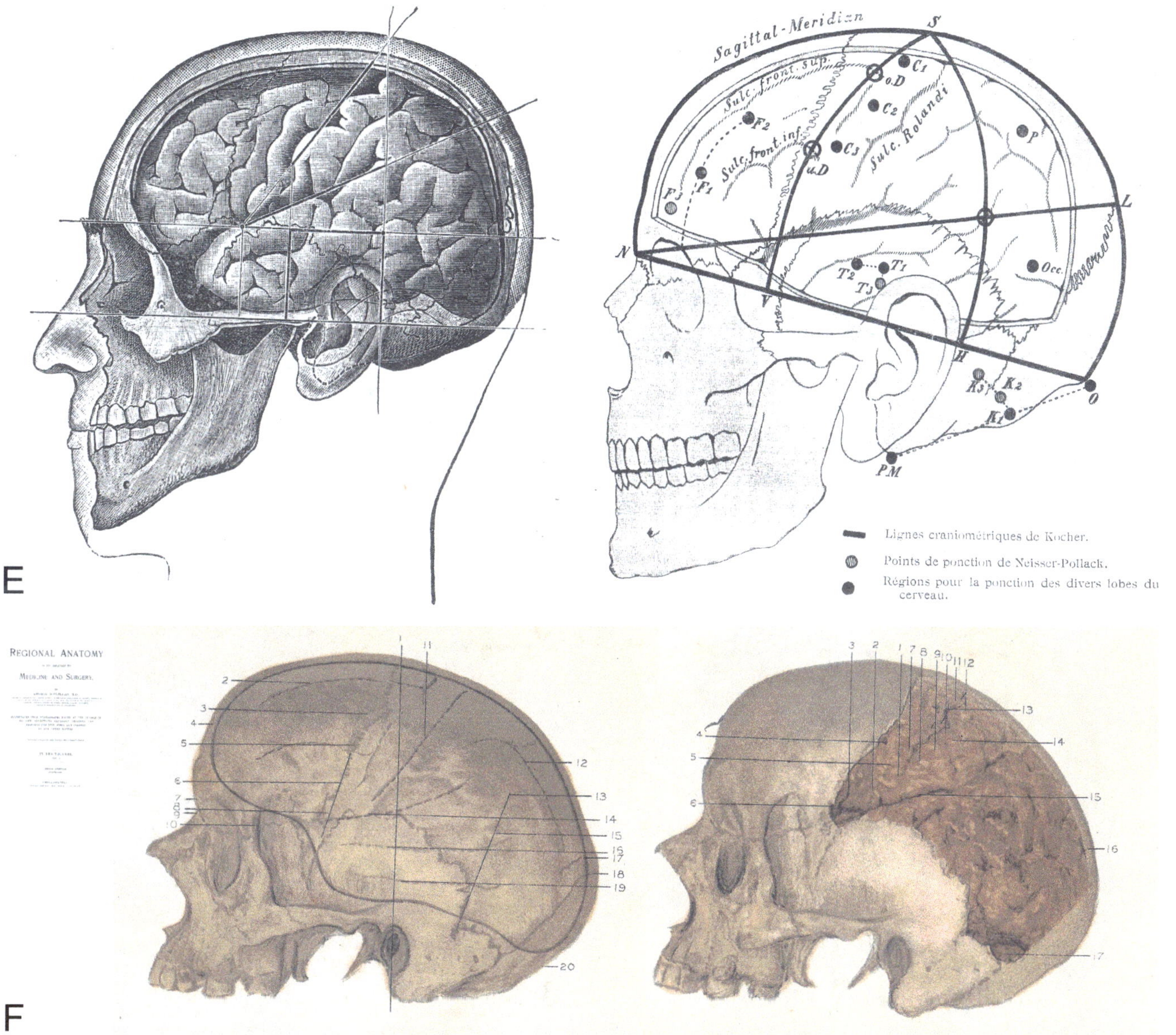

Figure 1.7 (cont.)

1.5 Technology and Cerebral Localization

With the advent of radiology after the discovery of X radiation by Wilhelm Konrad Röntgen (1845–1923) in 1895 (Anderson, 1999), correlation studies were also performed in order to determine coordinates that allowed the identification of brain structures on simple radiological images of the skull.

Among these, mention should be made of the study entitled "Radiographic relations between the cerebral sulci and gyri and the cranial sutures," carried out by Marie, Foix, and Bertrand during World War I and published in 1915 (Testut and Jacob, 1932). In that study, the authors introduced metal rods into cadavers through cranial perforations made at the points to be studied, obtained simple radiological images, and then removed the brains from the cranial boxes to study in detail the locations affected by the metal rods. The study aimed to allow the localization of encephalic structures from the superposition of radiographs of patients on a scheme of the brain surface obtained from the results of the study. Its text mentions conclusions like "the center of Broca relates with the upper edge of the sphenoid bone," "the supramarginal gyrus is above the frontolambdoid line and must be determined from the terminus of the Sylvian fissure," and "the curved fold (angular gyrus) is also arranged above the frontolambdoid line, 2 centimeters posterior to the end of the Sylvian fissure, but at a fairly variable distance from the Lambda." In relation to the lateral ventricles, these authors have already pointed out "the relation of the frontal horns with the coronal suture" and with "the anterior portions of the Sylvian valley" (Testut and Jacob, 1932).

The advent of radiology also led to the important development of neurosurgical stereotactic procedures. This concept was developed by Victor Horsley in association with the mathematician and engineer R. H. Clark in 1908 in experiments which aimed to place electrodes in animal nuclei. Horsley and

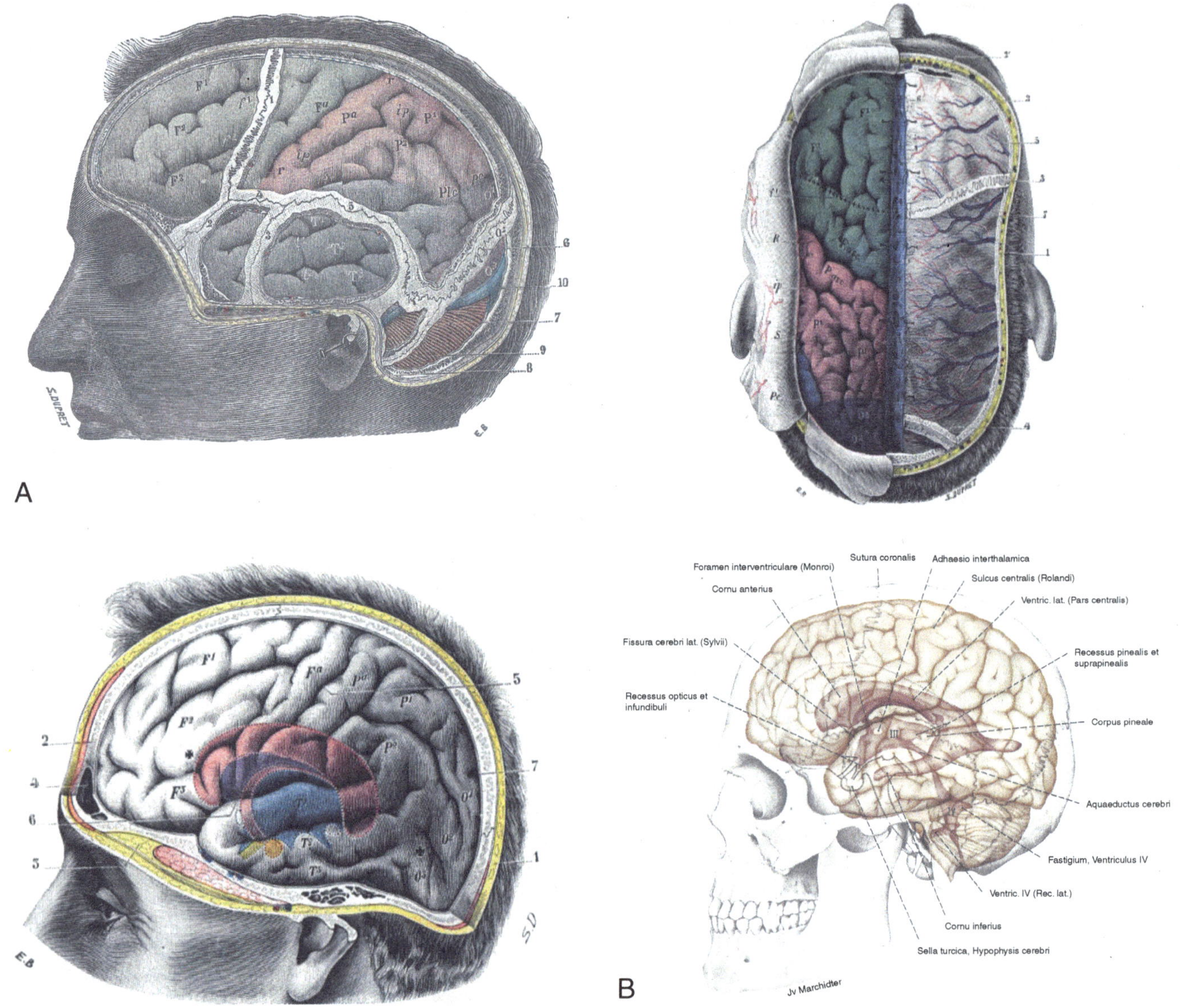

Figure 1.8 More recent atlases which disclose the relationships of the craniometric points and of the cranial sutures with the cerebral sulci and gyri: (A) by Testut and Jacob (1932); (B) by Pernkoff (1980).

Clark coined the term stereotaxia (from the Greek *stereo*: space, and *taxia*: arrangement), developed the first stereotactic instrument and published the first atlas on the subject, both pertinent to coordinates referring to skulls of rhesus monkeys (Chin *et al.*, 1999; Finger, 1994).

However, the stereotactic correlations of brain structures, more particularly of the deeper structures, with simple radiological images were not sufficiently precise, and the stereotactic method came to be much more precise with the discovery of pneumoencephalography in 1918 by Walter Dandy, disciple of Cushing and eminent neurosurgeon. The aerial contrast of the brain surface and ventricles obtained by injecting air into the subarachnoid space provided more precise radiological localization of neural structures and determination of the topography of intracranial lesions from the analysis of deformations and displacements of the air-filled natural intracranial spaces (Finger, 1994).

With the advent of pneumoencephalography, the concepts and initial development of the stereotactic technique could then be better elaborated for its practical and precise application in humans. The first stereotactic system for this purpose was developed by E .A. Spiegel and H. T. Wycis in 1947, and consisted of measured bars and cursors attached to a ring that, fixed around the patient's head, allowed three-dimensional coordinates to be obtained and then superimposed on pneumoencephalographic images. In 1952, the same authors published the first atlas of stereotactic coordinates of the human brain, and applied their method to the treatment of movement disorders, chronic pain, psychiatric disorders, and epilepsy (Chin *et al.*, 1999).

Another important contribution at this time for the location of encephalic structures, and particularly for the diagnosis of intracranial vascular lesions, was the development of angiography by the eminent Portuguese neurologist Egas Moniz, together with his neurosurgeon collaborator Almeida Lima, in 1927 (Finger, 1994).

Throughout the decade beginning in 1950, several other authors developed other systems and published other stereotactic atlases using angiographic images and neurophysiological stimuli. Among several published atlases, two that stand out were published by Talairach and collaborators in 1957, and by Talairach and Szikla in 1967, the latter of which includes the location of the main vessels, sulci, gyri, and subcortical structures (Chin *et al.*, 1999).

The stereotactic technique also allowed the development of the application of concentrated radiotherapy limited to a very precise and delimited intracranial volume, a technique idealized by Lars Leksell and collaborators in 1951 and named stereotactic radiotherapy, also known as radiosurgery.

The invention of computed tomography by G. Hounsfield (Breasted, 1930 apud Catani and Schotten, 2012) and its development throughout the second half of the 1970s revolutionized neurological and neurosurgical practice by allowing the direct observation of brain structures and intracranial lesions themselves. In addition to directly and precisely viewing the anatomical location of the structures and lesions, and their possible enhancement with the injection of iodinated contrast, computed tomography was also used as a basis for the acquisition of images of stereotactic systems. The Brown-Roberts-Wells, Cosman-Roberts-Wells, Leksell, Talairach, and Riechert-Mundinger (Chin *et al.*, 1999) systems are among several systems used, and their employment has also made possible the realization of biopsies of various lesions, as well as the treatment of functional disorders not capable of being performed by the older systems.

The use of stereotactic techniques based on images obtained by computed tomography also allowed the removal of brain tumors in a form directed by stereotactic coordinates, as proposed by Patrick Kelly in 1988 with the development of a stereotactic system specific for this purpose called "Volumetric Tumor Resection within a Stereotaxic Space" (Chin *et al.*, 1999; Kelly *et al.*, 1988).

The development of magnetic resonance imaging (MRI) in turn was the result of physical phenomena already known since the 1940s, but which were applied to obtain images in medicine developed during the 1970s from the contributions of Damadian in 1971, Lauterbur in 1973, and Mansfield and Grannell in 1973 (Sartor, 1992). The current images obtained by this method have an incredible anatomical definition and can be displayed in the three different planes (axial, coronal, and sagittal), thus providing a significantly greater understanding of the spatial arrangement of intracranial structures and lesions, and facilitating neurosurgical planning. In addition to providing information on the behavior of contrast-enhanced lesions with paramagnetic substances, the method also provides information on the behavior of normal intracranial structures and lesions with the variation of electromagnetic fields, according to the different systematically performed acquisitions.

Over the last decade, MRI has also provided imaging studies of several other physiological and pathophysiological phenomena. These studies have included those related to cerebrospinal fluid dynamics allowing the study of cerebrospinal fluid flow in the cerebral circulation using angioresonance and perfusion using diffusion studies; the study of the biochemical constitution of lesions using spectroscopic studies, and more recently, the study of cortical functions using functional magnetic resonance, and the study of the brain's own tracts by tractography (Witmer *et al.*, 2002).

From the surgical point of view, in addition to being able to constitute itself as the neuroimaging element coupled to the different stereotactic systems, its digital base of storage and manipulation of images allows the development of three-dimensional reconstructions which can be used as simulations of access routes and possible surgical visualizations.

The digital base of storage and manipulation of the different modalities of neuroimaging examinations, associated with the technology of light pulse transmission, culminated in the development of the so-called surgical neuronavigator, as originally conceived by Watanabe *et al.* (1987), and characterized as being a stereotactic neuronavigation system. With the aid of a computer station, with images obtained prior to surgery and at surgery guided by cranial repair points whose positioning is constantly updated during the surgical procedure, the neuronavigation system is able to identify, in the stored images, structures pinpointed in the surgical field (with the aid of a laser pointer) through a triangulation process similar to that used by known navigation instruments called Global Positioning System (GPS). Neuronavigation systems are made up of an antenna that has light emitting diodes (LED) and which are mobilized together with the patient's head, a bar with infrared sensors that picks up the pulses, and the computing station that stores the previously obtained images and which is connected to the bar with sensors. After initial registration of the chosen cranial repair points, which is done with a special sharpener connected to the system, any change in head position is informed to the system by the antenna attached to it, and any structure pinpointed by an instrument that also has light emitting diodes, which is suitably captured by the bar with sensors, is identified in relation to the images stored in the computing station. In some models of neuronavigators, the surgical microscope itself can be incorporated into the system so that the structure to be identified can be pinpointed by a laser beam in its own field of observation, and so that, in its own field of observation, it is possible to have the lesion itself and the route necessary for its access.

In practice, the neuronavigator is an instrument of immense help since anatomical identifications are greatly limited by restricted surgical exposure and by the overlap of different structural layers. In the case of the cerebral surface, even the anatomically more constant sulci and gyri are difficult to identify visually mainly due to the overlap of the arachnoid and vascular structures, and due to their frequent anatomical variations. In view of its features, the neuronavigator is particularly useful in the treatment of small subcortical lesions, but since it relies on previously obtained images, its accuracy becomes reduced in proportion to the removal of cerebrospinal fluid or any other intracranial volumes that cause displacements. The recent development of intraoperative imaging systems such as ultrasound and MRI which can update the previous data held by the neuronavigator is an alternative to remedy this limitation (Unsgaard *et al.*, 2002).

Transoperative identification and evaluation of intracranial structures and lesions in real time is currently possible with MRI during neurosurgical procedures (Black and Pikul,

1997; Black *et al.*, 1997; Wirtz *et al.*, 1997), and has recently become more feasible with the possible placement of resonance devices within the operating room.

Another innovative transoperative localization technique, which is still under development, consists of the use of instruments that allow optical visualization of light variations reflected in different cortical areas, thus allowing the identification of eloquent areas and also of pathological areas (Black and Pikul, 1997; Cannestra *et al.*, 1996; Haglund *et al.*, 1996).

The use of complementary magnetic resonance (MR) techniques such as MR angiography, diffusion, spectroscopy, functional MR, and MR imaging itself in conjunction with current stereotactic neuronavigation and with the developing transoperative MRI, will soon enable the intraoperative identification of vascular structures, evaluation of circulatory perfusion, identification of abnormal tissue composition, and recognition of functionally important cortical areas and tracts during surgical procedures.

However, the undoubted contribution of such technological advances is unfortunately accompanied by high costs for their widespread diffusion, and evidently does not replace the need for specialists to have a well-developed understanding of the three-dimensionality of the intracranial structures. Familiarity is essential for the perfect understanding of the spatiality of the central nervous system, of its lesions and for the planning of any intracranial procedure. Knowledge of the cranial-encephalic topographic relationships is the starting point for the constitution of this fundamental notion.

1.6 Microneurosurgical Anatomy

After about half a century of practice as a well-defined specialty worldwide, neurosurgery had its most important advance with the advent of microneurosurgery, mostly as a result of the contributions by M. Gazi Yasargil (1925–), a neurosurgeon of Turkish origin who developed most of his work in Zurich, Switzerland.

The surgical microscope was initially used by the otorhinolaryngologist William House (House, 1961 apud Yasargil, 1999) in 1961, and soon afterwards by the neurosurgeon Theodore Kurze (Kurze and Doyle, 1962; Yasargil, 1999), respectively, for the surgical treatment of acoustic schwannomas via the translabyrinthine and middle fossa routes. After reading the publications by these two authors, Yasargil began to use the surgical microscope in 1963. He undertook training in microsurgical techniques in the laboratory under the guidance of R. M. Peardon Donaghy, a neurosurgeon who was also a pioneer in microsurgery, in Burlington, Vermont, USA. On his return to Zurich in 1967, Yasargil began to use the microscope continuously in various types of neurosurgical procedures, thus definitively introducing the microscope into neurosurgical practice (Yasargil, 1999).

In parallel with the use of the microscope, microsurgery was only possible thanks to the use of bipolar microcoagulation, initially conceived by J. Greenwood in 1940 and later developed by the great and creative neurosurgeon Leonard Malis through successive models from 1960 onwards. The other surgical instrument fundamental to the application of these new techniques, and which would eventually allow the advent of skull base surgery proper, was the air drill, a system of high-speed bone drilling developed by several companies during the 1970s (Rhoton, 1999). The feasibility of more basal cranial access, made possible by its use, allowed better exposure of basal structures with less encephalic retraction and with greater viewing and working angles.

The magnification, and especially the illumination, provided by the surgical microscope, together with the use of delicate instruments, enabled the visualization and manipulation of the natural spaces that surround the central nervous system and that are contained in it. Dissections, particularly of the fissures and sulci, demonstrated that these natural spaces could be used as actual microneurosurgical corridors, greatly optimizing the exposure of structures and intracranial lesions. It was up to Yasargil himself to make the first studies and descriptions of this new anatomy demonstrated by the microscope from the surgical point of view, to design new instruments, and even to propose modifications to the surgical microscope itself (Yasargil, 1999).

After his classic descriptions of pterional craniotomy in 1975 (Yasargil *et al.*, 1975) and the surgical anatomy of the subarachnoid cisterns in 1976 (Yasargil *et al.*, 1976), Yasargil went on to study in detail the surgical microanatomy of the brain fissures, sulci, and gyri (Ono *et al.*, 1990; Yasargil, 1994; Yasargil *et al.*, 1988a) and through a voluminous surgical casuistry of vascular and tumoral lesions ended up systematizing several access approaches and techniques that today constitute the core of modern microneurosurgery (Yasargil, 1984a, 1984b, 1987, 1988, 1994, 1996).

In this new field of neurosurgical microanatomy, the Albert Rhoton Jr. school, initiated during the 1970s and productive until his death in 2016, stands out in parallel. Dozens of trainees passed through his laboratory at the University of Florida under his dedicated guidance, studied cranial and encephalic microanatomy through a vision fundamentally applied to neurosurgical practice, and disseminated it in numerous publications always illustrated with beautiful images of dissections of human cadaveric specimens with arteries and veins properly injected, and with particularly didactic texts.

These anatomical studies, pioneered by M. G. Yasargil and the school of A. Rhoton Jr. and disseminated worldwide through a vast number of publications and practical courses mostly by their fellows, not only opened up a new neuroanatomic dimension constituted by neurosurgical microanatomy, but also gave rise to a new radiological and neurosurgical philosophy (Yasargil, 1999). Observation and examination of the brain through normal and altered images are done from the brain sulci and ventricular surfaces, which now constitute the core of neurosurgical topographic reasoning. Throughout this philosophy and practice, the mere use of the microscope gave rise to the current modern microneurosurgery, and in parallel to its surgical and radiological importance, this anatomical knowledge also enriched clinical reasoning, guiding us towards a modern neurosurgical vision.

Chapter 2

The Cerebral Architecture

Anatomy is for physiology what geography is for history: it describes the scene of action.
Jean Fernel (1497–1558) (Haeger, 1988)

2.1 Developmental Aspects

The understanding of some evolutionary and embryological key features of central nervous system development can be very helpful, particularly for the comprehension of the final placements, shapes, and relationships of the cerebral hemispheric structures.

To some extent, the embryological development of the human central nervous system (CNS) mirrors the main changes that occurred during phylogeny (Sarnat and Netsky, 1981; Gould, 1977), and with regard to the morphological aspects of the CNS, bending and folding mechanisms predominate throughout both developments to yield an overall CNS enlargement without a proportional increase in its volume. The bending process of each developing cerebral hemisphere takes place around its center which corresponds to each thalamus, and this is responsible for the final C-shaped profile assumed by each hemisphere and by many of its inner structures. A similar folding process acting on its surfaces gives rise to the sulci, which delimit the cerebral convolutions, or gyri, significantly enlarging its cortical area.

Another important issue for the understanding of the complex anatomy of the human brain is to bear in mind that our whole body is composed of parts with roles that have changed since they first evolved, and that our nervous system in particular harbors many vestigial structures that were important for our ancestors but are currently less or even not functional for humans, with the olfactory structures probably representing the best example of this (Held, 2009; Gould, 1977; Sarnat and Netsky, 1981). The anterior commissure, which was the main commissure in ancient reptiles, now carries about 5 percent of all commissural fibers in the monkey (mainly connecting corresponding parts of the temporal lobes), and in humans only carries 1 to 2 percent (Brodal, 2010) with a uncertain functional importance.

2.1.1 Evolutionary Considerations

The primitive fishes left the oceans about 350 million years ago becoming amphibians and then reptiles (Gould, 2001; MacLean, 1973). According to evolutionary theory, among all of the tremendous body transformations they were submitted to, their primitive CNS, which was then characterized by a spinal cord segment with incipient brainstem, hypothalamus, and striatum on top, gained the olfactory lobes to perceive their new world and the hippocampus and amygdala, respectively, to identify their new perceptions and to direct their behavior in conjunction with the hypothalamus (MacLean, 1973; Sarnat and Netsky, 1981; Squire *et al.*, 2003; Oró, 2004; Park *et al.*, 2007). These new structures were arranged around the top of the ancient CNS and were called limbic structures, from *limbus* the Latin word for "ring." In order to perform different input and output combinations, their cells were arranged in a laminar pattern characterizing then the most primitive cortices, called the archicortex (amygdala and hippocampus) and paleocortex (olfactory piriform area) (Sarnat and Netsky, 1981) (Figure 2.1).

Regarding the cerebral hemispheres, and particularly their cortical surfaces, their ultimate development which began with these primitive structures came with the development of the neocortex. This started with the advent of the mammals about 230 million years ago, and proceeded particularly throughout

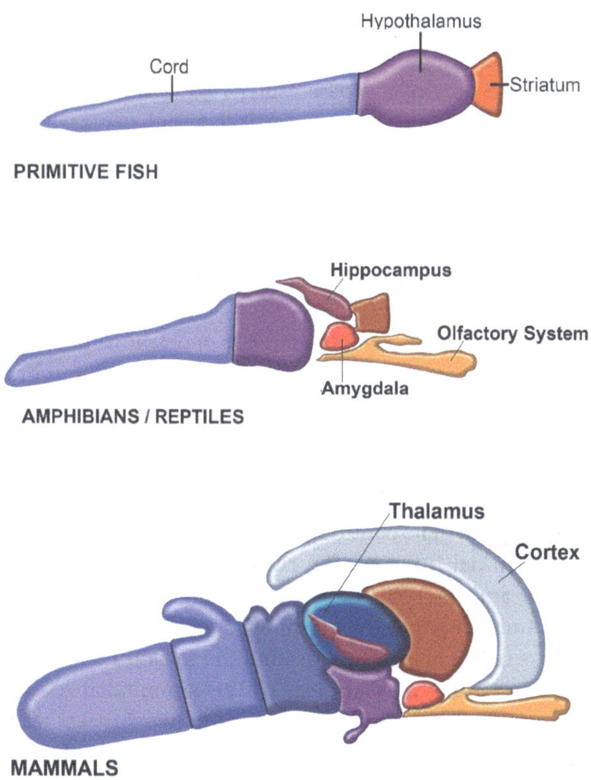

Figure 2.1 Evolutionary development of the neural structures.

Table 2.1 Mammalian cortical development

Primitive Cortex Allocortex **(3 layers)**	Medial Cortical Ring Mesocortex **(6 layers)**	Lateral Cortical Ring Isocortex **(6 organized layers)**
Limbic structures	Paralimbic structures and insula	Parainsular structures and neocortical structures
• Archicortex:		• Neocortex:
Amygdala	Parahippocampal gyrus	Motor cortex
Hippocampus	Cingulate gyrus	Sensory cortex
• Paleocortex:		Visual cortex
Olfactory or	Insula	Auditory cortex
Piriform cortex		Language cortices (humans)
		Rest of neocortex, associated areas

Adapted from Sarnat and Netsky (1981).

the evolution of the primates, culminating with the emergence of modern man about 50 000 years ago (Gould, 2001, 2002).

According to Sarnat and Netsky (1981), cytoarchitectonic evidence suggests that the generalized six-layered neocortex of primitive mammals evolved simultaneously from both the hippocampal archicortex and from the olfactory piriform paleocortex. As the first stage, with the archicortex forming the medial side and the paleocortex forming the lateral side of the cerebral hemisphere, both probably gave rise to a cortex with an architecture intermediate in complexity between three and six layers that surrounded the original primitive cortex. A second zone of further differentiated neocortex then formed as an additional concentric ring becoming the parahippocampal and the cingulate gyri on the medial side, and the insular cortex laterally. A third ring of further differentiated neocortex then appeared characterizing the paralimbic and parainsular cortices which became sites of specialized sensory and motor functions, with part of the parainsular region also becoming an auditory center and with a cortical visual center being developed in the paralimbic zone (Table 2.1).

The final shape and configuration of the human cerebral hemisphere itself is mostly given by the bending mechanism that takes place around its morphological center composed of its respective thalamus, throughout both evolution and human embryology (Figure 2.2).

In lower terrestrial vertebrates, the hippocampus develops as a dorsal structure forming the medial part of the cerebral hemispheres, and in advanced mammals, it is rotated back and down into a ventral position by the great expansion of the neocortex (Romer, 1970 apud Sarnat and Netsky, 1981). Further development of the parahippocampal gyrus along the hippocampus and of its continuous cingulate gyrus comprising the cortical initial inner medial ring, and of the paralimbic, parainsular, and the rest of the neocortex then occurred progressively and along the circular route generated by bending of the whole cerebral hemisphere around the thalamus.

The tremendous development of the mammalian cortex occurred throughout an extensive infolding process that made possible a significant increase in its surface without a proportional enlargement of its outer extent and total volume, and resulted in the final cortical human pattern given by its fissures, sulci, and their delimitated gyral convolutions. Considering also the interhemispheric fissure, this invagination process led by the evolutionary forces finally left in man approximately two-thirds of the cortical surface buried in the depths of the sulci and fissures (Williams and Warwick, 1980).

The first hemispheric sulcus to appear phylogenetically is the sulcus that separates the archicortex from its surrounding structures (namely the hippocampal sulcus that separates the dentate gyri of the hippocampus from the parahippocampal subiculum, and that arises medially along the phylogenetic and embryological caudal migration of the previous supracallosal hippocampus) (Sarnat and Netsky, 1981). The second is the sulcus that demarcates the paleocortex from the neocortex (namely the rhinal sulcus, secondary to the ventral displacement of the piriform cortex caused by neocortical development (Sarnat and Netsky, 1981), and that in man separates the parahippocampal uncus from the rest of the neocortical temporal pole). Both sulci were already present in early mammals (Sarnat and Netsky, 1981).

On the other hand, the Sylvian fissure was a result of the overlapping growth of the infolding opercula of the surrounding lobes onto the insula (Ribas, 2010; Sarnat and Netsky, 1981), and which became narrow only in man with the particular development of the frontoparietal operculum that is underdeveloped even in the highest anthropoid apes (Sarnat and Netsky, 1981; Squire *et al.*, 2003). The most notable development was the pars triangularis and the pars opercularis of the inferior frontal gyrus that in the dominant hemisphere of man correspond to the so-called Broca's speech area (Broca, 1876b).

2.1.2 Embryological and Fetal Considerations

The embryological development of the nervous system begins around the third week of intrauterine life with thickening of the ectoderm which generates the neural plate under the inducing influence of the notochord. The development of neural folds with a neural groove between them starts the formation of the neural tube, with the so-called neurulation proceeding with the cranial to caudal approximation and fusion of the neural folds along the midline, and with the subsequent

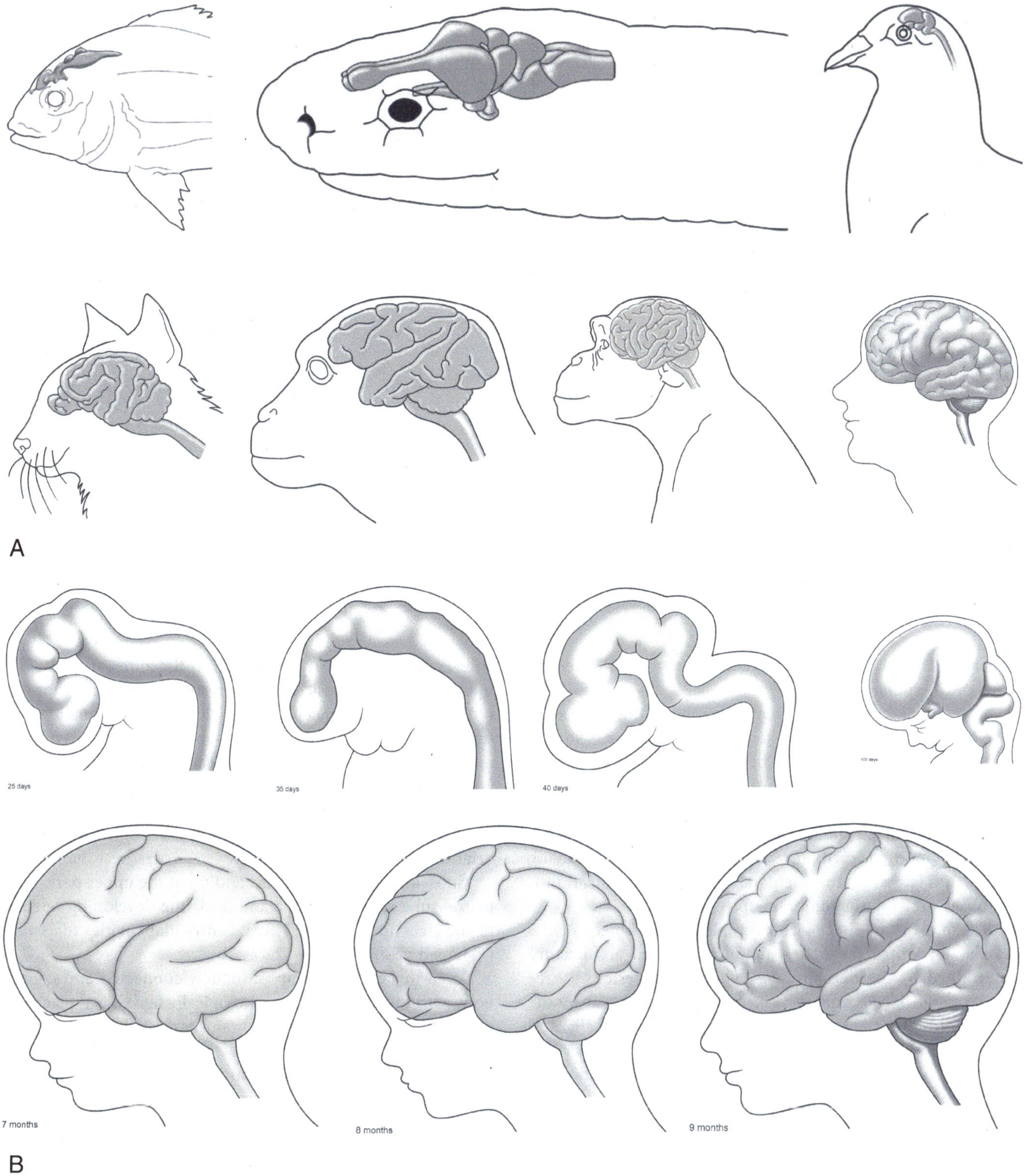

Figure 2.2 (A) evolutionary and (B) human embryological and fetal developments of the central nervous system.

closures of the cranial and posterior neuropores around the end the fourth week.

While the neural tube itself sinks from the surface of the ectoderm to generate the CNS, the remaining pluripotent cells of the neural crest migrate to form sensory and autonomic ganglia, Schwann cells, adrenal medulla, the pia matter, and the arachnoid among other structures (Borden *et al.*, 2016).

While the mantle layer of the neural tube forms the gray matter, its marginal layer gives rise to the white matter, and its

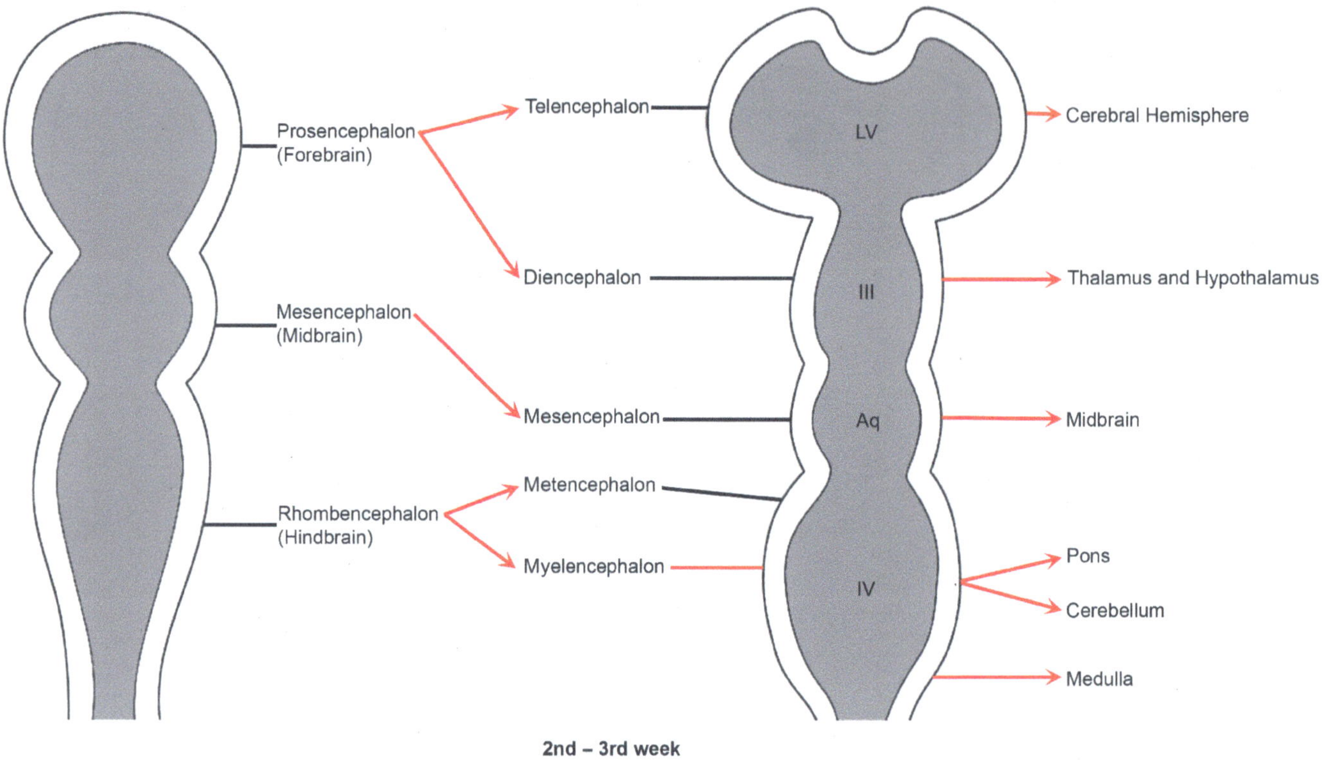

Figure 2.3 Embryological development of the neural tube and brain vesicles. III: third ventricle; IV: fourth ventricle; LV: lateral ventricle; Aq: aqueduct.

lumen the ventricular cavities, the aqueduct, and the central canal of the spinal cord.

The spinal cord and caudal portion of the brainstem develop according to a straightforward organization, with the mantle layer of the spinal cord developing in each side into a basal plate (future anterior horn) and an alar plate (future posterior horn). These become separated by an evident groove known as the sulcus limitans, and with the motor and sensory cranial nerves of the medulla oblongata and of the pons having a medial to lateral arrangement; however, this organization is not observed from the midbrain up.

The more pronounced and complex development of the cranial portion of the neural tube has its final architecture determined by the development of the brain vesicles (three primary and five secondary vesicles) (Figure 2.3) and by the cranial folding of the neural tube (cervical, mesencephalic, and pontine) (Borden *et al.*, 2016) (Figure 2.4).

Very early during embryogenesis, the prosencephalic vesicle (forebrain), the most superior of the three primary brain vesicles originating from the neural tube, is divided cranial-caudally by the development of the transverse fissure of the brain forming the endbrain (telencephalic) and the interbrain (diencephalic) vesicles. A superior midline depression of the endbrain starts forming the interhemispheric fissure giving rise to both cerebral hemispheres. While the cerebral structures are developed from the walls of the endbrain vesicle, its residual central lumen becomes the lateral ventricles.

The superior midline depression of the endbrain, which originally corresponds to the top of the neural tube, as well as forming the interhemispheric fissure, is also displaced anteriorly and inferiorly ending up as the anterior wall of the midline interbrain vesicle that corresponds to the inferior part of the original prosencephalic vesicle. The diencephalic structures (thalamus, hypothalamus, subthalamus, and epithalamus) originate from its walls on each side, and its residual lumen becomes the third ventricle in between both thalami and with its anterior wall then having a telencephalic origin and being very appropriately called the lamina terminalis due to its original position.

Subsequently, the circular bending of the upper part of the neural tube around the thalami leads the developing telencephalic structures and the lateral ventricular cavities to assume C-shaped profiles (Figure 2.4).

Each thalamus ends up intimately connected and continuous with the midbrain, morphologically like a head placed on top of each upper half of the brainstem, at the center of the brain (Figure 2.5).

Each hippocampus, which initially occupies a superior and medial position, slides posteriorly and inferiorly around the thalamus ending within the inferior (temporal) horn of the lateral ventricle, leaving a tail of fibers along its course which constitute the fornix. The virtual space between each fornix and each thalamus becomes the choroidal fissure. The two small longitudinal striae of gray matter that end over the corpus callosum, which are known as the indusium griseum (supracallosal gyri), are believed to be remnants of both ancient hippocampi (Sarnat and Netsky, 1981) (Figure 2.6).

Concomitantly, the callosal fibers develop over the top of the lateral ventricles from anterior to posterior, and the projection fibers, which connect the cortex with subcortical

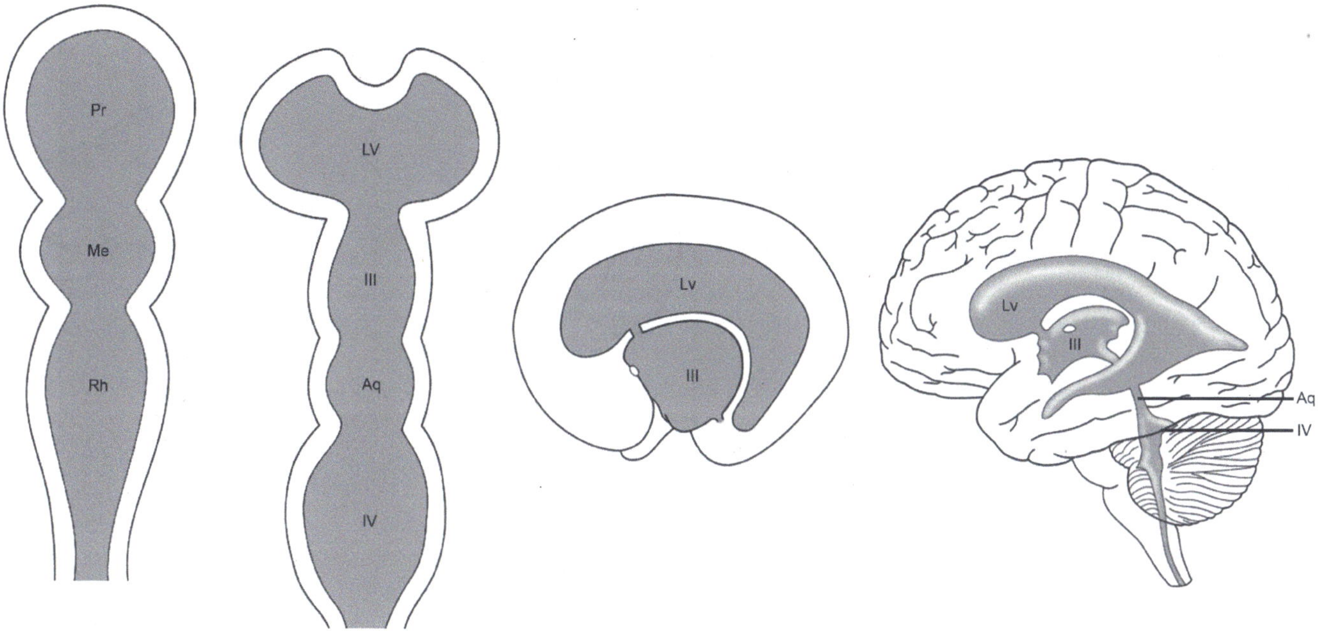

Figure 2.4 Embryological and fetal development of the ventricular system.
III: third ventricle; IV: fourth ventricle; Aq: aqueduct; Lv: lateral ventricle; Me: mesencephalon; Pr: proencephalon; Rh: rhombencephalon.

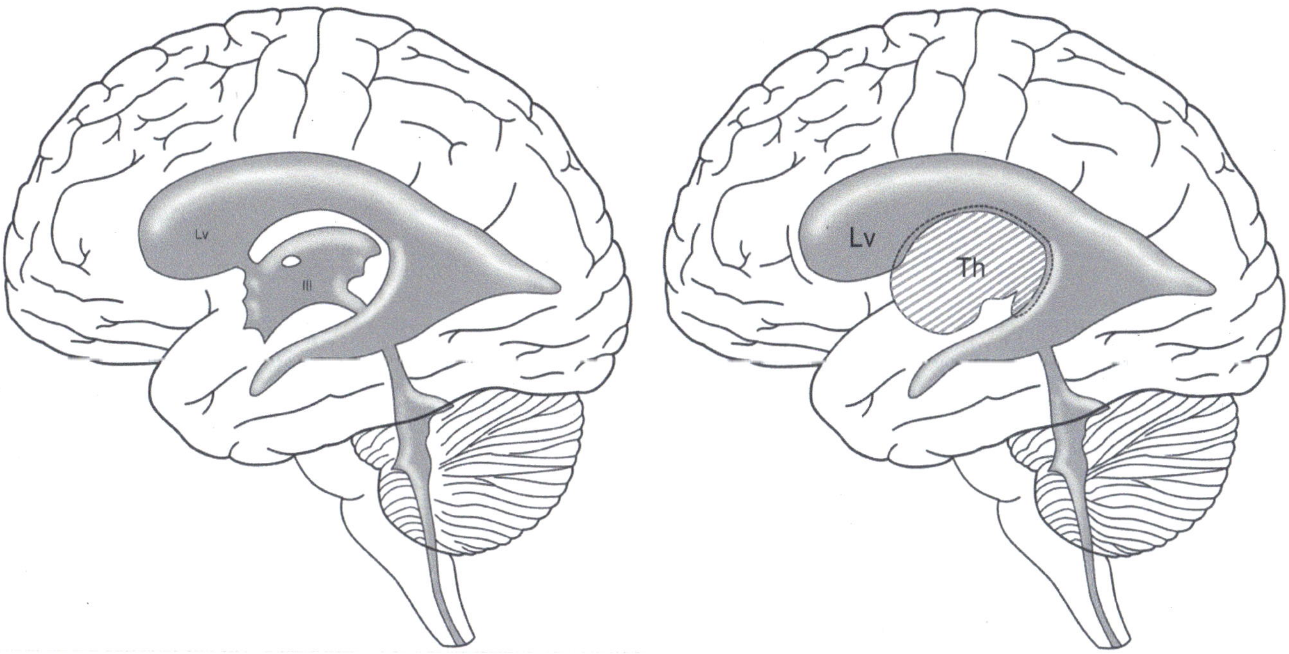

Figure 2.5 The ventricular system and the thalamus.
Th: thalamus; LV: lateral ventricle; III: third ventricle.

structures, develop splitting the previously formed corpus striatum on both sides.

Since the cranial-caudal projection fibers in each hemisphere assume a final fan-like shape, opening toward the cortical surface and converging toward the thalamus and brainstem, the dorsal aspect of each corpus striatum is divided generating the caudate nucleus medially and the putamen laterally. The ventral aspect of the striatum remains undivided still connecting the anterior and basal aspects of the caudate and putamen with the ventral striatum harboring the nucleus accumbens (Figure 2.7). Usually small residual nests of striatal cells can be found within the ascending and descending projection fibers, particularly within the most anterior groups of fibers (anterior limb of the internal capsule) where division of the corpus striatum can frequently be incomplete.

The globus pallidus has a different embryological origin but lies attached to the inferior and medial aspect of the putamen

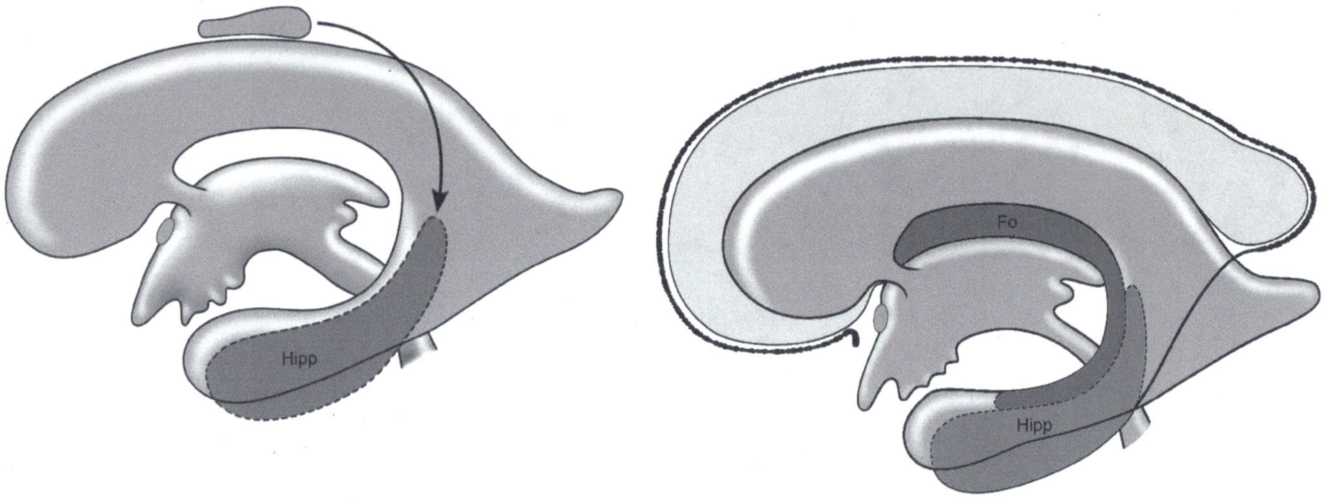

Figure 2.6 Migration of ancient hippocampus and human hippocampal formation structures.
Hipp: hippocampus; Fo: fornix.

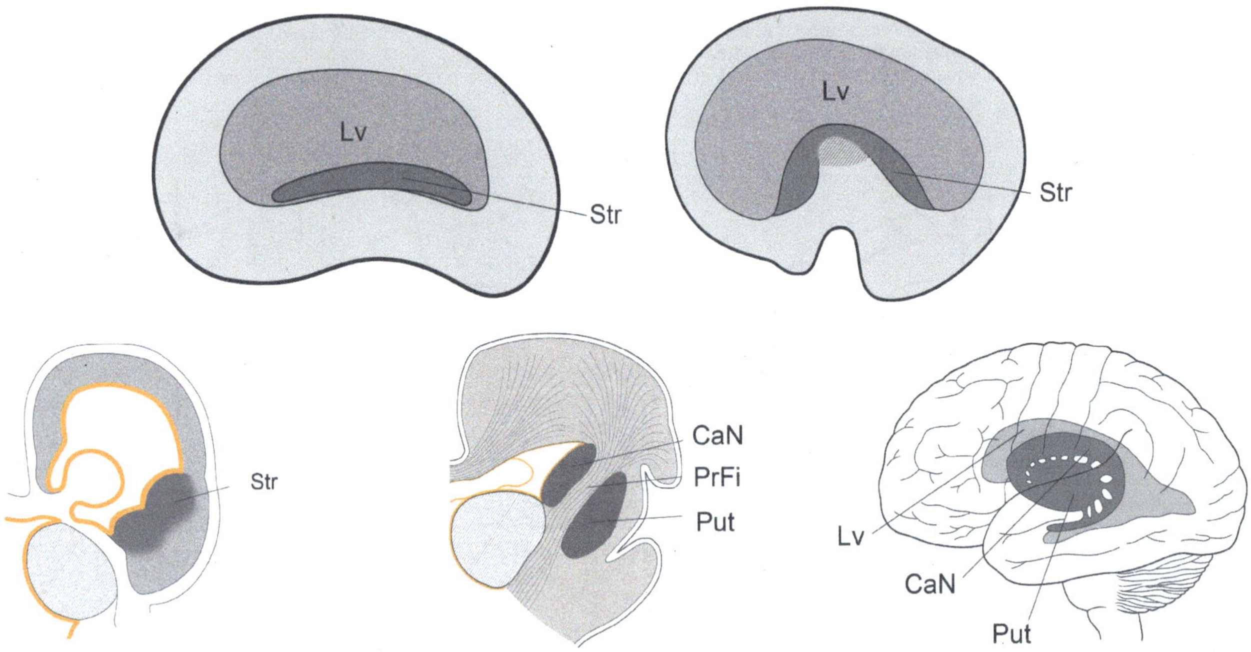

Figure 2.7 Embryological and fetal development of the caudate and putamen.
Lv: lateral ventricle; Str: striatum; CaN: caudate nucleus; Put: putamen; PrFi: projection fibers.

with both the globus pallidus and putamen constituting the lentiform nucleus. The projection fibers within its superior and inferior levels are referred to as the internal capsule of the lentiform nucleus.

The same evolutionary and embryological bending mechanisms also affect other deep structures such as the stria terminalis (which is a dorsal extension of the amygdala) ending up with these structures also encircling each thalamus in a C-shaped configuration, just like the lateral ventricle and the outer aspects of the cerebral hemisphere itself. The deeper structures in part become the walls of the lateral ventricles as discussed later, with each fornix wrapping around each thalamus medially and the caudate nucleus wrapping around each thalamus laterally.

Both the transverse fissure of the brain, which separates the endbrain (telencephalic) from the interbrain (diencephalic) vesicles, and the interhemispheric fissure, which starts as a superior midline depression dividing the endbrain vesicle, arise around the tenth week of gestation (Chi *et al.*, 1977).

Regarding the cerebral surface, a similar folding process gives rise to the fissures and sulci that delimit the cerebral convolutions or gyri, and this process significantly enlarges its cortical area without a proportional increase in brain volume.

Embryologically, the sulci are formed according to a sequence which reflects their phylogeny and a true hierarchy exists among them. Their formation begins with the appearance of the fissures, followed by the sulci related to eloquent

Table 2.2 Prenatal cerebral sulci development in weeks of gestation

	Chi *et al.*, 1977	Nishikuni, 2006
No. of fetuses	207	107
Gestational age range, weeks	10–44	12–40
Longitudinal cerebral fissure	10	12
Superolateral surface		
Lateral sulcus	14	17
Circular insular sulcus	18	17
Central insular sulcus		29
Central sulcus	20	21
Precentral sulcus	24	26
Superior frontal sulcus	25	25
Inferior frontal sulcus	28	30
Postcentral sulcus	25	29
Intraparietal sulcus	26	29
Transverse occipital sulcus		30
Lunate sulcus		24
Superior temporal sulcus	23	26
Inferior temporal sulcus	30	31
Transverse temporal sulcus	31	33
Inferior surface		
Olfactory sulcus	16	17
Orbital sulcus		22
Hippocampal sulcus	10	12
Rhinal sulcus		25
Collateral sulcus	23	29
Occipitotemporal sulcus	30	33
Medial surface		
Callosal sulcus	14	12
Cingulate sulcus	18	19
Marginal ramus		33
Paracentral sulcus		30
Paraolfactory sulcus		29
Subparietal sulcus		30
Calcarine sulcus	16	17
Parieto-occipital sulcus	16	19
Secondary sulcus	40	38

Adapted from Chi *et al.* (1977) and from Nishikuni and Ribas (2013).

areas of the brain, and finally by sulci of the secondary and tertiary cortical areas (Broca, 1876a apud Stone, 1991; Broca, 1877 apud Finger, 1994; Chi *et al.*, 1977; Nishikuni and Ribas, 2013) (Table 2.2) (Figure 2.8).

Between the eighth and tenth weeks, transitory furrows, which are not precursors of the definite sulci, appear in the cerebral hemispheric surfaces and last until the fifth month when the brain surfaces become smooth with only the insular area present as an evident depression (Ono *et al.*, 1990).

During the fourth to fifth months of fetal life, the first definite sulci (olfactory, calcarine, parieto-occipital, cingulate, and central) begin to appear initially as points or grooves, followed by further secondary and tertiary furrows, with some of these being developed only after birth (Chi *et al.*, 1977; Ono *et al.*, 1990; Nishikuni and Ribas, 2013).

Control of this process and of its relatively variable final result are to a large part genetically determined (Squire *et al.*, 2003); however in practical terms, it is interesting to point out that, given the mechanism of infolding in which the sulci are developed and given the concomitant circular curvature that the whole developing brain is submitted to such as wrapping the thalami at its morphological center, the sulci, particularly of the superolateral and inferior surfaces of the cerebral hemisphere, end up pointing toward the nearest part of the lateral ventricular cavity. The development of the sulcal pattern in the medial surfaces seems to be particularly influenced by the development of the corpus callosum since its congenital absence is linked to the absence of an arched cingulate gyrus and to the radial pattern of the sulci in the medial surfaces (Ono *et al.*, 1990).

Regarding the extensive variability of the basic arrangement of the cortical sulci and gyri, Régis *et al.* (2005) recently proposed that the occurrence of such variations might depend on the variable development of connecting gyri buried at depth in the sulci ("plis de passage"). Taking into account these buried gyri, and using a database of MR images from 20 healthy patients, these authors proposed an interesting generic model of folding patterns based on a constant number of indivisible units they termed "sulcal roots," and proposed a common constant protomap. According to this hypothesis, the burying process is believed to result from a trade-off between the various folding pressures that occur during brain growth, with the superficial variability resulting from the chaotic behavior given by the greater or lesser development of the buried gyral connections, with a major development of a given gyral connection causing an interruption to the sulcus located above this connection. As an example based on this hypothesis, the occasional interruption of the central sulcus is then due to a more significant development of the middle frontoparietal connection (of Broca) that lies between the precentral and postcentral gyri at the so-called omega region (Boling and Olivier, 2004; Yousry *et al.*, 1997).

The telencephalic insula, basal ganglia (lentiform and caudate nuclei) and its surrounding fibers (internal and external capsules of the lentiform nucleus), together with the diencephalic thalamus itself, morphologically comprise a rather well-defined anatomical block within each hemisphere, delimited medially by the lateral and third ventricular cavities. As discussed in more detail later, this block is referred to as the central core of the brain.

2.2 The Cerebral Hemispheres

The two cerebral hemispheres together constitute the most developed part of the human nervous system (Ribas, 2015), and each corresponds to a large mass of neuronal tissue with a C-shaped format which medially wraps the ipsilateral thalamus with the lateral ventricle in between (Figure 2.9).

Each cerebral hemisphere has the cerebral cortical mantle as its surface, anteriorly it is characterized by the frontal and temporal poles, and posteriorly by the occipital poles. It

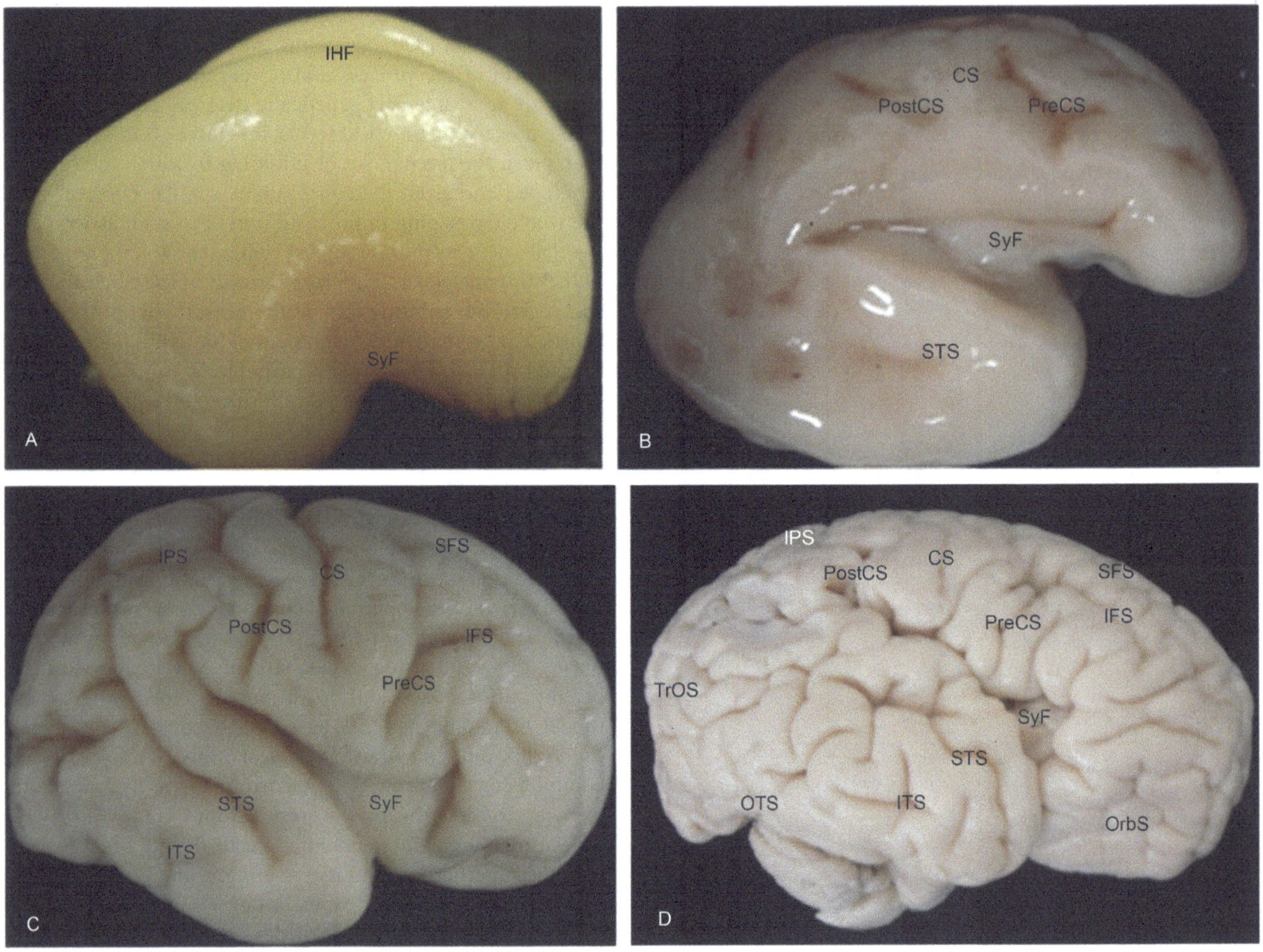

Figure 2.8 Development of sulci in the superolateral cerebral surface of the fetus at (A) 17, (B) 24, and (C) 36 weeks, and (D) at 1 postnatal week.
CS: central sulcus; IFS: inferior frontal sulcus; IHF: interhemispheric fissure (longitudinal cerebral fissure); IPS: intraparietal sulcus; ITS: inferior temporal sulcus; OrbS: orbital sulcus; OTS: occipitotemporal sulcus; PostCS: postcentral sulcus; PreCS: precentral sulcus; SFS: superior frontal sulcus; STS: superior temporal sulcus; SyF: lateral sulcus (Sylvian fissure); TrOS: transverse occipital sulcus. (Adapted from Nishikuni and Ribas (2013).)

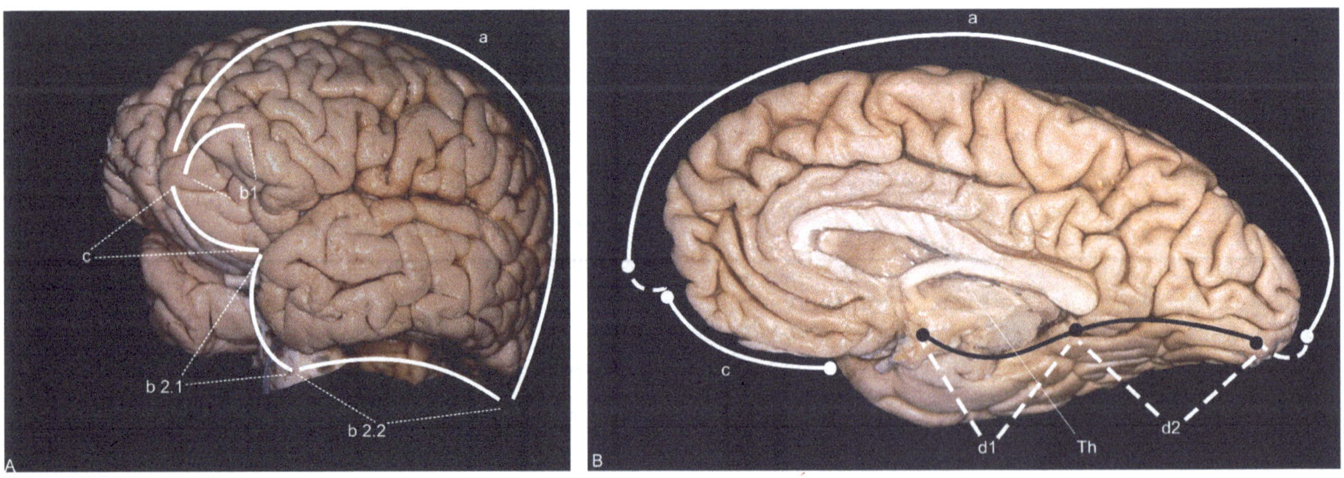

Figure 2.9 (A and B): The margins of the cerebral hemispheres.
a: Superomedial; b: inferolateral – b1: superciliary, b2.1: inferolateral-sphenoidal part, b2.2: inferolateral – basal temporal part; c: medial orbital; d1: medial perimesencephalic, d2: medial occipital; Th: thalamus.

harbors the basal ganglia (caudate nucleus, putamen, nucleus accumbens, globus pallidus amygdala, and claustrum) (Lockard, 1977), and the association, commissural, and projection fibers, with both hemispheres being connected mainly by the corpus callosum along the midline.

Each hemisphere has a superolateral surface (dorsal, cerebral convexity), a medial surface, and an inferior or basal surface, respectively separated by the superomedial, inferolateral (with its anterior part also known as superciliary), medial orbital, and medial occipital margins (Figure 2.9 A and B).

The superolateral or dorsal surface is concave and lies underneath the bones of the cranial vault, with the frontal, parietal, temporal, and occipital lobes approximately corresponding in surface extent to the overlying cranial bones from which they take their names. The frontal and parietal lobes are separated from the temporal lobe by the very evident lateral (Sylvian) sulcus.

The inferior or basal surface is divided by the anterior part of the lateral sulcus into a small anterior and a larger posterior part. The anterior part constitutes the orbital surface of the frontal lobe, and rests on the cribriform plate of the ethmoid, on the orbital plate of the frontal bone, and on the lesser wing of the sphenoid bone, which altogether constitute the floor of the anterior cranial fossa. The posterior part of the inferior surface is larger, composed of the basal aspects of the temporal and occipital lobes, and rests on the floor of the middle cranial fossa and on the posteriorly continuous upper face of the tentorium cerebri, which is a dural fold that covers the cerebellum.

The medial cerebral surface is flat and lies within the great longitudinal fissure, limited inferiorly by the commissural fibers of the corpus callosum which lie in the depths of the fissure. The surface is separated from the medial surface of the opposite hemisphere by a crescent-shaped fold of the dura mater, the falx cerebri.

The cerebral surface is excavated by the sulci which roughly separate the gyri, with the more pronounced and well-defined sulci generically referred to as fissures (Gusmão *et al.*, 2000; Gratiolet, 1854 apud Pearce, 2006).

2.2.1 The Meninges, the Subarachnoid Space, and the Main Cerebral Fissures

The CNS is surrounded externally by the three meninges: the pia mater, the arachnoid, and the dura mater.

The pia mater is firmly attached to the surface of the CNS along its whole extent, depressions, and recesses, and is responsible for the consistency and relative endurance of the CNS surface. The arachnoid completely covers the CNS as a tight envelope, harboring the subarachnoid space and with the cerebrospinal fluid (CSF) running underneath the arachnoid. Delicate trabeculae of the arachnoid stand out and bind to the pia mater, thus justifying its name.

The dura mater is the most superficial of the meninges, being the thickest and the only one that contains blood vessels and nerves. While the dura that covers the brain is formed by two leaflets, the spinal cord dura is composed of only one leaflet. The falx and the tentorium are thick dural folds. The falx separates the two cerebral hemispheres and the tentorium supports both temporo-occipital surfaces. The subdural space between the dura and the arachnoid is a virtual space throughout its whole extent.

Table 2.3 The supratentorial subarachnoid cisterns

Anterior (parasellar)
1) Carotid cistern
2) Chiasmatic cistern
3) Lamina terminalis cistern
4) Olfactory cistern
5) Sylvian cistern
Lateral (parapeduncular)
1) Crural cistern
2) Ambient cistern
Posterior (tentorial notch)
1) Quadrigeminal cistern
2) Velum interpositum cistern
Superior (callosal)
1) Corpus callosum cistern – anterior portion
2) Corpus callosum cistern – posterior portion
3) Interhemispheric cistern

Adapted from Yasargil (1984a).

On the superolateral surface of the brain, the subarachnoid space is very shallow over the crest of the gyri, and extends to the intrasulcal spaces. Along the lateral (Sylvian) fissure, it gradually expands toward the cerebral base giving rise to the subarachnoid cisterns (Key and Reteius, 1875 apud Yasargil, 1984a; Matsuno *et al.*, 1988; Yasargil *et al.*, 1976). The basal subarachnoid cisterns (Table 2.3) are CSF compartments that are anatomically relatively distinct, are separated by porous trabeculated walls, and harbor the basal vessels and cranial nerves (Yasargil, 1984a; Yasargil *et al.*, 1976). While the arteries lie loosely within the cisterns, attached only to the arachnoid trabeculae, the veins are always firmly adhering to the pial surface of the brain.

Given the anatomy of the arachnoid and of the pia, the brain sulci correspond to extensions of the superolateral subarachnoid space, and the brain fissures harbor the basal subarachnoid cisterns.

There are three major cerebral fissures which are particularly characteristic of each hemispheric brain surface, and which define much of the brain architecture: the lateral or Sylvian fissure along the superolateral surface, the interhemispheric or longitudinal fissure along the medial surface, and the transverse fissure of Bichat (Bouchet *et al.*, 1966; Testut and Jacob, 1932a; Yasargil, 1987) within the cerebral basal surface (Figure 2.10). These three fissures constitute well-defined and anatomically constant natural spaces, and they harbor the main supratentorial subarachnoid cisterns (Ono *et al.*, 1990; Yasargil, 1984a; Yasargil *et al.*, 1976; Yasargil *et al.*, 2002a) (Figure 2.10).

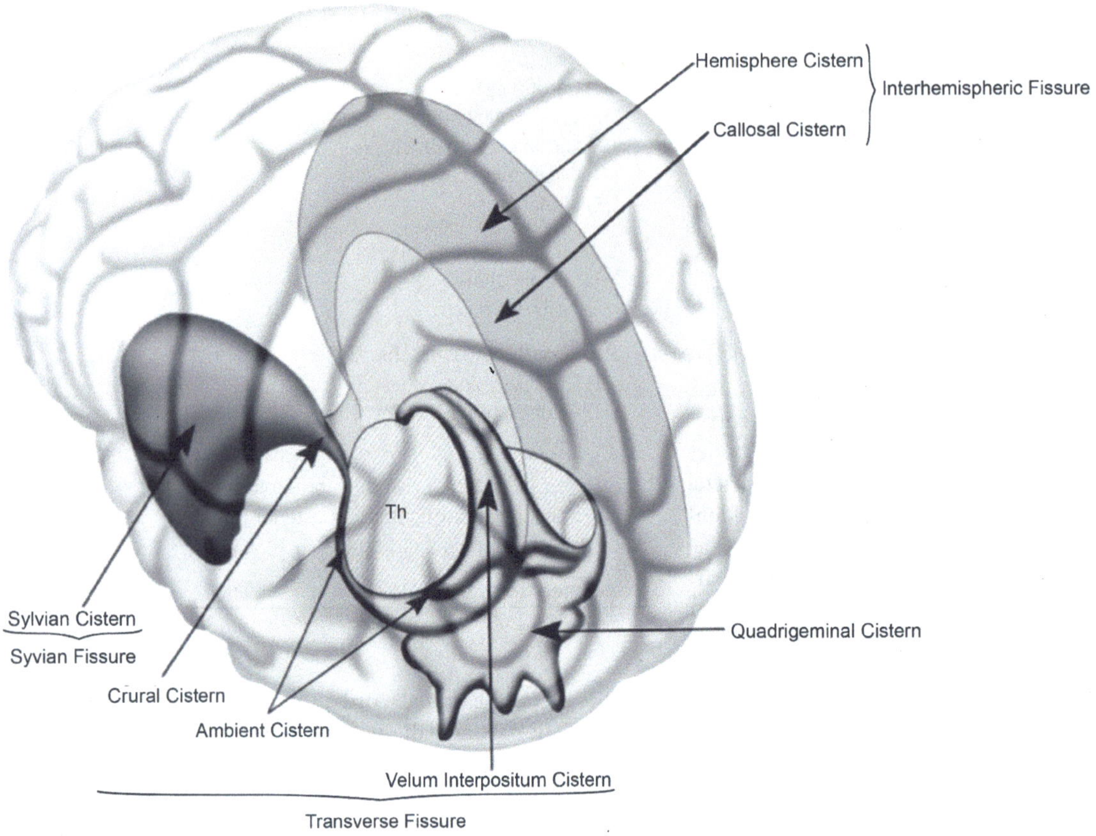

Figure 2.10 The concept of three main cerebral fissures and the cisterns which they harbor. Th: thalamus. (Adapted from Yasargil (1987).)

The lateral (or Sylvian) fissure is classically divided into an anterior part (also known as the sphenoidal part and as the stem of the Sylvian fissure) and into a lateral or posterior part (Ono *et al.*, 1990; Yasargil, 1984a; Yasargil *et al.*, 1976; Yasargil *et al.*, 2002a). The division occurs at the anterior Sylvian point, which corresponds to a usually evident enlargement of the fissure at the bottom of the triangular part of the inferior frontal gyrus (Ribas *et al.*, 2005a).

The anterior part of the Sylvian fissure lies anteriorly to the lateral aspect of the anterior perforated substance, ends at the level of the limen insulae, and harbors the most basal part of the Sylvian cistern with the initial segment of the middle cerebral artery (M1 segment) and with its temporal and perforating branches (Gibo *et al.*, 1981a; Gibo *et al.*, 1981b; Yasargil, 1984a).

The lateral or posterior part runs obliquely along the superolateral brain surface separating the surfaces of the frontal and temporal lobes, usually underneath the superficial Sylvian vein. It is composed of a thin superficial part located between the frontoparietal and the temporal opercular surfaces, and by a deep part that corresponds to a real fossa over the insular surface.

Sequentially along the superior aspect of the extent of the Sylvian point, first the horizontal and anterior ascending branches that delimit the triangular part of the inferior frontal gyrus, and then the anterior and posterior subcentral branches that delimit the subcentral gyrus originate from the anterior Sylvian point. The posterior ascending branch which ends inside the supramarginal gyrus, and, occasionally, a distal descending branch that penetrates inside the superior temporal gyrus originate from the posterior Sylvian point (Ono *et al.*, 1990; Ribas *et al.*, 2005a; Yasargil, 1984a; Yasargil, 1984b; Yasargil and Abdulrauf, 2003)(Figure 2.13 and Figure 3.9). Eventually, the most inferior segments of the precentral, central, and postcentral sulci can reach the lateral (Sylvian) fissure, but they cannot be considered Sylvian branches since these sulci always end inside U-shaped convolutions which may eventually lie inside the lateral (Sylvian) fissure (Ribas *et al.*, 2005a).

The lateral or posterior part of the Sylvian fissure harbors the largest part of the Sylvian cistern, with the superior and inferior branches of the middle cerebral artery at its base (M2 segments), and with its frontoparietal and temporal branches (M3 segments) looping around the respective opercula toward the brain surface. The most distal branches of the middle cerebral artery displayed on the frontoparietal and temporal superolateral surfaces (M4 segments) are already external to the lateral (Sylvian) fissure (Gibo *et al.*, 1981a; Yasargil, 1984a; Yasargil *et al.*, 2002a).

The interhemispheric or longitudinal fissure separates the medial surfaces of both cerebral hemispheres around and superiorly to the corpus callosum, and is divided longitudinally by the falx cerebri. Since the falx does not reach the superior surface of the corpus callosum, both cingulate gyri are usually attached along the midline. The interhemispheric or longitudinal fissure contains the callosal and the interhemispheric cisterns, which harbor the pericallosal and the callosomarginal arteries, and the distal branches of both anterior cerebral arteries (A2, A3, A4, and A5 segments of the anterior cerebral arteries) (Perlmutter and Rhoton, 1978; Rhoton, 2003).

The transverse fissure of Bichat (Bouchet *et al.*, 1966; Testut and Jacob, 1932a; Yasargil, 1987) is located around the inner basal aspects of both cerebral hemispheres, resembling two horseshoes with anterior concavities and with a common median part. While its lateral limbs lie along each side of the tentorial incisural region (Testut and Jacob, 1932a; Yasargil, 1987), its superior, median limb lies superiorly within the roof of the third ventricle (Testut and Jacob, 1932a; Yasargil, 1987; Williams and Warwick, 1980).

Each lateral limb of the transverse fissure is delimited medially by the cerebral peduncle, superiorly and anteriorly by the optic tract, superiorly and more posteriorly by the pulvinar of each thalamus (lateral and medial geniculate bodies), and inferiorly by the superior surface of each parahippocampal gyrus (the subiculum). Its most anterior aspect corresponds to the anterior perforated substance space from which it is continuous with the lateral (Sylvian) fissure, and its most posterior aspect corresponds to the subsplenial space that overlies the quadrigeminal plate, from where it is anteriorly continuous with its median limb along the roof of the third ventricle (Testut and Jacob, 1932a; Yamamoto *et al.*, 1981; Yasargil, 1987; Yasargil, 1994).

Each lateral limb of the transverse fissure harbors anteriorly and superiorly the crural cistern between the cerebral peduncle and the uncus, and this cistern contains the anterior choroidal artery (Fujii *et al.*, 1980; Rhoton *et al.*, 1979; Yasargil, 1987; Yasargil *et al.*, 1976). More inferiorly and posteriorly, between the cerebral peduncle and the subiculum, each lateral limb of the transverse fissure also harbors the ambient cistern, which contains the dentate gyri, the fimbria, the posterior cerebral artery, and the basal vein of Rosenthal (Ono *et al.*, 1984; Párraga *et al.*, 2011; Testut and Jacob, 1932a; Yasargil, 1984a; Yasargil, 1987). Posteriorly, both ambient cisterns are continuous with the quadrigeminal or pineal cistern.

The median limb of the transverse fissure lies below the splenium and above the superomedial surfaces of both thalami, and between the superior and inferior layers of the tela choroidea that run within the roof of the third ventricle. Whereas the superior layer of the tela choroidea is attached along and underneath both fornices and the hippocampal commissure, the inferior layer is attached along both thalamic striae and the superior surface of the pineal body (Testut and Jacob, 1932a; Williams and Warwick, 1980; Yamamoto *et al.*, 1981; Yasargil, 1987). The median limb of the transverse fissure harbors the cistern of the velum interpositum which extends from the quadrigeminal cistern as far as the posterior borders of both interventricular foramens (of Monro), and which contains both internal veins and the branches of both posteromedial choroidal arteries (Fujii *et al.*, 1980; Yamamoto *et al.*, 1981; Yasargil, 1987).

Since both the transverse fissure and the choroidal fissure encircle each thalamus, they are parallel and intimately related, being continuous throughout their whole extent. Nevertheless, whereas each transverse fissure is a broader space than the choroidal fissure delimited by part of the surface of each thalamus and by the surfaces of the neural structures that encircle the thalamus, each choroidal fissure is a narrow cleft between each thalamus and each fornix (Nagata *et al.*, 1988). The transverse fissure is continuous with the lateral ventricle along the choroidal fissure, which implies that any opening of the choroidal fissure from the lateral ventricle leads to the transverse fissure and to its subarachnoid cisterns. The opening of the choroidal fissure from the temporal horn will lead to the ambient cistern, from the atrium will lead to the quadrigeminal cistern, and from the body of the lateral ventricle will lead to the velum interpositum cistern within the roof of the third ventricle.

With regard to the other basal cisterns that are not contained within the three major brain fissures, anteriorly and inferiorly to the most anterior and basal aspect of the callosal cistern, there is the lamina terminalis cistern, which is anteriorly contiguous with the chiasmatic cistern. Inferiorly, the chiasmatic cistern is continuous with the interpeduncular cistern which has the Liliequist membrane as its anterior wall. More anteriorly, there are both olfactory cisterns. Lateral to these, there are on each side the parasellar carotid cistern which extends posteriorly to the parapeduncular crural and ambient cisterns. Laterally, these basal cisterns are contiguous with the most medial and inferior aspect of the Sylvian cistern (Yasargil, 1984a) (Figure 2.11).

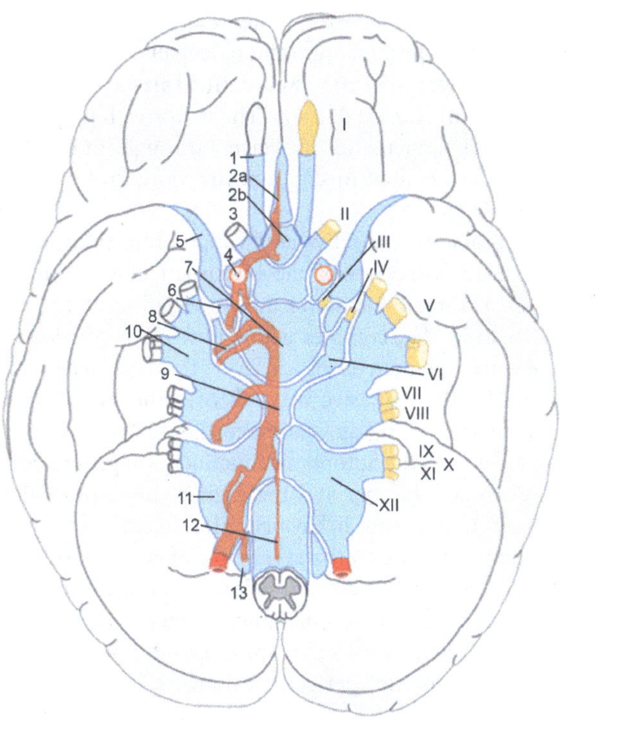

Figure 2.11 The basal cisterns (Arabic numbers), the anterior and posterior arterial systems (in red), and the cranial nerves (Roman numerals). (Adapted from Yasargil (1984a).)
1: Olfactory cistern; 2a: Callosal cistern; 2b: Lamina terminalis cistern; 3: Chiasmatic cistern; 4: Carotid cistern; 5: Sylvian cistern; 6: Crural cistern; 7: Interpeduncular cistern; 8: Ambient cistern; 9: Prepontine cistern; 10: Superior cerebellar-pontine cistern; 11: Inferior cerebellar-pontine cistern (lateral cerebello-medullary); 12: Anterior spinal cistern; 13: Posterior spinal cistern.

2.2.2 The Cerebral Surface, Its Sulci and Gyri

The evolutionary invagination process that produced the convoluted form of the cerebral surface increased its extent three-fold having generated a cortical area of approximately 2200 cm^2 (von Economo and Koskinas, 1925 apud Williams and Warwick, 1980). Only one-third is exposed on its surface with two-thirds buried inside the intrasulcal spaces, and with a thickness that varies between 3 and 5 mm (Brodal, 2010; Standring, 2008).

Although still a subject of debate (Azevedo *et al.*, 2009), it is believed that the human cerebral cortex harbors about 20 billion of the almost 100 billion neurons in the whole human brain, being also supported by up to 10 times as many neuroglial cells, and with each neuron being able to perform from some hundreds up to thousands of synapses. Within 1 mm^2, the cerebral cortex harbors about 100 000 neurons (Brodal, 2010; Henneberg, 1910 apud Catani and Schotten, 2012).

According to its structural differences, the cerebral surface or pallium (cerebral cortex and its underlying white matter) (Lockard, 1977) can be divided into the archipallium which still has white matter as its outer surface (hippocampal formation) and neopallium which has gray matter as its outer surface (Meynert, 1885 apud Catani and Schotten, 2012). The term paleopallium is related only to the intermediary cortex of the pyriform area (uncus and adjacent part of the parahippocampal gyrus) (Lockard, 1977).

The cerebral surface is comprised of a small proportion of phylogenetically old allocortex (unlaminated or partly laminated cortex) of the archipallium and paleopallium, and a huge proportion of newer isocortex (well-defined six-layered cortex of the neopallium) (Lockard, 1977). The isocortex has different organizational arrangements of its layers throughout its whole extent, which are related to different functional roles (Ribas, 2015).

The cerebral cortex is activated through projections arising in the reticular formation of the brainstem and within the thalami, and is directly or indirectly connected to all the subcortical structures. The complex neural physiology provided by the different arrangement of cortical layers throughout the brain surface, and by the extensive network of white matter fibers (with each neuron being able to make thousands of synaptic contacts), influences the autonomic functions and generates the basic (sensory and motor) and the higher cortical functions (cognition, emotion and behavior). The interactions of all these functions give rise to the experience of consciousness, to the notion of one's self, and to the tailoring of our personality.

According to Mesulam, anatomically there are five well-defined large-scale networks that are most relevant to clinical practice: a left-dominant perisylvian network for language; a right-dominant parietofrontal network for spatial cognition; an occipitotemporal network for face and object recognition; a limbic network for retentive memory; and a prefrontal network for attention and behavior (Catani *et al.*, 2005; Mesulam, 1987; Mesulam, 1990; Mesulam, 2011; Papez, 1937).

Anatomically, given their phylogenetic (Butler and Hodos, 2005; Park *et al.*, 2007; Sarnat and Netsky, 1981) and embryological (Chi *et al.*, 1977; Nishikuni and Ribas, 2013; Ono *et al.*, 1990; Williams and Warwick, 1980) development of folding, the cerebral sulci delineate the brain gyri and correspond to natural extensions of the subarachnoid space. When they are deep and anatomically more constant, they are also referred to generically as fissures (Broca, 1876b; Broca, 1861 apud Gusmão *et al.*, 2000; Gusmão *et al.*, 2000; Gratiolet, 1854 apud Pearce, 2006).

The main sulci have approximate depths ranging from 1 to 3 cm, and their walls harbor small gyri that face, adapt to, and connect with each other; those gyri are generically designated as transverse gyri. The sulci that separate the transverse intrasulcal gyri vary in length and depth, and, at the surface of the brain, they become visible as incisures. The indentations caused by cortical arteries can have an appearance similar to that of the incisures.

It is noteworthy that the timing of the embryological development of the sulci and their degree of variability (Chi *et al.*, 1977; Nishikuni and Ribas, 2013) define a true morphological hierarchy, at the top of which are the fissures and main sulci (Table 2.2). It is equally notable that this structural hierarchy is directly correlated with the functional importance of the areas to which the sulci are related, with the more anatomically constant sulci being those that are topographically related to areas that are more specialized (Penfield and Baldwin, 1952 apud Hansebout, 1977; Uematsu *et al.*, 1992).

On the brain surface, the sulci can be long or short as well as continuous (Sylvian fissure, callosal, calcarine, parieto-occipital, collateral, and generally the central sulcus)or interrupted. Ono *et al.* (1990) have described four main types of sulci: large primary sulci (e.g., central, precentral, postcentral, and continuous sulci); short primary sulci (e.g., rhinal, olfactory, lateral, and occipital sulci); short sulci composed of several branches (e.g., orbital and subparietal sulci); and short, free supplementary sulci (e.g., medial frontal and lunate sulci). Frequently, the sulci are composed of side branches that can be unconnected or connected (with end-to-side, end-to-end, or side-to-side connections that can also join two neighboring parallel sulci).

Due to their frequent variations and connections, the nomenclature of sulci varies among different authors according to their interpretations and designations (Duvernoy, 1991; Ono *et al.*, 1990; Ribas, 2010; Testut and Jacob, 1932a). For a better understanding, it is important to emphasize that the sulci can vary in size and shape from person to person. The brain gyri constitute a real continuum that present as a serpentine configuration on the surface of the brain due to their connections along the sulcal extremities and interruptions, and have their continuity mainly along the sulci depths and intrasulcal multiple connecting extension arms (Yasargil, 1994). The gyral separation is then only superficial and each gyrus should be understood in reality as a region and not as a well-defined structure (Ribas, 2010).

For practical surgical purposes, it is also interesting to note that, due to their origin by a process of infolding, the sulci of the superolateral and the inferior surfaces of the brain are usually oriented toward the nearest ventricular cavity, which does not apply to the medial cerebral face where the sulci are

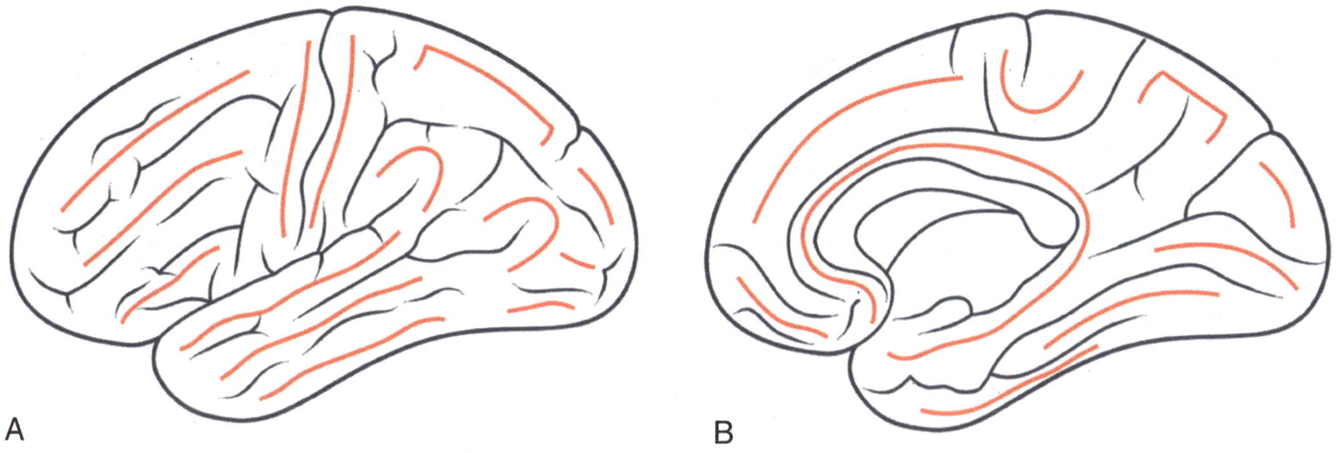

Figure 2.12 Basic organization of the brain gyri. (A) Superolateral surface and (B) medial and basal surfaces. Red lines indicate the constant arrangement of the main brain gyri. (Adapted from Ribas (2010).)

predominantly secondary to the development of the corpus callosum (Ono *et al.*, 1990).

Although appearing as having a labyrinthine disposition, the main cerebral sulci and gyri are arranged through a predominantly basic configuration, and their main points display fairly constant relationships with the cranial vault and with the deep neural structures (Ribas *et al.*, 2006). According to their anatomical uniformity, and to their related parallel cortical functional importance, both the gyri and sulci can be categorized as primary, secondary, or tertiary. The gyri that are more rounded or quadrangular are usually referred to as lobules.

On the superolateral surface of the brain, the frontal and temporal regions of each hemisphere are each composed of three horizontal gyri (superior, middle and inferior frontal, and temporal gyri); the central area is composed of two slightly oblique gyri (pre- and postcentral gyri); the parietal region is composed of two semicircular lobules (superior and inferior parietal lobules, with the inferior lobule composed of the supramarginal and angular gyri); the occipital region is composed of two or three less well-defined gyri (superior, middle, and inferior occipital gyri); and the insula, which lies deep in the floor of the very evident lateral (Sylvian) fissure, is composed of four to five diagonal gyri (short and long insular gyri) (Figure 2.12.A).

The superolateral gyri extend along its inferolateral border constituting the cerebral inferior surface with its orbital part (orbital gyri and basal aspect of rectus gyri) and its tentorial part (basal aspects of the inferior temporal, inferior occipital and lingual gyri, and fusiform gyrus). The gyri of the superolateral and inferior surfaces extend along their medial margins constituting the cerebral medial surface. This is characterized by a very well-defined C-shaped inner ring, primarily composed of two continuous gyri (cingulate and parahippocampal gyri), which is surrounded by a much less well-defined outer ring of gyri (medial aspects of rectus and superior frontal gyri, paracentral lobule, precuneus, cuneus, and medial aspect of lingual gyrus). Unlike the other gyri (neocortical), each parahippocampal gyrus (paleocortical) is harbored inside the more ancient hippocampus (archicortical) along the inferior horn of the lateral ventricle, with the amygdala anteriorly. Due to their disposition around each thalamus and hypothalamus, the structures of this inner ring are referred to as limbic structures (Figure 2.12.B).

Among all these features, the evident lateral (Sylvian) fissure and the uniquely oblique pre- and postcentral gyri with their related sulci predominantly show up as distinctive structures on the superolateral aspect of the brain. The macroscopic study of the sulci and gyri of each cerebral hemisphere should therefore begin with the identification of the lateral (Sylvian) fissure, which clearly separates the superolateral surfaces of the frontal and parietal lobes from the temporal lobe. This should be followed by identification of the precentral and postcentral gyri, which divide the portion of this surface that is superior and posterior to the Sylvian fissure into an anterior and a posterior half. On the cerebral medial surface, one should initially identify the cingulated and the parahippocampal gyri that constitute the very well-defined C-shaped inner ring, and then identify their surrounding gyri.

For practical purposes, Ecker (1869) identified the gyri through numbers. The superior, middle, and inferior frontal gyri were referred to as F_1, F_2, and F_3; the superior, middle, and inferior temporal gyri as T_1, T_2, and T_3, with T_4 and T_5 corresponding, respectively, to the fusiform (currently divided into T_4 and O_4 (Duvernoy, 1991)) and to the lingual gyri (currently O_5 (Duvernoy, 1991)); the superior parietal lobule and the precuneus to P_1, the supramarginal gyrus to P_2, and the angular gyrus to P'_2 (currently frequently referred to as P_3); and the occipital superior, middle, and inferior gyri, respectively, to O_1, O_2, and O_3.

The divisions of the cerebral hemispheres into lobes are described in detail in their specific sections.

2.2.3 The Cerebral Lobes and Related Regions

The arbitrary division of the cerebral hemispheres into lobes has been done through progressive editions of the *Nomina Anatomica*, which recently changed its denomination to *Terminologia Anatomica – International Anatomical Terminology* (Federative Committee on Anatomical Terminology, 1998), based on neural, morphological, and functional aspects and having as its main objective the establishment of a categorization that could help the medical practice in the fields of neurology, neurosurgery, and neuroradialogy.

The first version, known as the *Basle Nomina Anatomica* (BNA) was published in 1895 (His, 1895), dividing each cerebral hemisphere into frontal, parietal, occipital, and temporal lobes as already proposed by Gratiolet (1854 apud Pearce, 2006), and considering the insula as a separate addendum but not a lobe.

The following version did not change this division until the publication of the fourth edition of the *Paris Nomina Anatomica* (PNA) in 1975 (Excerpta Medica Foundation, 1975), which then considered the insula as another brain lobe, a notion that was also kept in the fifth edition published in 1980 (Excerpta Medica Foundation, 1980).

Finally, the *Terminologia Anatomica – International Anatomical Terminology* published in 1998 (Federative Committee on Anatomical Terminology, 1998) substituted the previous *Nomina Anatomica* adding a list of English terms in common usage to the revised Latin terminology, and included the limbic lobe as another subdivision of each cerebral hemisphere.

According to the official anatomical nomenclature, each cerebral hemisphere is then currently divided into six lobes: frontal, parietal, occipital, temporal, insular, and limbic lobes, which are described in the following sections.

In relation particularly to the pre- and postcentral gyri, some of the anatomists of the nineteenth century, such as Bischoff (Broca, 1876a apud Stone, 1991) and Taylor (Taylor and Haughton, 1900 apud Uematsu *et al.*, 1992), had already started proposing to group these two together given their morphologically unique character and juxtaposition. Although, respectively more related to the anterior frontal and posterior parietal cortical areas, the pre- and postcentral gyri do constitute a morphological and functional unit given their anatomical continuity, their own reciprocal connection, and the observation that both generate a rather similar amount of corticospinal fibers to constitute the pyramidal tract (Brodal, 1981; Jane *et al.*, 1967; Liu and Chambers, 1964 apud Brodal, 1981; Nyberg-Hansen and Brodal, 1963 apud Brodal, 1981; Standring, 2008). On clinical grounds, the vast dimensions and heterogeneity of the conventionally named frontal lobe justify its subdivision, and the pre- and postcentral gyri grouping was made more recently initially by Penfield (Penfield and Baldwin, 1952 apud Hansebout, 1977) who named these two gyri the Rolandic or sensorimotor cortex. Later, Rasmussen (1979, 1991a, 1991b) referred to them as the central region, and more recently, Yasargil (1994) designated these two gyri and their related sulci as the central lobe. Considering the criteria adopted by the previous *Nomina Anatomica* editions that progressively incorporated further divisions of the brain hemispheres into cerebral lobes, the pre- and postcentral gyri, and their related sulci could very well be grouped together as another cerebral lobe.

Parallel to the concept of cerebral lobes and to the knowledge of their underlying white matter fibers, the medical practice requires an understanding of the anatomy of the intracranial neural structures mainly regarding the three-dimensionality of these structures, the topographical relationships among them, their vascularization, and their relationships with the natural spaces containing the cerebrospinal fluid (CSF) and with the skull vault and base.

The identification of the encephalic structures, and of their occasional lesions, in all neuroimaging studies, always requires an initial recognition of the natural CSF spaces (subarachnoid space with sulci and fissures that constitute its outer limits, and inner ventricular cavities that delimit its deeper contours), and of the shape of its main and well-defined structures. Therefore, the anatomical characterization of well-defined regions is useful because it leads to a more specific understanding of their structures with their respective continuity, vascularization, and functions, and of their occasional harboring lesions.

For this reason, the main, well-defined cerebral topographic regions are described here together with their respective related cerebral lobes.

2.2.3.1 The Frontal Lobe

The frontal lobe corresponds to the rostral region of each cerebral hemisphere, and is the largest part of each hemisphere. It is delimited posteriorly by the central sulcus, anteriorly by the cerebral supracilliary margin, medially by the interhemispheric fissure, and laterally and inferiorly by the lateral (Sylvian) fissure (Figures 2.13 and 2.15).

Its superolateral (dorsal) surface underlies the frontal bone and is constituted posteriorly by the slightly oblique precentral gyrus that extends to the medial surface, and the area of the frontal lobe lying anteriorly to it is divided into the longitudinal superior, middle, and inferior frontal gyri, with the frontal pole lying in front of these gyri.

The frontal basal (ventral) surface lies over the orbital part of the frontal bone and over the cribriform plate of the ethmoid bone, and is composed of the orbital and rectus gyri.

The medial frontal surface faces the falx cerebri, extends from the frontal to the central sulcus within the paracentral lobule, and consists of the medial aspect of the superior frontal gyrus.

The frontal lobe harbors the primary motor area (MI) within the precentral gyrus, the supplementary motor area (SMA) anteriorly and medially, and the ventral and dorsal premotor areas anteriorly and laterally with the frontal eye field cortical area in between, and hence is functionally predominantly related to motor functions. While the movement itself is generated within MI, the supplementary motor and the lateral premotor areas are believed to instruct the MI area (Brodal, 2010).

The most anterior and basal aspects of the frontal lobes are bilaterally related to judgment and complex volitional aspects of behavior.

2.2.3.1.1 Frontal Lobe Sulci and Gyri

The precentral gyrus is disposed obliquely along the superolateral surface of the cerebral hemisphere, with its upper

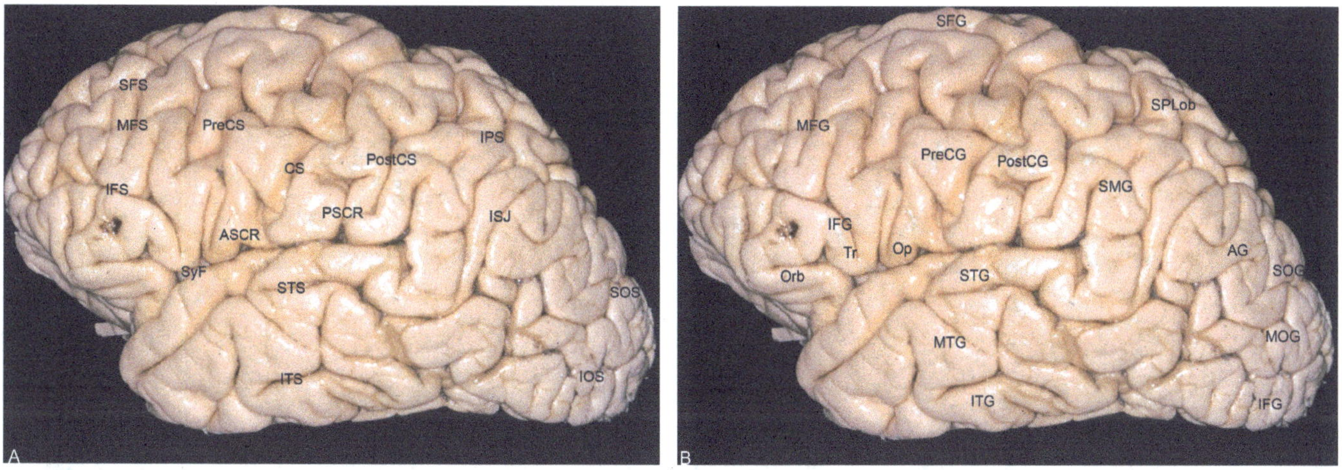

Figure 2.13 The main brain sulci (A) and gyri (B) of the superolateral surface of the brain.
AG: angular gyrus; ASCR: anterior subcentral ramus of Sylvian fissure; CS: central sulcus; IFG: inferior frontal gyrus; IFS: inferior frontal sulcus; IOS: inferior occipital sulcus; IPS: intraparietal sulcus; ISJ: intermediary sulcus of Jensen; ITG: inferior temporal gyrus; ITS: inferior temporal sulcus; MFG: middle frontal gyrus; MFS: middle frontal sulcus; MOG: middle occipital gyrus; MTG: middle temporal gyrus; OP: opercular part of inferior frontal gyrus; Orb: orbital part of inferior frontal gyrus; PostCG: postcentral gyrus; PostCS: postcentral sulcus; PreCG: precentral gyrus; PreCS: precentral sulcus; PSCR: posterior subcentral ramus of Sylvian fissure; SFG: superior frontal gyrus; SFS: superior frontal sulcus; SMG: supramarginal gyrus; SOG: superior occipital gyrus; SOS: superior occipital sulcus; SPaLob: superior parietal lobule; STG: superior temporal gyrus; STS: superior temporal sulcus; SyF: lateral or Sylvian fissure; Tr: triangular part of inferior frontal gyrus. (Adapted from Ribas (2010).)

aspect extending along its medial surface, and is delineated posteriorly by the central sulcus.

The central sulcus separates the frontal and parietal lobes and demarcates the primary motor and somatosensory areas of the cortex, located in the precentral and postcentral gyri, respectively. It starts in or near the superomedial border of the hemisphere, a little behind the midpoint between the frontal and occipital poles (Williams and Warwick, 1980), and runs, resembling a lengthened italic S (Talairach and Tornoux, 1993 apud Yousry *et al.*, 1997), downward and forwards, to end usually a little above the posterior ramus of the lateral sulcus. The central sulcus is usually a continuous sulcus (92 percent in both hemispheres (Ono *et al.*, 1990)).

Broca (Broca, 1888 apud Boling and Oliver, 2004; Testut and Jacob, 1932a) classically described the central sulcus as having two (superior and inferior) anteriorly convex genua, and one posteriorly convex middle genu. Cunningham (Cunningham, 1892 apud Yousry *et al.*, 1997), and more recently Ono (1990), considered the central sulcus as having only two genua, but described the superior one as being posteriorly convex probably then consisting of both the superior and middle genua classically previously described (Broca, 1888 apud Boling and Oliver, 2004; Déjérine, 1895; Testut and Jacob, 1932a), and disregarded the most superior one because of its small size (Yousry *et al.*, 1997).

Posteriorly, the precentral gyrus is superiorly and inferiorly connected and continuous with the postcentral gyrus along connections that encircle both extremities of the central sulcus, comprising altogether a lengthened and oblique ellipse excavated by the central sulcus.

The inferior connection corresponds to the subcentral gyrus which is delineated anteriorly and posteriorly by the anterior and posterior subcentral rami of the Sylvian fissure, respectively. It can be situated either completely over the Sylvian fissure or can be in part internal to the fissure, then giving the false impression that the central sulcus is a branch of the Sylvian fissure (Ribas *et al.*, 2005a).

The superior connection corresponds to the paracentral lobule of Ecker (Déjérine, 1895) already disposed along the medial surface of the cerebral hemisphere inside the interhemispheric fissure, delineated anteriorly by the paracentral sulcus and posteriorly by the ascending and distal part of the cingulated sulcus, that is, the marginal ramus of the cingulated sulcus.

Broca also described a middle connection between these two gyri ("plis de passage" moyen of Broca) characterized by a gyral bridge usually hidden within the central sulcus, and which in the cortical surface corresponds to the classic middle genu of the central sulcus that is posteriorly convex (Broca, 1888 apud Boling and Oliver, 2004). For Régis, this middle connection corresponds to a sulcal root, and when it is developed enough to reach the brain surface, it interrupts the central sulcus (Régis *et al.*, 2005).

Using functional resonance imaging, Yousry *et al.* (1997) described that the anatomical cortical location of the motor hand area is anatomically related to a knob-like structure of the precentral gyrus that, on the cortical surface, corresponds precisely to the classic middle knee of the central sulcus, which is topographically located at the level of the distal end of the superior frontal sulcus (Yousry *et al.*, 1997; Ribas *et al.*, 2006; Ribas, 2010). Having also studied cadaveric specimens, Yousry *et al.* observed that this posteriorly oriented protrusion of the precentral gyrus is delimited by two anteriorly directed fissures that deepen toward the base of the knob resulting in a characteristic inverted omega shape in the axial planes of the MRIs in 90 percent of the hemispheres. The occasional occurrence of a third fissure with a horizontal course between the two fissures is responsible for a horizontal epsilon shape in the other 10 percent of brain hemispheres (Yousry *et al.*, 1997) (Figure 2.14). In the sagittal plane, the

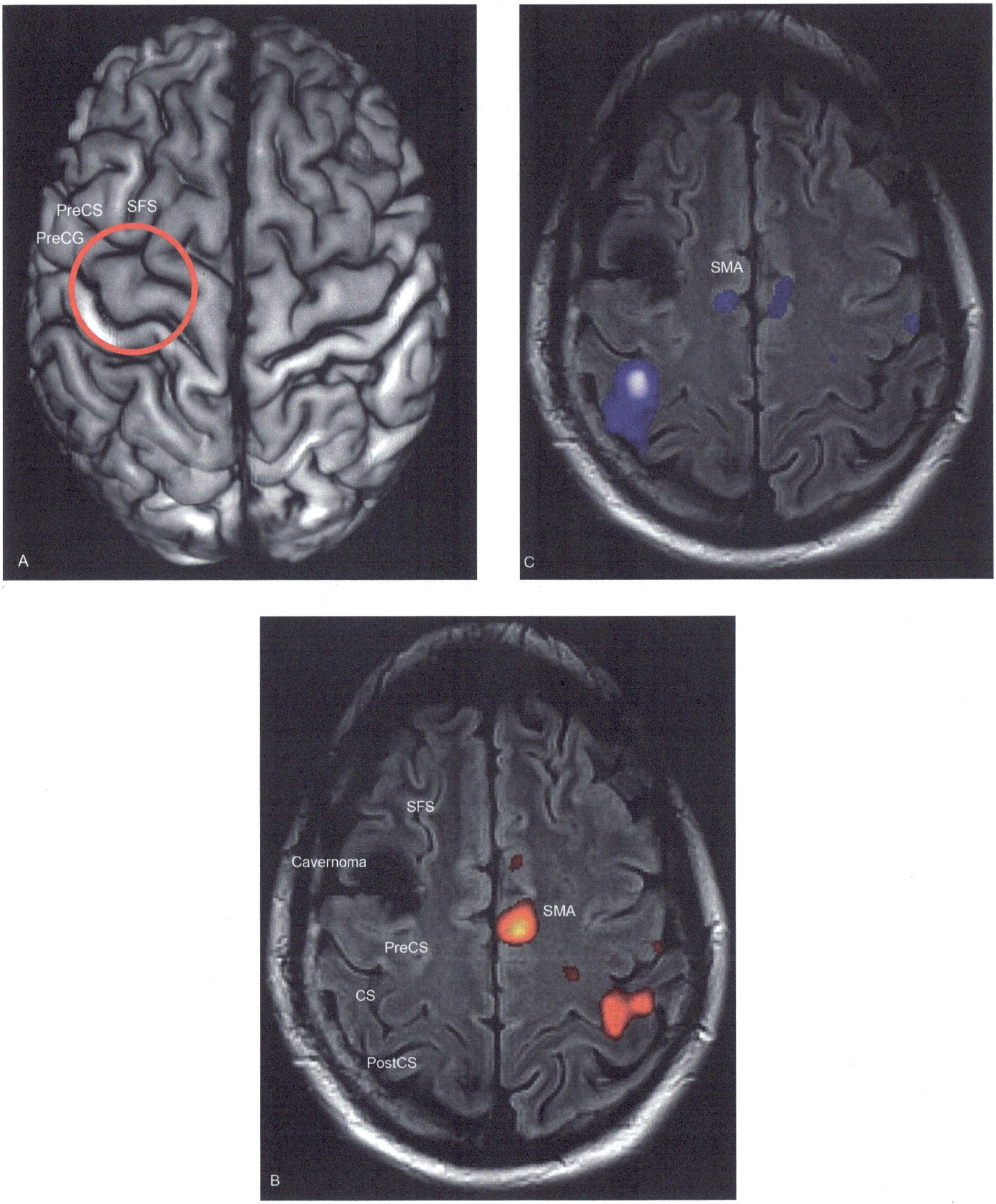

Figure 2.14 (A) The hand motor activation site corresponds to a knob-like cortical area of the contralateral precentral gyrus, which in MRI axial planes usually resembles an inverted omega with the posterior end of the superior frontal sulcus pointing towards it. Functional MRI of the right (B) and left hand motor (C) activity of a patient that harbors a cavernoma within the most posterior aspect of the right middle frontal gyrus, disclosing cortical activities of the omega region of each contralateral precentral gyrus and supplementary motor area.

Omega: within the red circle; PreCG: precentral gyrus; PreCS: precentral sulcus; SFS: superior frontal sulcus (non-continuous, interrupted) CS: central sulcus; PostCS: postcentral sulcus; PreCS: precentral sulcus, SFS: superior frontal sulcus; SMA: supplementary motor area. (Courtesy of E. Amaro, Department of Radiology, University of São. Paulo Medical School.)

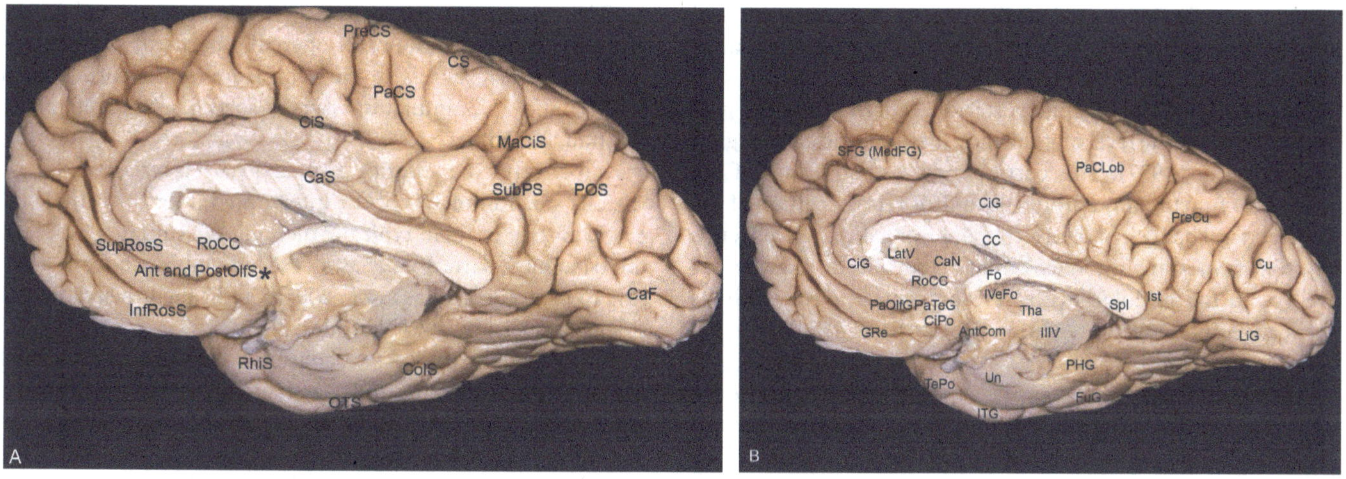

Figure 2.15 The main sulci (A) and gyri (B) of the medial and basal temporo-occipital surfaces.
AntComm: anterior commissure; Ant and PostOlfS: anterior and posterior paraolfactory sulcus; CaF: calcarine fissure; CaN: caudate nucleus; CaS: callosal sulcus; CC: corpus callosum; CiG: cingulate gyrus; CiPo: cingulate pole; CiS: cingulate sulcus; ColS: collateral sulcus; CS: central sulcus; Cu: cuneus; Fo: fornix; FuG: fusiform gyrus; GRe: gyrus rectus; IIIv: third ventricle; InfRosS: inferior rostral sulcus; Ist: isthmus of cingulate gyrus; ITG: inferior temporal gyrus; IVeFo: interventricular foramen of Monro; LatV: lateral ventricle; LiG: lingual gyrus; MaCiS: marginal ramus of the cingulate sulcus; MedFG: medial frontal gyrus; OTS: occipitotemporal sulcus; PaCLob: paracentral lobule; PaCS: paracentral sulcus; PaOlfG: paraolfactory gyri; PaTeG: paraterminal gyrus; PHG: parahippocampal gyrus; POS: parieto-occipital sulcus; PreCS: precentral sulcus; PreCu: precuneus; RhiS: rhinal sulcus; RoCC: rostrum of the corpus callosum; SFG: superior frontal gyrus; Spl: splenium of corpus callosum; SubPaS: subparietal sulcus; SupRosS: superior rostral sulcus; TePo: temporal pole; Th: thalamus; Un: uncus. (Adapted from Ribas (2010).)

appearance of the knob assumes the shape of a posteriorly directed hook (Yousry *et al.*, 1997).

Boling and Olivier (2004) studied the middle connection of the pre- and postcentral gyri (the "plis de passage" moyen of Broca), with positron emission tomography and MRI. Through fixed cadaveric brain dissections removing the precentral component of the "plis de passage" moyen (that corresponds to the cortical substratum of hand motor function), they demonstrated that hand sensory function is highly correlated with the postcentral component of this cortical fold. Utilizing cortical stimulation in a posterior study, Boling *et al.* (2008) identified a strong relationship among the "plis de passage" moyen, whole-hand sensory and motor stimulation responses, and functional magnetic resonance imaging (fMRI) hand activation.

The precentral gyrus is anteriorly delimited by the precentral sulcus which is systematically divided into a superior and an inferior precentral sulcus by an evident connection of the middle frontal gyrus with the precentral gyrus (Duvernoy, 1991; Ono *et al.*, 1990; Petrides, 2012). Further connections of the superior, middle, and inferior frontal gyri can divide the superior and inferior precentral sulcus into additional segments (Ono *et al.*, 1990).

The superior part of the precentral sulcus is very often interrupted superiorly due to a connection between the superior frontal and the precentral gyri. When interrupted, this gives rise to a more medial segment called the medial precentral sulcus, and this corresponds to the sulcus precentralis medialis of Eberstaller (Petrides, 2012). More dorsally and within the precentral region, there is frequently another short gyrus called the marginal precentral sulcus, which corresponds to the sulcus precentralis marginalis of Cunningham, and which may merge with the superior precentral sulcus or with the central sulcus (Petrides, 2012).

Inferiorly, the inferior segment of the precentral sulcus always ends inside the opercular part of the inferior frontal gyrus, giving rise to its U-shape (Ribas *et al.*, 2005a; Ribas, 2010; Ribas *et al.*, 2006).

In relation to the skull surface, the pre- and postcentral gyri are roughly parallel to the coronal suture, with the precentral sulcus placed slightly posterior to this suture (Ebeling *et al.*, 1987; Ebeling *et al.*, 1989; Ebeling and Steinmetz, 1995b; Gusmão *et al.*, 2001; Pernkoff, 1980; Ribas *et al.*, 2006).

The superior, middle, and inferior frontal gyri are then disposed longitudinally anteriorly to the precentral gyrus, and are, respectively, separated by the superior and inferior frontal sulci. These frontal gyri are frequently referred to as F_1, F_2, and F_3 (Ecker, 1869; Duvernoy, 1991) (Figure 2.17).

The superior frontal gyrus is continuous with the rectus gyrus anteriorly and inferiorly, and can also be connected to the orbital gyri and to the middle frontal gyrus. Posteriorly, the superior frontal gyrus is connected to the precentral gyrus by at least one fold, which more commonly lie medially along the interhemispheric fissure. Usually, the superior longitudinal gyrus is subdivided into two longitudinal portions by the so-called medial frontal sulcus, and its medial portion is also called the medial frontal gyrus by some authors (Ono *et al.*, 1990).

Along the most medial portion of the superior frontal gyrus and immediately facing the precentral gyrus is the important region known as the supplementary motor area (SMA). This corresponds to the medial premotor cortex, related to performing learned sequences of movements and which has poorly defined borders (Brodal, 1981; Williams and Warwick, 1980; Standring, 2008). Anteriorly to the SMA there is the Pre-SMA area believed to be involved in learning sequential movements (Figure 2.14B).

The superior frontal sulcus that separates the superior and middle frontal gyri is a very deep and frequently continuous sulcus (40 percent in the right side, 32 percent in the left side (Ono *et al.*, 1990)), and ends posteriorly encroaching the precentral gyrus at the level of its already mentioned omega region (Yousry *et al.*, 1997). This corresponds to the portion of the gyrus that functionally harbors the motor representation of the contralateral hand. Therefore, the superior frontal sulcus tends to point toward the middle frontoparietal "plis de passage," as well as to the middle knee of the precentral gyrus, with its respective motor representation of the hand (Boling *et al.*, 1999).

The most caudal aspect of the superior frontal gyrus anterior to the precentral gyrus, corresponds to the dorsal premotor (dPM) cortical area which is involved with planning movements.

The middle frontal gyrus is typically the largest of the frontal gyri and harbors a complex of multiple shallow sulcal segments known altogether as the middle (Duvernoy, 1991; Petrides, 2012) or intermediate frontal sulcus (Ono *et al.*, 1990). Usually the middle frontal gyrus is superficially connected to the precentral gyrus by a prominent root that lies between the extremities of a marked interruption in the precentral sulcus. Within its caudal portion are the frontal eye fields (FEF), the cortical area responsible for saccadic eye and voluntary gaze movements.

The inferior frontal sulcus is always interrupted, due to the multiple connections between the middle frontal gyrus and the inferior frontal gyrus.

The constant emergence of the horizontal and anterior ascending rami of the lateral (Sylvian) fissure from the anterior Sylvian point (Ribas *et al.*, 2005a), which divides this fissure into anterior and posterior branches (Yasargil *et al.*, 2002a; Yasargil, 1984a; Yasargil *et al.*, 1976; Yasargil and Abdulrauf, 2003; Ono *et al.*, 1990), characterizes the triangular part of the inferior frontal gyrus in between its orbital and opercular parts (Figure 2.13).

The orbital part is the most prominent of the three parts that constitute the inferior frontal gyrus. The triangular part is usually more retracted causing the small widening of the lateral (Sylvian) fissure that corresponds to the anterior Sylvian point at its base. The opercular part is always U-shaped harboring the inferior aspect of the precentral sulcus and is posteriorly continuous with the basal aspect of the precentral gyrus over the anterior subcentral ramus of the lateral (Sylvian) fissure. In some cases, the anterior basal portion of the opercular part is more developed and is divided by another branch of the lateral fissure that runs from front to back and is called the diagonal sulcus of Eberstaller. When the diagonal sulcus of Eberstaller is present, it divides the anterior portion of the opercular part into two triangular portions that are positioned inversely to each other.

In the dominant hemisphere, the opercular and triangular parts of the inferior gyrus correspond to the Broca area, which is responsible for the production of spoken language (Broca, 1861 apud Finger, 1994; Brodal, 1981; Heimer, 1995; Quiñones-Hinojosa *et al.*, 2003; Williams and Warwick, 1980).

The most posterior aspect of the inferior frontal gyrus, given by the connection of its opercular part with the precentral gyrus, corresponds to the ventral premotor cortical area (vPM), and its stimulation causes speech arrest bilaterally (Duffau, 2011b).

Superiorly, the inferior frontal gyrus is crisscrossed by various small branches of the interrupted inferior frontal sulcus, with one of them typically piercing the superior aspect of the triangular part, usually as a descending branch from anterior to posterior (Ribas *et al.*, 2005a) and called the triangular sulcus (Duvernoy, 1991; Petrides, 2012).

Inferiorly, the orbital part continues with the lateral orbital gyrus, at times passing under a shallow sulcus known as the fronto-orbital sulcus. The basal apex of the triangular part is always above the lateral (Sylvian) fissure, and the base of the opercular part can be located either superiorly or within the fissure (Ono *et al.*, 1990; Ribas, 2005b).

Anteriorly, the inferior frontal gyrus terminates merging with the anterior portion of the middle frontal gyrus and all the frontal gyri together are anteriorly delineated by the appropriately named frontomarginal sulcus, which lies superior and parallel to the supraciliary margin, separating the superolateral and orbital frontal surfaces (Ono *et al.*, 1990; Yasargil, 1994). Very frequently, this so-called frontomarginal sulcus of Wernicke (Duvernoy, 1991) is interrupted and composed of three segments (Petrides, 2012).

Posteriorly, the inferior frontal gyrus is connected to the precentral gyrus along the posterior aspect of its opercular part as already mentioned.

On the frontobasal or orbital surface of each frontal lobe, the deep olfactory sulcus lies longitudinally in a paramedian position harboring the olfactory tract and bulb. Posteriorly, the olfactory tract is divided into its medial and lateral striae, which delineate the anterior-most aspect of the anterior perforated substance (Figure 2.16).

Medial to the olfactory sulcus is the long and narrow gyrus rectus, considered the most anatomically constant of the cerebral gyri, which is continuous with the superior frontal gyrus.

Lateral to the olfactory sulcus are the orbital gyri, which account for the greatest proportion of the frontobasal surface. The anterior, posterior, medial, and lateral orbital gyri are delineated by the H-shaped orbital sulci, which are composed of the lateral and medial orbital sulci united by the transverse orbital sulcus, with all the segments corresponding together to the cruciform sulcus of Rolando. The posterior orbital gyrus is situated anterior to the anterior perforated substance and typically presents a configuration similar to a tricorner or "Napoleon" hat. This can facilitate its identification in anatomical specimens in which the H-shaped orbital sulcus presents variations.

While the anterior orbital gyrus is traversed by small intermediate orbital sulci, the posterior orbital gyrus is traversed by small posterior orbital sulci.

The posterior orbital gyrus is connected medially to the medial orbital gyrus, characterizing the posteromedial orbital lobule (Yasargil, 1994) situated posterior and along the olfactory tract and the lateral olfactory striae, which is in turn

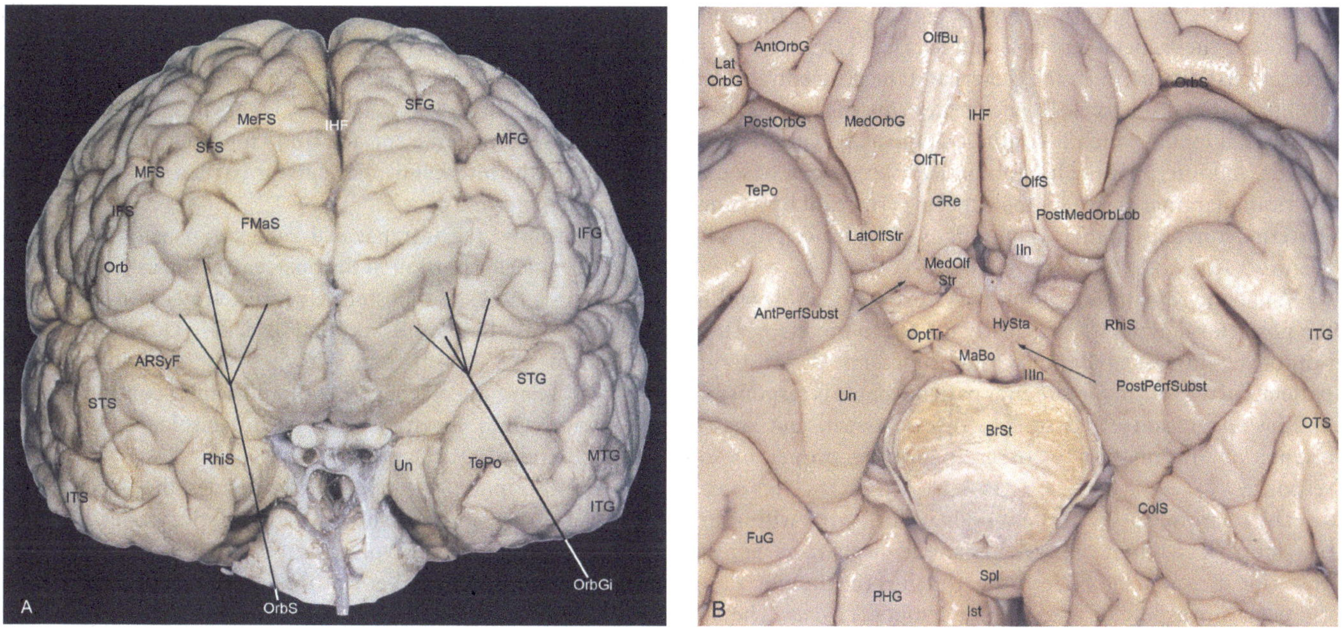

Figure 2.16 Anterior view of the cerebral hemispheres (A) and a view of the basal frontotemporal surface (B).
AntOrbG: anterior orbital gyrus; AntPerfSubst: anterior perforated substance; ARSyF: anterior ramus or stem of lateral or Sylvian fissure; BrSt: brainstem (pons); ColS: collateral sulcus; FMaS: frontomarginal sulcus; FuG: fusiform gyrus; GRe: gyrus rectus; HySta: hypophyseal stalk; IFG: inferior frontal gyrus; IFS: inferior frontal sulcus; IHF: interhemispheric fissure; Ist: isthmus of cingulate gyrus; ITG: inferior temporal gyrus; ITS: inferior temporal sulcus; LatOlfStr: lateral olfactory striae; LatOrbG: lateral orbital gyrus; MaBo: mammillary body; MedOlfStr: medial olfactory striae; MedOrbG: medial orbital gyrus; MeFS: medial frontal sulcus; MFG: middle frontal gyrus; MFS: middle frontal sulcus; MTG: middle temporal gyrus; OlfBu: olfactory bulb; OlfS: olfactory sulcus; OlfTr: olfactory tract; OptTr: optic tract; Orb: orbital part of inferior frontal gyrus; OrbGi: orbital gyri; OrbS: orbital sulcus; OTS: occipitotemporal sulcus; PHG: parahippocampal gyrus; PostMedOrbLob: posteromedial orbital lobule; PostOrbG: posterior orbital gyrus; PostPerfSubst: posterior perforated substance; RhiS: rhinal sulcus; SFG: superior frontal gyrus; SFS: superior frontal sulcus; Spl: splenium of corpus callosum; STG: superior temporal gyrus; STS: superior temporal sulcus; TePo: temporal pole; Un: uncus; IIn: optical nerve; IIIn: oculomotor nerve.

connected to the anterior portion of the insula via the transverse insular gyrus. The remaining orbital gyri are connected to the superior, middle, and inferior frontal gyri, along the frontal pole.

On its medial surface, the frontal lobe is inferiorly delimited by the cingulated sulcus, which starts within the subcallosal region and extends over the cingulated gyrus ending along an upward and curved segment known as the marginal ramus of the cingulated sulcus. Frequently, the cingulated sulcus ends anteriorly between the anterior aspect of the cingulate gyrus and a connection of this gyrus with the medial and anterior aspect of the superior frontal gyrus, and frequently shows inferiorly directed side branches (Ono *et al.*, 1990) (Figure 2.15).

The paracentral lobule is bounded posteriorly by the marginal ramus, and anteriorly by the paracentral sulcus, a branch of the cingulate sulcus. The paracentral lobule harbors the distal part of the central sulcus, and inferiorly to it, the so-called paracentral fossa (Petrides, 2012).

Anteriorly to the paracentral lobule, the medial aspect of the superior frontal gyrus lies over the cingulated sulcus and the cingulated gyrus, merging inferiorly with the rectus gyrus (Duvernoy, 1991).

The rectus gyrus is bounded superiorly by the superior rostral sulcus, and harbors along its surface the shallower inferior rostral sulcus.

Around the posterior end of the superior rostral sulcus the cingulated gyrus systematically connects with the rectus gyrus through a very evident U-shaped cortical fold known as the cingulate pole (Yasargil, 1994), located immediately anteriorly to the subcallosal gyri (paraolfactory gyri, paraterminal gyrus) (Figure 2.15B).

Superiorly to the superior rostral sulcus, small supra-orbital sulci (Petrides, 2012) can be observed within the medial surface of the frontal pole, at the level of the knee of the corpus callosum.

2.2.3.2 Parietal Lobe

Each parietal lobe lies posteriorly to each central sulcus on the superolateral and on the medial surface of each cerebral hemisphere (Figures 2.13, 2.15, and 2.17).

Posteriorly, the parietal lobe is delineated medially by the parieto-occipital sulcus, and along the lateral aspect of the hemisphere by an imaginary line running from the point from which the parieto-occipital sulcus emerges on the superomedial border to the preoccipital notch, which is an evident incisure situated on the inferolateral border approximately 5 cm anterior to the occipital pole.

Its inferior boundary is the posterior ramus of the lateral (Sylvian) fissure and its imaginary posterior prolongation.

The anatomy of the parietal lobe is more complex in the sense that it is composed of gyri morphologically less well defined and particularly serpiginous and curved, which are referred to as lobules. It is comprised of the postcentral gyrus, the inferior and superior parietal lobules, and the precuneus.

The lateral aspect of the parietal lobe is divided into three areas by the postcentral sulcus that lies parallel to the central sulcus, and by the intraparietal sulcus that lies predominantly longitudinally and slightly ventrally concave along the midportion of the parietal superolateral surface. While the postcentral gyrus lies between the central and the postcentral sulci, the intraparietal sulcus clearly delineates superiorly the superior parietal lobule which is continuous medially with the precuneus, and inferiorly the inferior parietal lobule, composed of the supramarginal gyrus, by the angular gyrus, and by a more posterior convolution that is continuous with the occipital lobe (Figure 2.13).

While the somatosensory primary cortical area (SI) within the postcentral gyrus is particularly related to the discrimination of the different types of sensory functions, the posterior parietal cortex within the superior parietal lobule is responsible for the integration of all somatosensory, visual, and spatial orientation information in order to provide proper motor responses.

The inferior aspects of the supramarginal gyrus within the inferior parietal lobule of the dominant hemisphere harbor the posterior speech area of Wernicke, which is continuous along the posterior aspect of the superior temporal gyrus. The so-called Wernicke's area is a poorly defined area that belongs to the complex language network, and is more related to its sensory or comprehension aspects. Posteriorly to the supramarginal gyrus, in the dominant hemisphere, the cortex of the angular gyrus is related to the functions of reading and writing given its nearness to the occipital visual cortex.

2.2.3.2.1 Parietal Lobe Sulci and Gyri

The postcentral gyrus lies posteriorly and connected to the precentral gyrus along the superior and inferior extremities of the central sulcus, constituting the posterior aspects of the paracentral lobule and of the subcentral gyrus, respectively, as already described in the section dealing with the frontal lobe (Section 2.2.3.1).

The postcentral gyrus is usually narrower than the precentral gyrus, and morphologically, both of them are distinctively obliquely disposed on the superolateral surface of the brain just superiorly to the lateral (Sylvian) fissure, with their mid portions corresponding approximately to the center of each cerebral hemisphere. Since they are disposed obliquely, the superior portions of the precentral and postcentral gyri, which constitute the paracentral lobule on the medial surface of the cerebral hemisphere, are topographically related to the ventricular atrium, which is situated posteriorly to the thalamus (Ribas, 2005b). In contrast, the inferior portions of both gyri cover the posterior half of the insula and are topographically related to the body of the lateral ventricle, which is situated above the thalamus. The portion of the subcentral gyrus that corresponds to the base of the postcentral gyrus consistently lies over the transverse gyrus of Heschl, which is situated on the opercular surface of the temporal lobe (Wen *et al.*, 1999).

The postcentral sulcus delineates the postcentral gyrus posteriorly, and is frequently interrupted (56 percent in the right hemisphere, and 52 percent in the left hemisphere (Ono *et al.*, 1990)) due to connections between this gyrus and the posteriorly adjacent superior and inferior parietal lobules. The inferior segment of the postcentral sulcus inferiorly always ends inside a basal connection between the postcentral and the supramarginal gyri (Ribas, 2010).

The intraparietal sulcus, which originates from around the midpoint of the postcentral sulcus, is very prominent along the parietal superolateral surface and, in general, runs almost parallel to the interhemispheric fissure with a slightly arciform inferiorly concave course.

Anteriorly, the intraparietal sulcus is usually continuous with the inferior portion of the postcentral sulcus (Ribas, 2010; Duvernoy, 1991), and posteriorly it penetrates into the occipital lobe as the intra-occipital sulcus (Duvernoy, 1991; Mesulam, 1987), also then known as the superior occipital sulcus (Testut and Jacob, 1932a), and which continues more posteriorly into the transverse occipital sulcus (Ono *et al.*, 1990; Petrides, 2012).

The intraparietal sulcus clearly divides the superolateral parietal surface into the superior and inferior parietal lobules, and along its length, it typically gives rise to a superior and to an inferior vertical smaller sulcal branch (Figure 2.13).

The superior vertical branch constitutes the transverse parietal sulcus of Brissaud, and partially divides the superior parietal lobule, anteriorly to the parieto-occipital incisures.

The inferior vertical sulcal branch of the intraparietal sulcus corresponds to the intermediate sulcus of Jensen (or sulcus intermedius primus of Jensen), which separates the supramarginal gyrus anteriorly from the angular gyrus posteriorly (Testut and Jacob, 1932a; Testut and Jacob, 1932a; Duvernoy, 1991; Petrides, 2012).

The supramarginal gyrus is always a very well-defined curved gyrus which surrounds the distal portion of the lateral (Sylvian) fissure, namely, its posterior ascending branch (Ono *et al.*, 1990), becoming inferiorly and anteriorly always continuous with the posterior portion of the superior temporal gyrus. Above the distal end of the lateral (Sylvian) fissure, the supramarginal gyrus is anteriorly connected to the postcentral gyrus through a fold that runs underneath the inferior aspect of the postcentral sulcus, and posteriorly, it occasionally rounds the inferior extremity of the intermediate sulcus, connecting to the angular gyrus.

The angular gyrus is also a curved gyrus, very often not very well-defined morphologically, but which always surrounds one of the distal segments of the superior temporal sulcus, usually the middle one, also known as the angular sulcus (Ono *et al.*, 1990), and with its most inferior portion then becoming always anteriorly continuous with the middle temporal gyrus.

The configuration of the angular gyrus is very much defined by the distal branching of the superior temporal sulcus, which usually ends forming three continuous or interrupted caudal branches (Petrides, 2012).

The most superior distal branch of the superior temporal sulcus has an ascending course, and can either penetrate the supramarginal gyrus or be coincident with the intermediate sulcus of Jensen which separates the supramarginal gyrus from the angular gyrus (Ono *et al.*, 1990; Petrides, 2012).

The second branch is usually less ascending and more horizontal, and systematically enters the angular gyrus constituting the angular sulcus (Ono *et al.*, 1990; Petrides, 2012; Duvernoy, 1991), then having the curved angular gyrus encircled around its distal end and continuous anteriorly with the middle temporal gyrus.

The most inferior caudal branch of the superior temporal sulcus is less evident and less constant, courses underneath a frequent posterior fold that connects the angular gyrus with the most lateral aspect of the occipital lobe, and is usually continuous with the anterior occipital sulcus (Ono *et al.*, 1990; Petrides, 2012) that lies predominantly vertically along the anterior edge of the middle occipital gyrus.

Basing his ideas on the work of Gratiolet, Broca considered the supramarginal and angular gyri to be folds connecting the parietal lobe with the temporal lobe. From Broca's perspective, the supramarginal gyrus, which wraps around the distal portion of the lateral (Sylvian) fissure, corresponded to Gratiolet's parietotemporal superior marginal fold, and the angular gyrus, which wraps around a distal portion of the superior temporal sulcus, corresponded to the parietotemporal inferior marginal fold, or curved fold of Gratiolet (Testut and Jacob, 1932a; Testut and Jacob, 1932a; Déjérine, 1895).

The bulge of the supramarginal and of the angular gyri is responsible for the cranial parietal tuberosity or bossa.

The superior parietal lobule has a quadrangular shape, is anteriorly delineated by the superior aspect of the postcentral sulcus, laterally by the intraparietal sulcus, and is medially continuous with the precuneus gyrus along the superomedial border (Figure 2.17).

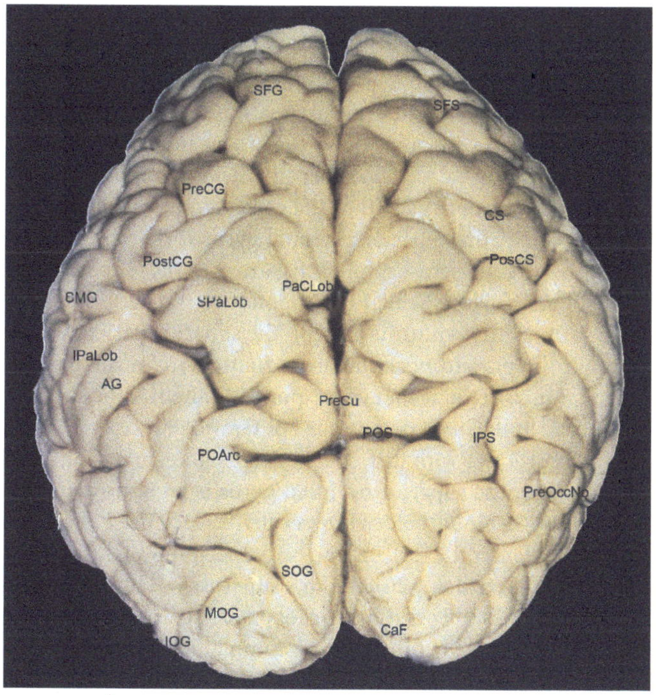

Figure 2.17 Superior view of the cerebral hemispheres.
AG: angular gyrus; CaF: calcarine fissure; CS: central sulcus; IOG: inferior occipital gyrus; IPaLob: inferior parietal lobule; IPS: intraparietal sulcus; MOG: middle occipital gyrus; PaCLob: paracentral lobule; POArc: parieto-occipital arch; POS: parieto-occipital sulcus seen on the superolateral surface, which corresponds to the parieto-occipital incisure within the parieto-occipital arch; PosCS: postcentral sulcus; PostCG: postcentral gyrus; PreCG: precentral gyrus; PreCu: precuneus; PreOccNo: pre-occipital notch; SFG: superior frontal gyrus; SFS: superior frontal sulcus; SMG: supramarginal gyrus; SOG: superior occipital gyrus; SPaLob: superior parietal lobule. (Adapted from Ribas (2010).)

Anteriorly, the superior parietal lobule is typically connected to the postcentral gyrus via a connection that transects the most superior portion of the postcentral sulcus and, occasionally, via another fold which interrupts the postcentral sulcus more inferiorly.

Posteriorly, the superior parietal lobule continues to the superior occipital gyrus via the prominent parieto-occipital arcus that surrounds the parieto-occipital incisure, which corresponds to the depth of the parieto-occipital sulcus over the superolateral cerebral surface.

Occasionally, there is also a small sulcus emerging from the interhemispheric fissure over the superior parietal lobule, between the postcentral sulcus and the parieto-occipital incisure, designated the superior parietal sulcus (Ono *et al.*, 1990).

On the medial surface of each hemisphere, the precuneus gyrus lies posteriorly to the paracentral lobule as a medial extension of the superior parietal lobule along the superomedial border of the brain, and together with the medial aspect of the postcentral gyrus corresponds to the medial portion of the parietal lobe (Figure 2.15). The precuneus is also quadrangular (quadrangular lobule of Foville (Déjérine, 1895)), delineated anteriorly by the marginal branch of the cingulate sulcus, posteriorly by the parieto-occipital sulcus, and inferiorly by multiple Y-shaped sulcal segments that constitute the subparietal sulcus. Inferiorly to the subparietal sulcus, the precuneus is connected to the isthmus of the cingulate gyrus which is continuous with the parahippocampal gyrus.

The parieto-occipital sulcus that separates the precuneus from the cuneus is a deep and wide sulcus when opened, and constitutes a deep fossa which harbors many small sulci and gyri resembling the lateral (Sylvian) fissure (Petrides, 2012). Along the most superficial aspects of its superior and inferior margins within the hemispheric surface, there are the precuneal limiting sulcus and the cuneal limiting sulcus, which, respectively, delineate the inferior (or posterior) limit of the precuneus and the superior (or anterior) limit of the cuneus (Petrides, 2012). Along its inner surfaces there are small cuneal gyri.

The depth of the most distal aspect of the parieto-occipital fissure within the superolateral hemispheric surface creates the parieto-occipital incisure, which is surrounded by the parieto-occipital arcus (Ebeling *et al.*, 1987; Petrides, 2012) that connects the superior parietal lobule with the superior occipital gyrus (Figure 2.17). This particular fold consists of an anatomically very constant U-shaped convolution, which corresponds to the first or superior parieto-occipital "plis de passage" of Gratiolet. It is delimited anteriorly by the superior parietal sulcus of Brissaud which is a superior vertical branch of the intraparietal sulcus, laterally by the transition of the intraparietal into the intra-occipital sulcus, and posteriorly by the medial part of the transverse occipital sulcus (Petrides, 2012).

The parieto-occipital incisure is always very evident within the medial margin of the hemispheric superolateral surface, and corresponds to the previous external perpendicular fissure. It received this name from Gratiolet in accordance with the fact that the parieto-occipital fissure itself had previously been named the internal perpendicular fissure by Ecker, due to its perpendicularity to the calcarine fissure (Déjérine, 1895).

The superior parietal lobule and the precuneus are also referred to as P_1, and the supramarginal and the angular gyri, respectively, as P_2 and P_c (Déjérine, 1895) or P_3 (Ecker, 1869; Duvernoy, 1991).

2.2.3.3 The Occipital Lobe

On the superolateral cerebral surface, the occipital lobe is situated posteriorly to the imaginary line that connects the point of emergence of the parieto-occipital fissure of the superomedial border of the cerebral hemisphere with the preoccipital notch of Meynert (Déjérine, 1895). The preoccipital notch is located about 5 cm from the occipital pole. On the medial surface, the occipital lobe is limited anteriorly by the parieto-occipital fissure itself and by its prolongation toward the tentorium. Along the inferior cerebral surface, the base of the occipital lobe is continuous with the temporal lobe base (Figure 2.13, 2.15, 2.17, 2.18).

While the superolateral surface of the occipital lobe lies mostly underneath the squamous part of the occipital bone, its medial surface faces the most posterior aspect of the falx, and the occipital base lies over the superior surface of the tentorium.

The sulci and gyri of the occipital lobe, particularly of its superolateral surface, have a greater anatomical variation compared with other lobes, and its cortex as a whole is particularly related to visual function. The striate cortex of the primary visual area lies along the cuneal and lingual margins of the posterior half of the calcarine fissure.

Experimental studies in monkeys led to the concept that there are two distinct projection systems, originating within different areas of the striate cortex, that deal with two different aspects of visual perception (Schneider, 1969 apud Goodale and Milner, 1992; Ungerleider and Mishkin, 1982 apud Goodale and Milner, 1992; Gross, 1973 apud Goodale and Milner, 1992; Livingstone and Hubel, 1988 apud Goodale and Milner, 1992). While a ventral stream of projections from the striate cortex toward the inferotemporal cortex is more particularly related to visual pattern discrimination and recognition (corresponding to a "what" visuomotor system), a dorsal stream of projections toward the posterior parietal regions interferes with neural mechanisms more related to spatial perception, mediating the required sensorimotor transformations for visually guided actions directed at such objects (corresponding to a "where" and "how" visuomotor system) (Goodale and Milner, 1992).

2.2.3.3.1 Occipital Lobe Sulci and Gyri

Despite being less well defined and less anatomically constant than the gyri in other dorsal cortical areas, the occipital gyri of the superolateral cerebral surface tend to consist of two or three gyri which converge posteriorly to form the occipital pole of each hemisphere. As is the case for the other lobes, the occipital gyri of the superolateral surface are usually designated superior, middle, and inferior (Duvernoy, 1991; Testut and Jacob, 1932a), or O1, O2, and O3, respectively (Figure 2.17).

While the superior and inferior occipital gyri are anatomically more constant, the middle one is much more variable with regard to its characterization. The inferior occipital gyrus is always placed horizontally along the inferolateral margin of the cerebral hemisphere, with its base lying over the tentorium. Anteriorly, it is mostly continuous with the inferior temporal gyrus, and posteriorly it extends medially around the occipital pole becoming continuous with the lingual gyrus within the medial surface of the hemisphere. Superiorly, the inferior occipital gyrus is delimited by the lateral or inferior occipital sulcus.

The lateral occipital sulcus (Duvernoy, 1991; Ono *et al.*, 1990) is a very evident horizontal sulcus, usually also known as the inferior occipital sulcus (Ono *et al.*, 1990; Testut and Jacob, 1932a), and is anteriorly more frequently connected directly to the inferior temporal sulcus (Ono *et al.*, 1990). A shorter accessory lateral occipital sulcus frequently runs below the main one (Petrides, 2012), and both of them can also be connected to a sulcal complex known as the anterior occipital sulcus which is then related to the distal segments of the inferior (Duvernoy, 1991) or the superior temporal sulcus (Petrides, 2012). When evident, the anterior occipital sulcus in itself is usually an ascending sulcus placed along the anterior aspect of the middle occipital gyrus region (Ono *et al.*, 1990; Petrides, 2012).

For other authors, the inferior occipital sulcus is a distinct and very small sulcus located near the inferior margin of the inferior occipital gyrus (Duvernoy, 1991; Petrides, 2012). In this text, we consider the lateral and the inferior occipital sulcus as the same sulcus.

The superior occipital gyrus is always very well defined, arranged more vertically along the interhemispheric fissure, and is continuous along the superomedial margin of the hemisphere with the cuneus within the cerebral medial surface.

Superiorly, the superior occipital gyrus is delimited by the depth of the parieto-occipital fissure on the superolateral hemispheric surface, which corresponds to the parieto-occipital incisure, and is continuous with the superior parietal lobule through the parieto-occipital arcus that encircles the parieto-occipital incisure and that corresponds to the first or superior parieto-occipital "plis de passage" of Gratiolet.

In accordance with different concepts, interpretations, and terminology, the superior occipital gyrus is laterally delimited by the intra-occipital sulcus (Duvernoy, 1991; Türe *et al.*, 2000; Testut and Jacob, 1932a), or transverse occipital sulcus (Ono *et al.*, 1990; Petrides, 2012), or superior occipital sulcus (Duvernoy, 1991; Testut and Jacob, 1932a), with these three sulci being partially coincident or complementary.

The intraparietal sulcus systematically extends longitudinally and inferiorly into the occipital lobe (Ono *et al.*, 1990), becoming then the intra-occipital sulcus (Duvernoy, 1991; Türe *et al.*, 2000; Testut and Jacob, 1932a) and delimiting the superior occipital gyrus laterally. The intra-occipital sulcus can occasionally descend as far as the occipital pole (Alves *et al.*, 2012), in that case characterizing a long and vertical sulcus also called the superior occipital sulcus (Duvernoy, 1991; Testut and Jacob, 1932a), but most frequently the intra-occipital sulcus terminates as a T end when reaching the transverse occipital sulcus (Ono *et al.*, 1990; Alves *et al.*, 2012) (Figure 2.17).

The transverse occipital sulcus is usually an evident occipital sulcus, generally related to the posterior end of the intra-occipital sulcus which divides it into a lateral part and a medial part that penetrates the superior occipital gyrus (Ono *et al.*, 1990; Alves *et al.*, 2012; Petrides, 2012). More rarely, it can be just a side branch of the intra-occipital sulcus, or completely separated from it (Ono *et al.*, 1990).

Since the lateral (or inferior) occipital sulcus is always present and clearly divides the superolateral occipital surface into an inferior part, composed of the inferior occipital gyrus, and a superior part, Alves *et al.* (2012) observed that the gyral pattern of the superior part depends mainly and particularly on the morphology of the lateral aspect of the transverse occipital sulcus. When this sulcal segment descends toward the occipital pole, as an inferior extension of the intra-occipital sulcus and comprising the also called superior occipital sulcus (Duvernoy, 1991; Testut and Jacob, 1932a), it divides the upper occipital lateral convexity into two distinct gyri, namely the superior and middle occipital gyri, while its absence or smaller lateral extension does not permit its division into two gyri. According to their findings, these authors concluded that the superolateral surface of the occipital lobe is then composed of three gyri (superior, middle, and inferior) in 30 percent of their studied specimens, and by only two gyri (superior and inferior) in 70 percent (Alves *et al.*, 2012). The area corresponding to the middle occipital gyrus then lies in between the inferior extension of the intra-occipital (or superior occipital or transverse occipital) sulcus and the lateral (or inferior occipital) sulcus.

The lunate sulcus is a very evident sulcus in monkeys and apes clearly separating the occipital lobe and delineating the visual striate cortical area laterally (Duvernoy, 1991; Alves *et al.*, 2012). In humans, it is evident as a well-defined vertical and backward curved sulcus anterior to the occipital pole in less than 40 percent of the brain hemispheres (Duvernoy, 1991; Ono *et al.*, 1990; Alves *et al.*, 2012). More frequently it is absent, only vestigial, or may stem from any of the other main superolateral occipital sulci (Duvernoy, 1991; Ono *et al.*, 1990).

Although disclosing significant anatomical variations, the superolateral occipital convolutions are systematically connected to the parietal and temporal convolutions along rather constant cortical folds.

According to the classic description given by Gratiolet, the parietal and temporal lobe connections with the occipital lobe are made via four folds (two parieto-occipital and two temporo-occipital): 1) the first and more superior parieto-occipital fold, currently known as the parieto-occipital arcus (Duvernoy, 1991; Petrides, 2012), surrounds the parieto-occipital incisure (Petrides, 2012; Duvernoy, 1991) and connects the superior parietal lobule with the superior occipital gyrus; 2) the second and more inferior parieto-occipital fold, composed of a posterior extension of the angular gyrus, connects it with the middle occipital gyrus and occasionally also with the superior occipital gyrus; 3) the first temporo-occipital fold, characterized by the connection of the middle temporal gyrus with the inferior occipital gyrus; and 4) the second temporo-occipital fold, composed of the continuation of the inferior temporal gyrus with the inferior occipital gyrus (Testut and Jacob, 1932a).

In their study, Alves *et al.* (2012) recognized the first or superior temporo-occipital fold in only 40 percent of their studied specimens, but identified the other three occipital connections in all specimens.

Posteriorly, the three occipital gyri converge to form the occipital lobe. Nevertheless, similarly to the temporal pole, the middle occipital gyrus is frequently shorter and the occipital pole is constituted by the convergence of the superior and inferior occipital gyri (Alves *et al.*, 2012).

On the medial surface, the occipital lobe is anatomically particularly well defined and constant. It is separated from the parietal lobe by the parieto-occipital fissure (already fully described in Section 2.2.3.2 on the parietal lobe) and is composed of the cuneus and lingual gyri, which are separated by the calcarine fissure (Figure 2.15).

The calcarine fissure starts anteriorly underneath the splenium of the corpus callosum delineating the inferior aspect of the isthmus of the cingulate gyrus, and runs posteriorly just above the inferomedial margin of the cerebral hemisphere with a gentle and superior convex curvature separating the cuneus from the lingual gyrus. From the apex of the calcarine curvature, around its midpoint, the parieto-occipital fissure emerges superiorly separating the cuneus from the precuneus of the parietal lobe and dividing the calcarine fissure into an anterior and a posterior part. The parieto-occipital and calcarine fissures appear continuous on the surface, but when their borders are retracted, it becomes clear that they are separated by one or more small gyri.

While the anterior part of the calcarine fissure is classified as a complete sulcus because its depth creates a rise in the medial wall of the occipital horn of the lateral ventricle, designated the calcar avis, the posterior part is considered to be an axial sulcus given that its axis runs along the visual cortex (Williams and Warwick, 1980). Only the posterior part includes the primary visual cortical areas, which are located on its superior (cuneal) and inferior (lingual) surfaces. Frequently, this part of the calcarine fissure harbors the cuneolingual gyrus linking both gyri.

At the level of the occipital pole, the calcarine fissure branches usually in a T or Y shape (Ono *et al.*, 1990) forming the retrocalcarine sulcus, sometimes already over the superolateral surface of the cerebral hemisphere. Posteriorly to and along the retrocalcarine sulcus lies the gyrus descendens of Ecker, occasionally bounded posteriorly by the occipitopolar sulcus (Duvernoy, 1991). The gyrus of Ecker is a small lobule still composed of the striate cortex, and its limits correspond to the real lateral limits of this type of cortex in humans (Duvernoy, 1991). For some authors, the retrocalcarine sulcus and its variations are referred to as external calcarine sulci (Petrides, 2012).

Given the anatomical evidence and constancy of the calcarine and of the parieto-occipital fissure on the medial occipital surface, the cuneus is then always a very well-defined wedge-like convolution.

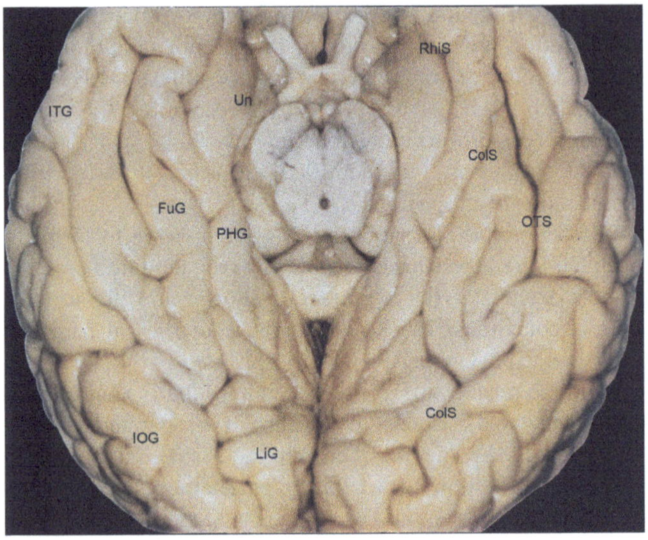

Figure 2.18 The basal temporo-occipital surface.
ColS: collateral sulcus; FuG: fusiform gyrus; IOG: inferior occipital gyrus; ITG: inferior temporal gyrus; LiG: lingual gyrus; OTS: occipitotemporal sulcus; PHG: parahippocampal gyrus; RhiS: rhinal sulcus; Un: uncus. (Adapted from Ribas (2010).)

The real anterior border of the cuneus is the cuneal limiting sulcus which lies within the parieto-occipital fissure (Petrides, 2012), and posteriorly the cuneus rests over the posterior part of the calcarine fissure and over the posterior aspect of the lingual gyrus.

Superior to the posterior part of the calcarine fissure, the cuneus harbors within its surface the paracalcarine (Duvernoy, 1991) or cuneal sulcus (Petrides, 2012) (which corresponds to the inferior sagittal sulcus of the cuneus of Retzius), and further dorsally the occipital paramedial sulcus (which corresponds to the paramesial sulcus of Elliot Smith or the superior sagittal sulcus of Retzius) (Petrides, 2012).

The basal or inferior surface of the occipital lobe is continuous with the basal surface of the temporal lobe and is constituted, from medial to lateral, by the lingual, fusiform, and inferior occipital gyri (Figure 2.18).

The lingual gyrus, also known as the medial temporo-occipital gyrus, lies inferiorly and along the entire length of the calcarine fissure, constituting the mediobasal portion of the occipital lobe and being anteriorly continuous with the parahippocampal gyrus. The basal surface of the lingual gyrus rests over the cerebellar tentorium.

The lingual gyrus is laterally bounded by the collateral sulcus, which is a deep and generally continuous sulcus situated at the cerebral base, extending from the occipital pole to the temporal lobe and running parallel to the calcarine fissure. The lingual gyrus frequently harbors an intralingual sulcus (Duvernoy, 1991; Ono *et al.*, 1990) which divides it into a superior and an inferior part (Duvernoy, 1991), and which can be a posterior and medial ramus of the collateral sulcus (Ono *et al.*, 1990).

The fusiform or lateral temporo-occipital gyrus lies along the temporo-occipital transition, with its posterior or occipital part bounded medially by the collateral sulcus and laterally by the occipitotemporal sulcus, hence it lies between the lingual (medially) and the inferior occipital (laterally) gyri.

The occipital part of the fusiform gyrus lies over the tentorium just posteriorly to the petrous part of the temporal bone, and topographically corresponds to the floor of the ventricular atrium while its temporal part lies underneath the temporal or inferior horn of the lateral ventricle.

While the occipital part of the fusiform gyrus is referred to as O_4, the lingual gyrus corresponds to O_5, and the cuneus to O_6 (Duvernoy, 1991).

The occipitotemporal sulcus rarely extends posteriorly as far as the occipital pole, and both the collateral and the occipitotemporal sulci frequently have secondary side branches and merge anteriorly (Ono *et al.*, 1990).

The inferior or basal aspect of the inferior occipital gyrus lies laterally to the fusiform gyrus, and constitutes the inferiormost portion of the lateral aspect of the occipital lobe.

Along the inferolateral border of each cerebral hemisphere, the inferior temporal gyrus is continuous with the inferior occipital gyrus over the preoccipital notch, and posteriorly the inferior occipital gyrus is medially continuous with the lingual gyrus along the occipital pole.

Along the parietal and occipital aspects of the superomedial border of each cerebral hemisphere, the superior parietal lobule is continuous with the precuneus, and the superior occipital gyrus is continuous with the cuneus above the calcarine fissure and with the lingual gyrus below the calcarine fissure.

2.2.3.4 The Temporal Lobe

Each temporal lobe has a lateral surface which is situated inferior to the lateral (Sylvian) fissure and that lies underneath the squamous portion of the temporal bone, a basal surface that lies over the floor of the cranial middle fossa posteriorly to the great wing of the sphenoid bone, and an opercular surface which lies inside the lateral (Sylvian) fissure (Figure 2.13, 2.15, 2.18, 2.19).

Along the superolateral surface of each cerebral hemisphere, each temporal lobe is arbitrarily limited posteriorly by an imaginary line which runs from the superomedial portion of the parieto-occipital sulcus to the preoccipital notch or incisure. The preoccipital notch is located approximately 5 cm from the occipital pole, and by a posterior prolongation line of the lateral (Sylvian) fissure.

Functionally, the temporal lobe is bilaterally related to auditory functions and in the dominant hemisphere mostly with comprehension aspects of language.

2.2.3.4.1 The Temporal Lobe Sulci and Gyri

The lateral surface of the temporal lobe is composed of the superior, middle, and inferior temporal gyri, also known as T1, T2, and T3, respectively, and which are separated by the superior and inferior temporal sulci, both parallel to the lateral (Sylvian) fissure. Anteriorly, the middle temporal gyrus is generally shorter, causing the superior and inferior temporal gyri to come together forming the temporal pole which lies posteriorly to the great wing of the sphenoid bone (Figure 2.13, 2.16).

The superior temporal sulcus, so named by Ecker (Déjérine, 1895; Ochiai *et al.*, 2004), is always a very well-defined and deep sulcus very much parallel to the lateral (Sylvian) fissure, reason why it was called the parallel scissure by Gratiolet (Déjérine, 1895; Ochiai *et al.*, 2004). The superior temporal sulcus is continuous in about one-third of the human brains (Ono *et al.*, 1990), and, when interrupted, it can be constituted up to four segments (Ono *et al.*, 1990; Ochiai *et al.*, 2004).

Whereas the posterior portion of the lateral (Sylvian) fissure typically terminates as an ascending curve that penetrates the supramarginal gyrus, the superior temporal sulcus always terminates at a point posterior to the end of the lateral (Sylvian) fissure, already within the inferior parietal lobule. In general, the superior temporal sulcus then trifurcates into an ascending sulcal segment, which enters or separates the supramarginal gyrus from the angular gyrus being then coincident with the intermediate sulcus of Jensen, into a distal and horizontal segment that penetrates the angular gyrus and that corresponds to the angular sulcus (Ono *et al.*, 1990; Ribas, 2005a; Ribas *et al.*, 2006), and into an inferior branch that runs toward the occipital lobe (Petrides, 2012).

Given this configuration of the sulci, the superior temporal gyrus always continues posteriorly to the supramarginal gyrus encircling the terminal portion of the lateral (Sylvian) fissure. The middle temporal gyrus is always connected to the angular gyrus beneath the distal and horizontal portion of the superior temporal sulcus that penetrates the angular gyrus proper, and inferiorly it is often connected to the inferior occipital gyrus.

The inferior temporal sulcus, which separates the middle and the inferior temporal gyri, is usually discontinuous and composed of various parts. Inferiorly to it, the inferior temporal gyrus is posteriorly continuous with the inferior occipital gyrus over the preoccipital notch, and inferiorly it extends basally along the inferolateral margin of the cerebral hemisphere. The inferior temporal gyrus is much more developed along its width than along its height.

Both superior and inferior temporal sulci start at the most anterior aspect of the temporal pole and end posteriorly to the temporal lobe arbitrary border. Both have their depths directed toward the inferior or temporal horn of the lateral ventricle. The depth of the posterior part of the superior temporal sulcus is topographically particularly related to the atrium.

The basal surface of the temporal lobe is constituted laterally by the inferior surface of the inferior temporal gyrus, and medially by the anterior or temporal portion of the fusiform or lateral temporo-occipital gyrus, with the temporo-occipital sulcus separating both of them. Medially, the fusiform gyrus is delimited by the collateral sulcus (inferior longitudinal sulcus of Huschke (Déjérine, 1895)) that separates it from the parahippocampal gyrus that already belongs to the limbic lobe (Federative Committee on Anatomical Terminology, 1998) (Figure 2.18).

Although not long, the fusiform gyrus has an anterior or temporal part located between the inferior (laterally) and the parahippocampal (medially) gyri, and a posterior or occipital part located between the inferior occipital (laterally) and the lingual (medially) gyri. While the fusiform temporal part is referred to as T_4, its occipital part is referred to as O_4 (Ecker, 1869; Duvernoy, 1991). Within their surfaces, short and secondary sulci known as fusiform sulci (Petrides, 2012) can be found.

The anterior or temporal part of the fusiform gyrus is typically curved or pointed resembling an arrow, since the anterior-most portion of the temporo-occipital sulcus usually presents a medial curvature toward the collateral sulcus, and its anterior border, in general, corresponds medially to the level of the mesencephalic peduncle.

Anterior to the fusiform gyrus, the collateral sulcus can be continuous with the rhinal sulcus, or frequently separated from it by the so-called temporo-limbic passage (Petrides, 2012). The rhinal sulcus separates the uncus from the rest of the temporal pole, delimiting the entorhinal cortex medially and the neocortex laterally. The most anterior and shallowest aspect of the rhinal sulcus used to be known as the temporal incisure by classic anatomists (Petrides, 2012).

The temporal portion of the fusiform gyrus lies over the posterior aspect of the middle fossa floor and over the upper surface of the petrous part of the temporal bone, underneath the inferior or temporal horn of the lateral ventricles (Ribas, 2007a, 2010). Anteriorly, it presents a slight basal prominence due to its adaptation to the concavity of the middle cranial fossa. Posteriorly, the whole basal surface of the temporal lobe is continuous with the basal occipital surface which already lies over the superior surface of the cerebral tentorium, with the occipital part of the fusiform gyrus lying underneath the ventricular atrium.

The superior or opercular surface of the temporal lobe is formed by the superior surface of the superior temporal gyrus, which lies within the lateral (Sylvian) fissure and is composed of multiple transverse gyri (Figure 2.19).

Among these gyri of the temporal opercular surface, there is a much more voluminous transverse gyrus that originates around the midpoint of the superior temporal gyrus, and is oriented diagonally toward the posterior vertex of the floor of the Sylvian fissure with its longest axis oriented toward the ventricular atrium. This gyrus can be single or double when divided by a secondary sulcus, and is designated the transverse gyrus of Heschl. Together with the posterior-most aspect of the superior temporal gyrus, its cortex constitutes the primary auditory cortical area (Türe *et al.*, 1999; Williams and Warwick, 1980).

Heschl's gyrus is bounded anteriorly by the first transverse sulcus, and posteriorly by the more evident sulcus of Heschl (Petrides, 2012). It divides the temporal opercular surface into two planes: an anterior plane called the polar plane, and a posterior plane known as the temporal plane.

A small superior extension of the superior temporal sulcus anterior to Heschl's gyrus, known as the sulcus acusticus, is sometimes present indicating the anterior aspect of Heschl's gyrus on the superolateral surface of the temporal lobe. The transverse temporal sulcus, which lies posterior to Heschl's sulcus within the temporal plane, may reach the lateral surface of the superior temporal gyrus indicating the posterior aspect of Heschl's gyrus.

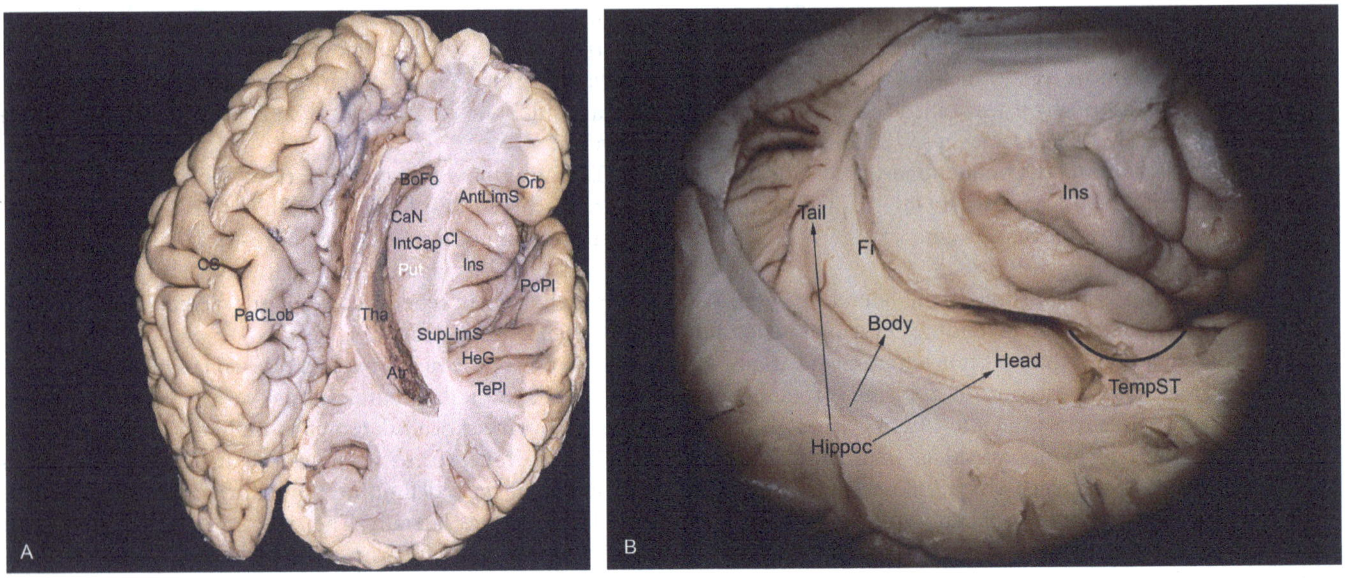

Figure 2.19 (A) The temporal opercular surface, the insula, and the central core of the brain. (B) The hippocampus lies along the temporal horn. AntLimS: anterior limiting sulcus of insula; Atr: atrium of lateral ventricle; BoFo: body of fornix; CaN: caudate nucleus; Cl: claustrum; CS: central sulcus; HeG: Heschl's gyrus; Ins: insula; IntCap: internal capsule fibers; Orb: orbital part of inferior frontal gyrus; PaCLob: paracentral lobule; PoPl: polar plane of the opercular temporal surface; Put: putamen; SupLimS: superior limiting sulcus of insula; TePl: temporal plane; Tha: thalamus. (Adapted from Ribas (2010).): Fi: fimbria of the fornix; Hippoc: hippocampus; Ins: insula; TempSt: temporal stem.

The surface of the polar plane is composed of multiple transverse gyri directed obliquely toward the inferior part of the circular insular sulcus (inferior limiting sulcus) (Türe *et al.*, 1999; Wen *et al.*, 1999), and which are generically known as Schwalbe gyri and separated by the sulci of Schwalbe.

The temporal plane that lies within the lateral (Sylvian) fissure posteriorly to Heschl's gyrus is flat, perpendicular to the brain surface, and has a triangular shape with its internal vertex corresponding to the posterior vertex of the bottom of the lateral (Sylvian) fissure, where the superior part of the insular circular sulcus (superior limiting sulcus) meets the inferior part of the insular circular sulcus (inferior limiting sulcus), hence immediately over the atrium. The temporal plane is usually larger in the dominant hemisphere, supposedly due to its involvement with language functions (Geschwind *et al.*, 1968).

Topographically, while the oblique polar plane actually covers the insular surface, Heschl's gyrus underlies the opercular surface of the postcentral gyrus (Wen *et al.*, 1999). The flat surface of the temporal plane underlies the opercular surface of the supramarginal gyrus. Given these configurations, whereas the lateral (Sylvian) fissure appears oblique in coronal slices taken in the polar plane, it appears horizontal in those taken in the temporal plane.

Heschl's gyrus is systematically pointing toward the ventricular atrium.

The posterior cortical area of the dominant hemisphere responsible for language, called Wernicke's area, is intrinsically related to the auditory cortex. This area is more particularly responsible for the comprehension aspect of language, but its stimulation also causes speech arrest. Anatomically not well defined, Wernicke's area mainly occupies the posterior aspect of the superior temporal gyrus and the basal aspect of the supramarginal gyrus, but it can extend inferiorly along the middle temporal gyrus and anteriorly until 3 cm from the temporal pole as demonstrated by Ojemann *et al.* (1989).

2.2.3.5 The Insular Lobe and the Central Core

On the publication of the fourth edition of the *Paris Nomina Anatomica* in 1975 (Excerpta Medica Foundation, 1975), the insula came to be considered to be a cerebral lobe.

Embedded between the frontal and temporal lobes of each cerebral hemisphere and constituting the base of each Sylvian cistern, the insula has an anterior and a lateral surface that are encased in their respective opercular (from the Latin *operculum* meaning curtain (Ferreira, 1966)) convolutions, which correspond to the most recently developed regions of the cerebral hemispheres (Figure 2.19A, 2.20).

Based on many clinical and experimental studies, the insula has been related to many different functions such as olfactory, gustatory, higher autonomic control, and memory among others. However, its full physiological role is still obscure (Türe *et al.*, 1999).

Morphologically, in each cerebral hemisphere, the insula constitutes an external shield of a very well-defined block comprised of the insular lobe itself, the lenticular and the caudate nucleus, the thalamus, and with the internal capsule in between (Rhoton, 2003; Ribas and Rodrigues, 2007).

2.2.3.5.1 Insular Lobe Sulci and Gyri

The anterior surface of the insula is covered by the fronto-orbital operculum (comprising the posterior portion of the posterior orbital gyrus and the orbital part of the inferior frontal gyrus). Its lateral surface is covered superiorly by the frontoparietal operculum (triangular and opercular parts of the inferior frontal gyrus, subcentral gyrus, and anterior and

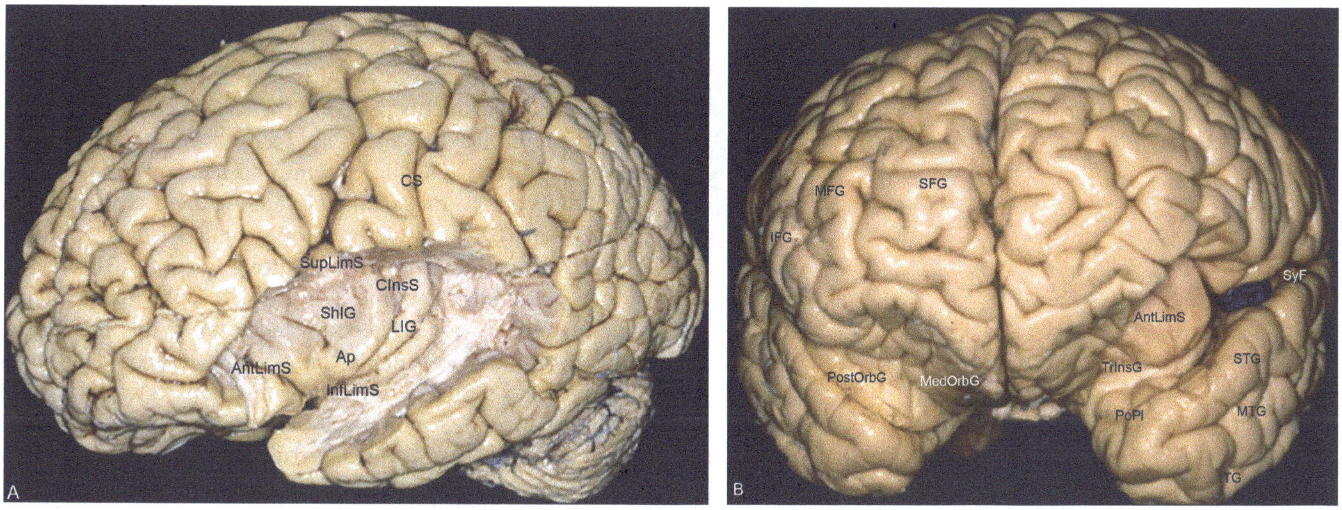

Figure 2.20 The lateral (A) and anterior (B) surfaces of the insula.
AntLimS: anterior limiting sulcus of insula; Ap: insular apex; ClnsS: central insular sulcus; CS: central sulcus; IFG: inferior frontal gyrus; InfLimS: inferior limiting sulcus; ITG: inferior temporal gyrus; LIG: long insular gyri; MedOrbG: medial orbital gyrus; MFG: middle frontal gyrus; MTG: middle temporal gyrus; PoPl: polar plane of the opercular temporal surface; PostOrbG: posterior orbital gyrus; SyF: lateral or Sylvian fissure; SFG: superior frontal gyrus; ShIG: short insular gyri; STG: superior temporal gyrus; SupLimS: superior limiting sulcus of insula; TrInsG: transverse insular gyrus. (Adapted from Ribas (2010).)

basal part of the supramarginal gyrus) and inferiorly by the temporal operculum (polar plane of the superior temporal gyrus) (Türe *et al.*, 1999; Williams and Warwick, 1980; Yasargil *et al.*, 1985).

The lateral surface of the insula is characterized as a pyramid with a triangular base, with its anteroinferior vertex constituting the limen insulae and with its summit referred to as the insular apex. The limen insulae consists of a narrow strip of olfactory cortex and extends along the lateral aspect of the lateral olfactory stria, cojoining the insular cortex and the anterior perforated substance (Türe *et al.*, 1999) (Figure 2.20).

The insular lateral surface is divided by the central sulcus of the insula into a smaller anterior part and a larger posterior part. The insular central sulcus is located posteriorly to the insular apex located within its anterior part, is the main and deepest sulcus of the insula, and courses obliquely from the limen insulae with a similar direction and toward the central sulcus of each cerebral hemisphere (Türe *et al.*, 1999).

The anterior part of the lateral insular surface is composed of the transverse, the accessory, and by three short insular gyri (anterior, middle, and posterior short insular gyri), all arising from the insular apex region. The middle and posterior short insular gyri are separated by the precentral insular sulcus (Petrides, 2012).

The transverse insular gyrus runs along the limen insulae connecting the anterior insula with the posteromedial orbital lobule, which is composed of the connection of the posterior portion of the medial orbital gyrus with the posterior orbital gyrus (Türe *et al.*, 1999; Yasargil, 1984a), and which is located anterior to and along the lateral olfactory stria. The accessory gyrus extends from the anterior portion of the anterior short gyrus superiorly to the transverse insular gyrus, beneath the fronto-orbital operculum (Türe *et al.*, 1999). Both gyri constitute the insular pole within the insular anterior aspect (Türe *et al.*, 1999; Türe *et al.*, 2000).

The posterior part of the insula is located behind its central sulcus, and is composed of the anterior and posterior insular long gyri that can be easily identified as they do not originate at the insular apex. Both gyri are separated by the postcentral insular sulcus, the anterior long gyrus is usually larger, and occasionally it is single and divided at its upper end.

The insular surface is delineated peripherally by the circular sulcus of Reil (Duvernoy, 1991; Taveras and Wood, 1976), or periinsular sulcus (Testut and Jacob, 1932a; Türe *et al.*, 1999), which is interrupted by the transverse insular gyrus running across the limen insulae. Given the triangular shape of the insula, its circular or periinsular sulcus is usually divided into three parts, that is, the anterior, superior, and inferior periinsular sulci (Türe *et al.*, 1999), also called the anterior, superior, and inferior limiting sulci of the insula (Rhoton, 2003).

To understand the periinsular spaces more fully, one should remember that the insula has a lateral and an anterior surface. The superior and inferior limiting sulci are morphologically categorized as true sulci that delineate the respective transitions and deflections occurring among the lateral insular surface and the frontoparietal operculum, and the lateral insular surface and the temporal operculum. The anterior limiting of the insula, on the other hand, is considerably deeper and morphologically characteristic of a true fissure or space that separates the anterior surface of the insula from the fronto-orbital operculum.

The upper half of the fundus of the anterior limiting sulcus is separated from a true anterior recess of the lateral ventricle, anterior to the head of the caudate nucleus, only by the fibers of the thin anterior limb of the internal capsule, whereas the fundus of the lower half continues to the ventral-striato-pallidal or anterior perforated substance region.

Underneath the insular cortex, there is the extreme capsule that corresponds to the subcortical white matter of the insular cortex, and which covers the claustrum laterally.

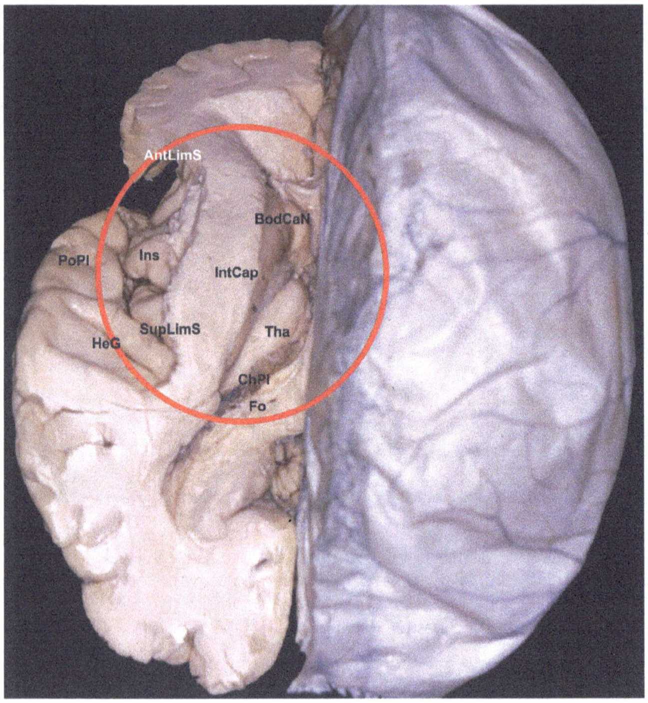

Figure 2.21 The insular lateral surface corresponds to an external shield of the central core of the brain.

AntLimS: anterior limiting sulcus of insula; BodCaN: body of the caudate nucleus; ChPl: choroid plexus; Fo: fornix; HeG: Heschl's gyrus; Ins: insula; IntCap: internal capsule fibers; PoPl: polar plane of the opercular temporal surface; SupLimS: superior limiting sulcus of insula; Tha: thalamus. (Adapted from Ribas (2010).)

2.2.3.5.2 The Insula and the Cerebral Central Core

From a topographical point of view, the surface of the insula is clearly characterized as the external shield of an anatomically well-defined cerebral core, which is constituted, in each hemisphere, by the insula itself, by the basal nuclei, the thalamus, and with the internal capsule between these structures (Rhoton, 2003; Ribas and Rodrigues, 2007; Choi *et al.*, 2011) (Figures 2.19 and 2.21).

The cerebral central core is located between the Sylvian cistern within the lateral (Sylvian) fissure, the parapeduncular cisterns around the brainstem (crural, ambient, and quadrigeminal cisterns), and the supratentorial ventricular cavities. When seen from above, this block has a biconvex configuration, with its lateral aspect given by the insular cortex and its medial aspect by the intraventricular surfaces of the caudate nucleus and of the thalamus. Whereas the anterior portion of the insula corresponds internally to the head of the caudate nucleus, its posterior portion is topographically related to the thalamus.

Each thalamus is morphologically characterized as the top of each side of the brainstem due to the intimate connections and anatomical continuity existing between the thalami and the tegmental portion of the mesencephalon. Each central core is morphologically equivalent to a true head of each half of the brainstem, surrounded by the ventricles and by the supratentorial cisterns, and encircled by the telencephalon. The C-shaped choroidal fissure, positioned between each thalamus and each fornix (Yasargil, 1984a; Brodal, 1981; Meneses, 1999; Yasargil *et al.*, 1985; Nagata *et al.*, 1988), constitutes an important avenue of communication between the ventricular and cisternal compartments linked to the central core.

Under the insular cortex, its respective subcortical white matter, also known as the extreme capsule, is composed of U fibers that connect the insular gyri among themselves and with the frontoparietal and temporal operculi, respectively, underneath the superior and inferior limiting sulci of the insula.

Underneath the extreme capsule, there is the fine lamina of gray matter that constitutes the claustrum. While the ventral portion of the claustrum is thinner and composed of small islands of gray matter within the white matter, its dorsal portion is thicker and much more well defined. The external capsule, which lies underneath the claustrum, is composed mainly of fibers originating within the claustrum and anteriorly, it is intermingled with the uncinate fasciculus and with the inferior occipitofrontal fasciculus (Fernández-Miranda *et al.*, 2008).

Externally, the external capsule covers the putamen, a large mass of gray matter that together with the smaller globus pallidus constitutes the lenticular nucleus, so called because of its lens-shaped format. The globus pallidus lies medially and basally in relation to the putamen. Regarding its consistency, it is much more pale and firm, and both of them are covered medially by internal capsule fibers.

Medially, the caudate nucleus forms an arch around the thalamus and a bulge in the lateral wall of the lateral ventricle. Its large anterior head constitutes the lateral wall of the anterior horn, its narrower body corresponds to the lateral wall of the ventricular body, and its tail encircles the pulvinar of the thalamus posteriorly and laterally, and then runs along the roof of the inferior horn (Figure 2.19).

The putamen and the caudate nuclei together correspond to the striatum, and while dorsally they are separated by fibers of the internal capsule, their ventral aspects are continuous underneath the anterior and inferior edge of the internal capsule constituting the ventral striatum which corresponds to the nucleus accumbens. The striatal nuclei and globus pallidus together correspond to the basal ganglia.

The external and internal capsules are capsules of the lenticular nucleus, and, whereas the thin external capsule is composed of fibers that cover only the lateral portion of the putamen and do not have any major functional importance, the internal capsule consists of important projection fibers that originate in, and are directed toward, the cerebral cortex as a whole. Above the superior aspect of the lenticular nucleus, the internal capsule is continuous as the centrum ovale or corona radiata, and inferiorly to the lenticular nucleus, it is continuous as the cerebral peduncle. The internal capsule has a V-shaped format, and, in relation to the lenticular nucleus, it is divided into an anterior limb (between the head of the caudate and the putamen), a genu (that corresponds to the medial apex of the V, adjacent to the interventricular foramen), a posterior limb (between the body of the caudate together with the thalamus and the putamen), and retrolenticular and sublenticular parts.

The central core is attached to the rest of the cerebral hemisphere by isthmi composed of these different internal capsule parts. Anteriorly and under the anterior limiting insular sulcus, there are the fibers of the anterior limb of the internal capsule. Superiorly and under the superior limiting sulcus, there are the remaining anterior limb fibers, as well as the genu and posterior limb fibers that harbor the corticonuclear and corticospinal tracts. Posteriorly and inferiorly to the insular inferior limiting sulcus, there are the retrolenticular and sublenticular internal capsule fibers that enclose the auditory and optic radiations.

Since the lateral surface area of the insula is greater than the area of the putamen (Ebeling *et al.*, 1992a; Türe *et al.*, 1999), its anterior, superior, and inferior limiting sulci lie very close, respectively, to these three internal capsule isthmi. Because the internal capsule is V-shaped with a medial vertex, the insular surface sites that are closest to the internal capsule fibers are precisely the insular areas that correspond to the existing angles between the anterior and superior limiting sulci (anterior insular point (Türe *et al.*, 1999)), and the superior and inferior limiting sulci (posterior insular point (Türe *et al.*, 1999)). Whereas the fibers that constitute the anterior limb of the internal capsule, located under the anterior insular angle, do not have any major functional importance, the capsular fibers located under the angle formed by the superior and inferior limiting sulci, as well as under the entire inferior limiting sulcus itself, are of great functional importance, since they correspond, respectively, to the corticospinal motor fibers, to the superior thalamic radiation, and to the auditory and optical radiations.

Medially, each cerebral central core is delimited by the structures that compose the walls of each lateral ventricle and the walls of the third ventricle (Tables 2.4 and 2.5).

While the anterior aspect of the central core is medially related to the head of the caudate nucleus, its posterior aspect is medially related to the body of the caudate nucleus and the thalamus. The head of the caudate nucleus corresponds to the lateral wall of the anterior horn, and the body of the caudate nucleus corresponds to the lateral wall of the body of the lateral ventricle.

The posterior surface of the central core, in turn, comprises the surface of the pulvinar of the thalamus, whose superior portion is seen in the atrium of the lateral ventricle and whose inferior portion appears within the ambient and pineal or quadrigeminal cisterns located around and posteriorly to the brainstem.

Laterally and inferiorly, the base of the central core is delineated by the lateral wing of the ambient cistern, which is located within the transverse fissure of the brain, between the pulvinar of the thalamus above and the subiculum of the parahippocampal gyrus below.

Superiorly, the cerebral central core is covered by fibers of the corpus callosum and by the subcortical white matter in each cerebral hemisphere. Anteriorly and inferiorly, this block is

Table 2.4 Brain structures that delineate each lateral ventricle

Frontal or anterior horn	Floor		Rostrum of the campus callosum
	Anterior wall		Genu of the corpus callosum
	Roof		Trunk of the corpus callosum
	Walls	Medial	Septum pellucidum
		Lateral	Head of the caudate nucleus
Ventricular body	Floor	Medial	Body of the fornix
		Lateral	Superior surface of the thalamus
	Roof		Trunk of the corpus callosum
	Walls	Medial	Septum pellucidum
		Lateral	Body of caudate nucleus
Atrium or ventricular trigone	Anterior walls	Medial	Crura fornicis
		Lateral	Pulvinar thalamus and tail of caudate nucleus
	Roof		Splenium of the corpus callosum
	Walls	Lateral	Hemispheric white matter/sagittal stratum
		Medial	Hippocampus, bulb of the corpus callosum, calcar avis
	Floor		Collateral trigone, splenium of the corpus callosum
Occipital or posterior horn	Roof		Splenium of the corpus callosum
	Walls	Medial	Splenium of the corpus callosum
		Lateral	Splenium of the corpus callosum/sagittal stratum
	Floor		Splenium of the corpus callosum
Temporal or inferior horn	Floor	Medial	Hippocampus
		Lateral	Collateral eminence
	Roof	Medial	Tail of the caudate nucleus, stria terminalis
		Lateral	Hemispheric white matter, sagittal stratum, amygdala
	Walls	Anterior	Amygdala, hemispheric white matter
		Medial	Fimbria fornix
		Lateral	Hemispheric white matter/sagittal stratum

Table 2.5 Brain structures that delineate the third ventricle

Roof	Bodies of the fornices Cistern of velum interpositum (with superior and inferior choroid plexus, posteromedial choroidal arteries, and internal cerebral veins)	
Anterior wall	Pillars or columns of the fornices Anterior commissure Lamina terminalis Optic chiasm	
Lateral walls	Thalami (stria medullaris of the thalamus) Hypothalamic sulcus Hypothalamus	
Posterior wall	Epithalamus	Habenulas Commissure of the habenulas Pineal gland
	Posterior commissure	
Floor	Hypothalamus	Optic chiasm Median eminence/pituitary stalk Tuber cinereum Mammillary bodies
	Mesencephalon	Posterior perforated substance/roof of interpeduncular fossa Mesencephalic tegmentum

contiguous with the basal forebrain, which corresponds, from lateral to medial, to the medial extension of the temporal stem, to the ventral pallidal-striatum region, and to the septal region.

The insular surface is a paralimbic structure that is composed of the so-called mesocortex. The mesocortex is anatomically situated between the allocortex, which is older and topographically more medial (comprising the amygdala and hippocampus), and the isocortex, which is phylogenetically younger and topographically more lateral (comprising the neocortex of the cerebral hemispheres).

2.2.3.6 The Limbic Lobe and Correlated Areas

The *International Anatomical Terminology*, published in 1998 (Federative Committee on Anatomical Terminology, 1998) and which replaced the previous *Nomina Anatomica*, introduced the limbic lobe as another of the cerebral lobes and described it as comprising the cingulate and parahippocampal gyri.

The term limbic was first used in the nineteenth century by Broca (Broca, 1877 apud Finger, 1994) who observed that certain cerebral structures constituted a continuum arranged in the shape of a C surrounding the diencephalic region. Broca originally described the cingulate and parahippocampal gyri as continuous, naming them together the greater limbic lobe, and considered the different sulci that limited these two gyri as parts of a single sulcus named by him the limbic sulcus (Broca, 1877 apud Finger, 1994; Heimer, 1995; Heimer, 2003).

Since then the term limbic (meaning border, ring, or surround (Ferreira, 1966)) came to be definitively established in the neuroanatomical literature, and subsequent studies introduced the notion that the so-called limbic system is composed of telencephalic and diencephalic structures that, despite their anatomical and functional diversity, are predominantly responsible for the physiology of emotions, memory, and learning (Heimer, 1995; Heimer *et al.*, 2008; Ribas, 2006; Ribas, 2007a; Williams and Warwick, 1980).

The structures that are related to this system and with its functions, but do not belong to the strict concept of limbic lobe, are discussed at the end of Section 2.2.3.6.4.

2.2.3.6.1 Limbic Lobe Sulci and Gyri

Within the inner aspect of the medial surface of each cerebral hemisphere, the cingulate gyrus wraps around the corpus callosum and continues posteriorly and inferiorly to the parahippocampal gyrus, forming the shape of a C around the diencephalon (Figure 2.15).

The cingulate gyrus is situated above the callosal sulcus and below the cingulate sulcus. It starts within the subcallosal area below the rostrum of the corpus callosum, and, as it ascends around the genu of the corpus callosum, it frequently presents an ascending connection with the medial aspect of the superior frontal gyrus. Over the body of the corpus callosum, the cingulate gyrus is connected to the paracentral lobule, and more posteriorly it is connected to the precuneus. These connections, which vary in number, are arrayed from front to back and from bottom to top and are particularly visible after removing the most cortical aspect of the cingulate gyrus.

Posterior to the splenium of the corpus callosum, the cingulate gyrus consistently becomes narrower, at which point it is referred to as the isthmus, and continues to the parahippocampal gyrus. The site of transition between these two gyri is identified by the emergence of the anterior branch of the calcarine fissure, which originates beneath the isthmus of the cingulate gyrus.

Anteriorly and basally, the cingulate sulcus can be continuous with the anterior paraolfactory sulcus underneath the rostrum of the corpus callosum (Ono *et al.*, 1990), causing the cingulate gyrus to be continuous with the paraolfactory or subcallosal gyri (Duvernoy, 1991). In about one-quarter of the human brain hemispheres, the cingulate sulcus is double and parallel (Ono *et al.*, 1990), and the superior additional fold was called the paracingulate sulcus by Elliot Smith (Petrides, 2012).

The terminal ascending branch of the cingulate sulcus delineates the paracentral lobule posteriorly and the precuneus anteriorly, whereas the usually interrupted subparietal sulcus is located inferior to the precuneus, separating it from the cingulate gyrus and appearing to be a posterior continuation of the cingulate sulcus after a short interruption of the latter. The connections between the cingulate and the precuneus gyri are anterior, posterior, and in between the multiple typically Y-shaped segments of the subparietal sulcus.

The parahippocampal gyrus forms the lower half of the C that wraps around the diencephalic region, lying laterally to the cerebral peduncle. Anteriorly, the parahippocampal gyrus folds back on itself medially constituting the uncus, with the uncal sulcus within (Figure 2.16B), and posteriorly it is continuous with the isthmus of the cingulated gyrus and also corresponds to the anterior continuation of the lingual gyrus, which lies under the calcarine fissure (Figure 2.18).

Along its axial extension, the basal and medial surface of the parahippocampal gyrus curves laterally constituting a flat superior surface known as the subiculum. The subiculum is slightly triangular with an anterior vertex, and corresponds to the floor of the lateral part of the transverse fissure, whose roof is formed by the lateral geniculate body anteriorly and by the pulvinar of the thalamus posteriorly (Duvernoy, 1998). This portion of the transverse fissure harbors the so-called lateral wing of the ambient cistern, which harbors the posterior cerebral artery.

The hippocampus proper is situated laterally and along the subiculum, within the parahippocampal gyrus already inside the inferior or temporal horn of the lateral ventricle. The hippocampus itself consists of Ammon's horn, which is characterized as an intraventricular prominence, and of the small dentate gyri, which lie medially and along Ammon's horn. Given the greater magnitude of Ammon's horn, the term hippocampus is commonly used in reference to this structure.

Within the inferior or temporal horn of the lateral ventricle, the hippocampus is characterized as a convex elevation approximately 5 cm long, placed along its floor, and, macroscopically, it can be divided into a head, a body, and a tail (Duvernoy, 1998) (Figure 2.19B). Its most anterior part or head is clearly expanded and presents two or three shallow grooves that give a paw-like appearance, known as the pes hippocampi. Its body lies along the inferior horn topographically encircling the cerebral peduncle, and macroscopically its tail partially ends posteriorly joining the medial of the ventricular atrium and is partially continuous as the gyrus fasciolaris around the splenium and toward the indusium griseum.

The surface of the hippocampus is called the alveus due to its clear white coloration, and is covered by the ependyma inside the ventricular cavity. The alveus is a thin layer composed of the fibers originating within the trilaminar cortex of the hippocampus.

The dentate gyrus is composed of small cortical prominences that form a chain along the medial aspect of the hippocampus forming the margo denticulatus (Duvernoy, 1998), which continues anteriorly into the notch of the uncus and posteriorly is continuous with the fasciola cinerea around the splenium, and thus with the indusium griseum over the corpus callosum. Along its medial margin, the dentate gyrus is separated from the subiculum of the parahippocampal gyrus by the hippocampal sulcus, which is usually a shallow sulcus that terminates anteriorly also within the uncus. More superiorly and also medially, the dentate gyrus is separated from the fimbria of the fornix by the fimbriodentate sulcus, which is parallel to the hippocampal sulcus (Duvernoy, 1998; Wen *et al.*, 1999).

The fornix constitutes the main bundle of the efferent fibers of the hippocampus, and is comprised of fimbria, crura, body, and column or pillar. Each fornix wraps each thalamus, with the choroidal fissure in between and with the choroid plexus inserted along the whole choroidal fissure (Nagata *et al.*, 1988).

The fornix begins along the hippocampus with convergence of the fibers of the alveus, which form the fimbria of the fornix along the medial portion of the floor of the inferior horn. The fimbria continues posteriorly becoming the crura of the fornix, which wraps the posterior aspect of the thalamus, called the pulvinar of the thalamus. The crura of the fornix has the shape of a tape which is attached to its corresponding contralateral portion through the commissure of the fornix, or hippocampal commissure, disposed beneath the lower surface of the splenium of the corpus callosum. Anteriorly and medially, the fornix continues constituting the body of the fornix, juxtaposed to its corresponding contralateral part along the midline and within the roof of the third ventricle (Figure 2.19B, 2.22).

The most anterior segment of the body of the fornix detaches from the thalamic surface, adopting an anterior-lateral-inferior course and therefore moving away from its corresponding contralateral part, constituting the column or pillar of the fornix which penetrates the hypothalamic parenchyma toward the ipsilateral mammillary body of the hypothalamus. When detaching from the thalamus, each column of the fornix delimits the anterior margin of the interventricular foramen of Monro on each side, which then has as its posterior margin the most anterior aspect of the ipsilateral thalamus that harbors the anterior thalamic nuclei.

The choroidal fissure extends between the whole fornix and thalamus, from the inferior choroidal point situated between the head and the body of the hippocampus, as far as the interventricular foramen, which then corresponds to an enlargement of the choroidal fissure at its superior end. The inferior choroidal point corresponds to the point of entrance of the anterior choroidal artery and exit of the inferior ventricular vein (Nagata *et al.*, 1988).

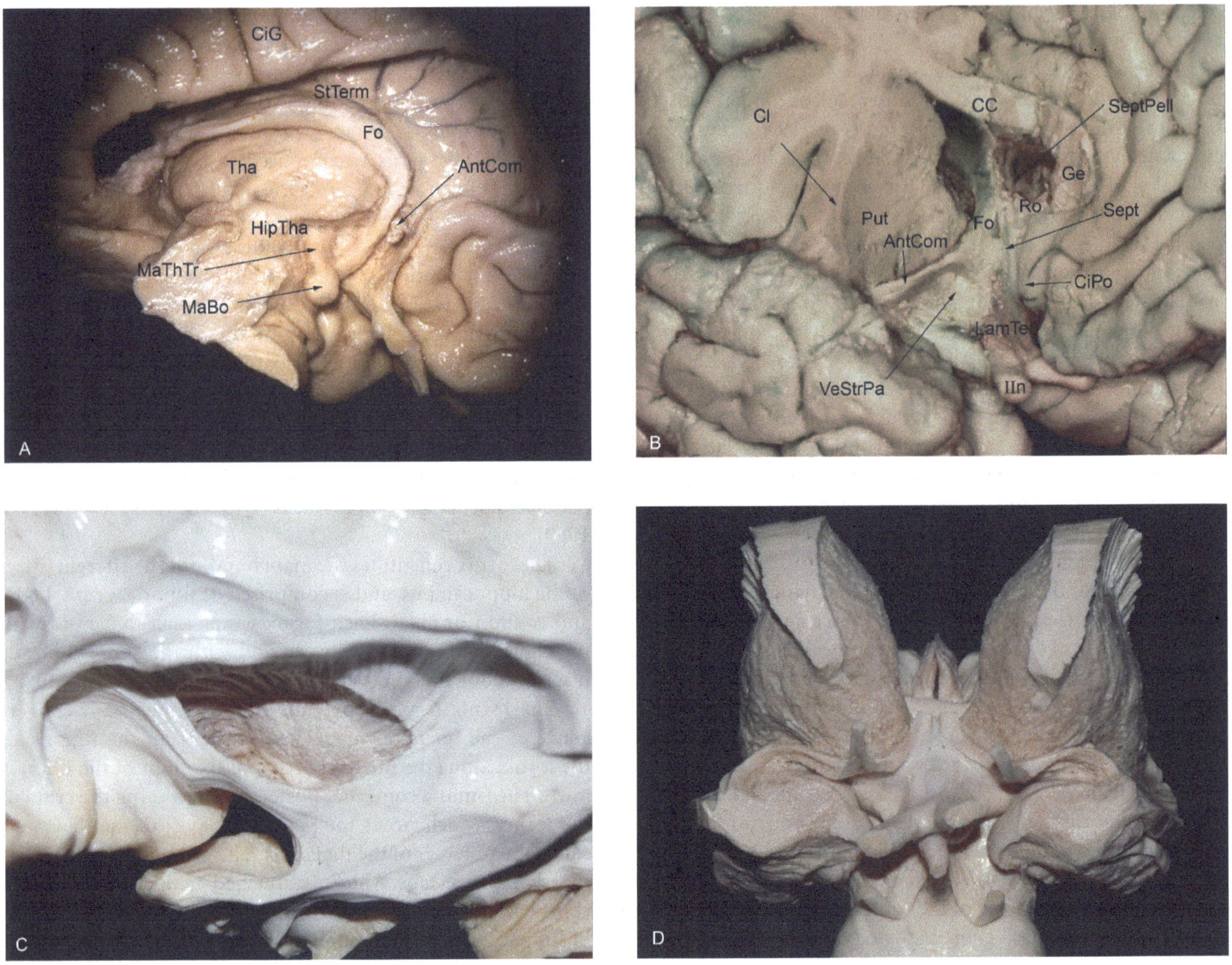

Figure 2.22 Limbic and related structures.
(A) Medial structures after removal of the corpus callosum, disclosing neural structures related to limbic circuits.
(B) The ventral-striato-pallidal or substantia innominata region (VeStrPa) lies inferiorly and anteriorly to the anterior commissure (AntCom). The septal region (Sept) lies anteriorly to the anterior commissure (AntCom) and posteriorly to the cingulate pole (CiPo). The column of the fornix (Fo) runs posteriorly to the anterior commissure (AntCom).
(C) The ventral-striato-pallidal or substantia innominata region has as its basal and anterior wall, the anterior perforated substance, as its roof, fibers of the anterior limb of the internal capsule, as its posterior wall, the central aspect of the globus pallidus which harbors the anterior commissure within its channel of Gratiolet, and as its medial wall, the nucleus accumbens; laterally, this region is contiguous with the temporal stem and medially, it is contiguous with the septal region.
(D) Anterior view of the nucleus accumbens or ventral striatum, which corresponds to the basal connection of the caudate and putamen, with the internal capsule in between.
AntComm: anterior commissure; CiG: cingulate gyrus; Fo: fornix; HipTha: hypothalamus; MaBo: mammillary body; MaThTr: mammillothalamic tract; StTerm: stria terminalis; Tha: thalamus.CC: corpus callosum; Cl: claustrum; Ge: genu of corpus callosum; LamTer: lamina terminalis; Put: putamen; SeptPell: septum pellucidum; Ro: rostrum of corpus callosum; IIn: optic nerve.

Anteriorly to the inferior choroidal point, the anterior and mesial parts of the temporal lobe and of the parahippocampal gyrus are incorporated in the basal and lateral aspect of the frontal lobe through a neural peduncle that constitutes the so-called temporal stem. Posteriorly to the inferior choroidal point, the choroidal fissure lies within the inferior horn between the fimbria of the fornix and the inferior aspect of the thalamus, along the parapeduncular space which harbors the ambient cistern. More posteriorly, the choroidal fissure within the atrium lies between the crura and the pulvinar of the thalamus, laterally to the quadrigeminal or pineal cistern, and, more superiorly and anteriorly, the choroidal fissure lies in between the body of the fornix and the superior surface of the thalamus, hence between the body of each lateral ventricle and the third ventricle (Nagata *et al.*, 1988).

The indusium griseum is classically described as being composed of a thin layer of gray matter situated on each side over the corpus callosum, and covered by its medial and lateral longitudinal striae that run within the callosal sulcus underneath each cingulate gyrus (Duvernoy, 1991; Williams and Warwick, 1980). Anteriorly, the indusium griseum is connected to the paraterminal gyrus via the prehippocampal rudiment. Posteriorly, it circles the splenium of the corpus callosum and, on each side, it runs along the fasciolar gyri (posterior extension of Ammon's horn) and the fasciola cinerea (posterior extension of the dentate gyrus). Some small hippocampal protrusions, known as gyri of Andreas Retzius, are also occasionally visible in the subsplenial area (Duvernoy, 1991).

To ease the understanding of these anatomical features, it is interesting to remember that, phylogenetically, the hippocampus is supracallosal in origin, and subsequently migrates posteriorly and inferiorly finally presenting as a structure that runs along the floor of the inferior horn of the lateral ventricle (Sarnat and Netsky, 1981). Considering these observations, the indusium griseum can be understood as a remnant of the supracallosal hippocampus, and the fornix as its tail that was left behind during its inferior migration.

The uncus of the parahippocampal gyrus is triangular with a medial vertex, such that its anteromedial surface faces the carotid cistern and its posteromedial surface faces and encircles the mesencephalic peduncle (Figure 2.16B).

The anterior half of the uncus is more voluminous, corresponds to the piriform lobe (Duvernoy, 1991), and harbors the amygdala, whereas its posterior half harbors the head of the hippocampus (Wen *et al.*, 1999; Duvernoy, 1991).

On its medial and anterior surface, there are two small prominences: the more superior is the semilunar gyrus, which is a lateral extension of the lateral olfactory stria, and the more inferior is the ambient gyrus. Both cover the amygdala and are separated by the semiannular sulcus, which harbors the anterior choroidal artery. More inferiorly there is frequently another depression, caused by the pressure of the free edge of the tentorium cerebelli.

The most rostral and anterior aspect of the uncus corresponds to the entorhinal cortical area, an ancient olfactory cortical area that can be recognized by its speckled superficial aspect attributed to the discontinuity of its most superficial cell layer that harbors islands of large, multipolar neurons. The entorhinal area lies within the lower part of the piriform lobe, and encroaches upon the posterior segment of the parahippocampal gyrus (Duvernoy, 1991; Duvernoy, 1998).

Anteriorly, the centromedial and larger part of the amygdala gives rise to a ventral bundle of fibers named the ansa peduncularis, composed of amygdalofugal fibers going to the septal, thalamic, and hypothalamic regions, which runs underneath the ventral aspect of the lenticulate nucleus and along the basal forebrain, and a dorsal extension named the stria terminalis, which wraps the thalamus dorsally. Within the inferior horn, the stria terminalis runs along its roof medially to the gray matter at the tail of the caudate nucleus, and within the ventricular body, it runs between the thalamus and the caudate nucleus underneath the thalamostriate vein.

Superiorly, the amygdala runs toward the base of the globus pallidus so that, in a coronal slice, the base of the lentiform nucleus and the amygdala form a figure-eight or an hourglass shape (Türe *et al.*, 2000; Wen *et al.*, 1999; Williams and Warwick, 1980).

The posterior half of the uncus contains the head of the hippocampus, and is separated inferiorly from the parahippocampal gyrus by the uncal sulcus. It has a medial surface which faces the crural cistern, and an inferior surface hidden inside the uncal sulcus.

Within the uncal sulcus the posterior half of the uncus harbors anteriorly the uncinate gyrus and posteriorly the uncal apex, both separated by the band of Giacomini and with all these structures corresponding to the extraventricular part of the head of the hippocampus (Duvernoy, 1991; Duvernoy, 1998). The band of Giacomini itself corresponds to the tail of the dentate gyrus which vanishes on the medial aspect of the uncus, and the uncal apex is also known as the intralimbic gyrus and as the hippocampus inversus (Duvernoy, 1998).

Along the cerebral base, the parahippocampal gyrus is laterally delineated by the collateral sulcus, which separates it from the fusiform gyrus, and more anteriorly by the rhinal sulcus, which is occasionally continuous with the collateral sulcus.

The collateral sulcus is a long and deep sulcus that extends along the basal temporal and occipital surface, constituted then by a temporal and by an occipital segment (Duvernoy, 1991), and has multiple side branches (Ono *et al.*, 1990). While its temporal depth bulges along the ventricular floor as the collateral eminence placed laterally to the hippocampus, its occipital depth corresponds to the collateral trigone which constitutes the triangular and flat surface of the atrium and of the posterior horn. The rhinal sulcus, which is not always readily identifiable, is consistently the sulcus that separates the uncus from the rest of the temporal pole.

The subcallosal, cingulate, subparietal, anterior calcarine, collateral, and rhinal sulci are altogether frequently referred to as the limbic fissure (Duvernoy, 1991; Duvernoy, 1998).

The parahippocampal gyrus is then laterally contiguous with the fusiform gyrus underneath the depths of the collateral sulcus. Posteriorly, it is continuous with the lingual gyrus and with the cingulate gyrus along its isthmus. Medially, it lies under the thalamus along the choroidal fissure. Anteriorly, it has its uncal portion superiorly incorporated into the lateral-most aspect of the frontobasal region via a well-defined neural peduncle anterior to the inferior horn of the lateral ventricles. Superiorly, it is attached along the inferior aspect of the insular lobe through fibers that cover the inferior horn.

The structures within the parahippocampal gyrus correspond to the so-called mesial temporal structures, and their upper insertions in the lateral aspect of the cerebral hemisphere, anterior to the inferior horn of the lateral ventricle, and underneath the inferior limiting sulcus of the insula, are frequently referred to as the temporal stem (Horel, 1978; Choi *et al.*, 2010; Kier *et al.*, 2004; Yasargil *et al.*, 2004; Türe *et al.*, 1999; Ebeling *et al.*, 1992a; Wang *et al.*, 2008) and sagittal stratum (Ludwig and Klinger, 1956; Türe *et al.*, 2000).

2.2.3.6.2 The Temporal Stem and the Sagittal Stratum

The term temporal stem is derived from the pictorial appearance of the temporal lobe fibers on coronal sections of the brain, which converge into a stem that is inserted into the temporal lobe medially in the central core of the brain hemisphere along the inferior aspect of the inferior limiting sulcus of the insula (Figure 2.23). It resembles the stem of an inclined tree, and, apparently, this designation was initially employed

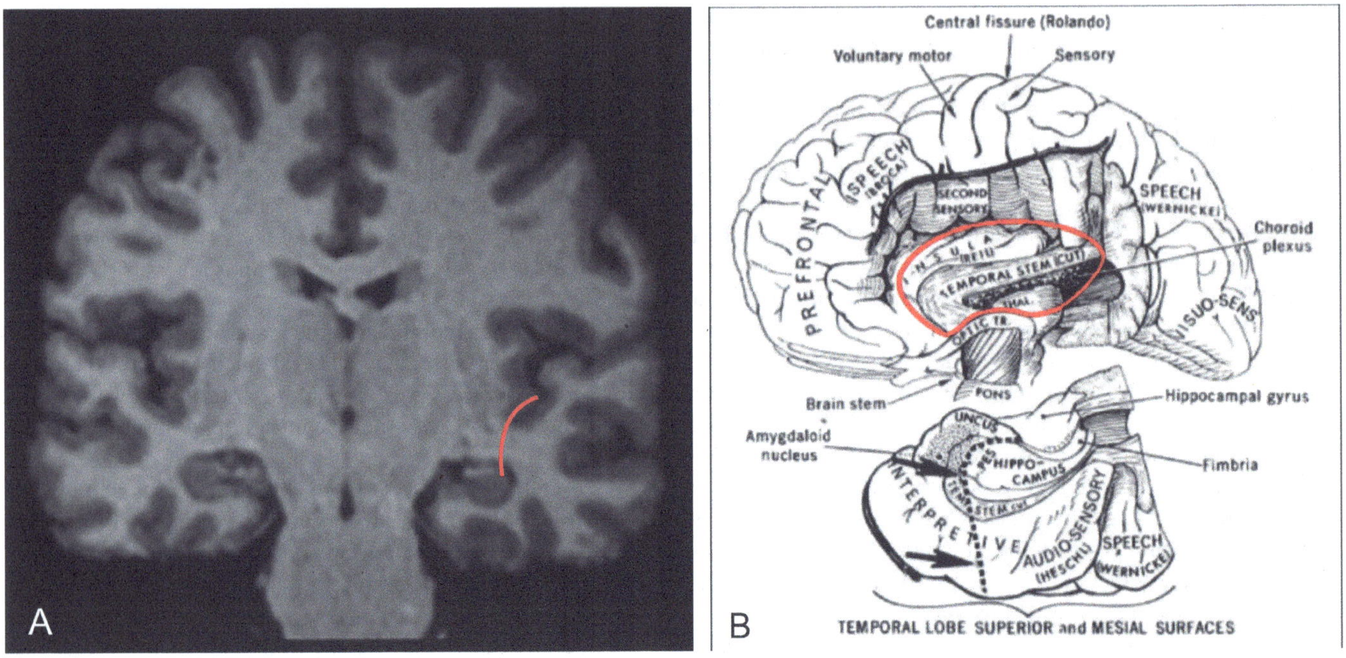

Figure 2.23 (A) Pictorial view of the so-called temporal stem in a coronal MRI view, and (B) conception of the temporal stem by Feindel and Rasmussen (1991).

by Horel (Horel, 1978; Choi *et al.*, 2010; Horel and Misantone, 1974; Horel and Misantone, 1976).

The importance of the temporal stem concept is mainly due to evidence from neuroimaging studies and to its frequent partial severing in temporal lobe microneurosurgery, since this group of fibers also includes optic radiation fibers.

Nevertheless, this heterogeneous contingent of fibers is morphologically constituted by at least two distinct sets of structures partially continuous among each other, which has generated different interpretations regarding its concept.

The most anterior set of fibers which is inserted medially into the temporal lobe corresponds to the upper extension of the posterior aspect of the anterior half of the uncus, which characterizes a true neural peduncle located between the limen insulae and the inferior horn of the lateral ventricle (Figure 2.19B). This peduncle has as its external surface the transverse insular gyrus along the limen insulae connecting the insula to the posteromedial orbital lobule (Yasargil, 1994). It harbors, from anterior to posterior, the anterobasal aspect of the extreme capsule that corresponds to the subcortical insular white matter, the uncinate fasciculus that joins the mesial temporal structures with the fronto-orbital region, the inferior fronto-occipital fasciculus which runs immediately posteriorly to the uncinate fasciculus, the ventral amygdalofugal fibers that comprise the ansa peduncularis, the anterior commissure, and, more medially, the superior extension of the amygdala which extends toward the globus pallidus.

Regarding the amygdalofugal fibers and the further extensions of the amygdala that join this anterior and mesial peduncle, the ansa peduncularis is a well-defined white matter bundle which sweeps around the cerebral peduncle, the reason for its name, and it is composed of the amygdaloseptal, amygdalohypothalamic, and amygdalothalamic fibers (Gloor, 1997; Peuskens *et al.*, 2004).

Immediately posteriorly and superiorly to this amygdalofugal bundle of fibers is the extracapsular thalamic peduncle originating within the amygdala and the cortex of the anterior temporal region, and directed to the medial thalamic nucleus and to the hypothalamus. This tract is known as the extracapsular thalamic peduncle because it runs within the ventral-striato-pallidal region and not through the internal capsule itself (Peuskens *et al.*, 2004; Heimer, 1995). Posteriorly to it there is the ansa lenticularis (Peuskens *et al.*, 2004) connecting the globus pallidus to the thalamus, already within the central core of the cerebral hemisphere.

The amygdala itself extends posteriorly partially covering the head of the hippocampus (Wen *et al.*, 1999), and gives rise to its dorsal extension known as the stria terminalis (Johnston, 1923 apud de Olmos and Heimer, 1999; Heimer, 1995; Heimer, 2003), which runs along the roof of the inferior horn medially to the tail of the caudate nucleus (Párraga *et al.*, 2012) toward the bed nucleus of the stria terminalis. Anteriorly, the tail of the caudate nucleus also merges with the amygdala (Párraga *et al.*, 2012; Choi *et al.*, 2010), still within the roof of the inferior horn. A ventral extension of the centromedial amygdala, which runs along the basal forebrain also toward the bed nucleus of the stria terminalis, has also been described (de Olmos and Heimer, 1999; Heimer, 1995; Heimer, 2003).

Superiorly, the amygdala is continuous with the globus pallidus (Figure 2.24).

Since the amygdala is situated inside the anterior half of the uncus, all these extensions of the amygdala and its overlying fibers, already mentioned, and cortex have to be surgically severed in order to completely disconnect the anterior part of the temporal lobe, which corroborates the inclusion of all these structures within this anterior and medial temporal peduncle.

This anterior insertion of the mesial temporal lobe is posteriorly contiguous with another set of fibers that clearly cover

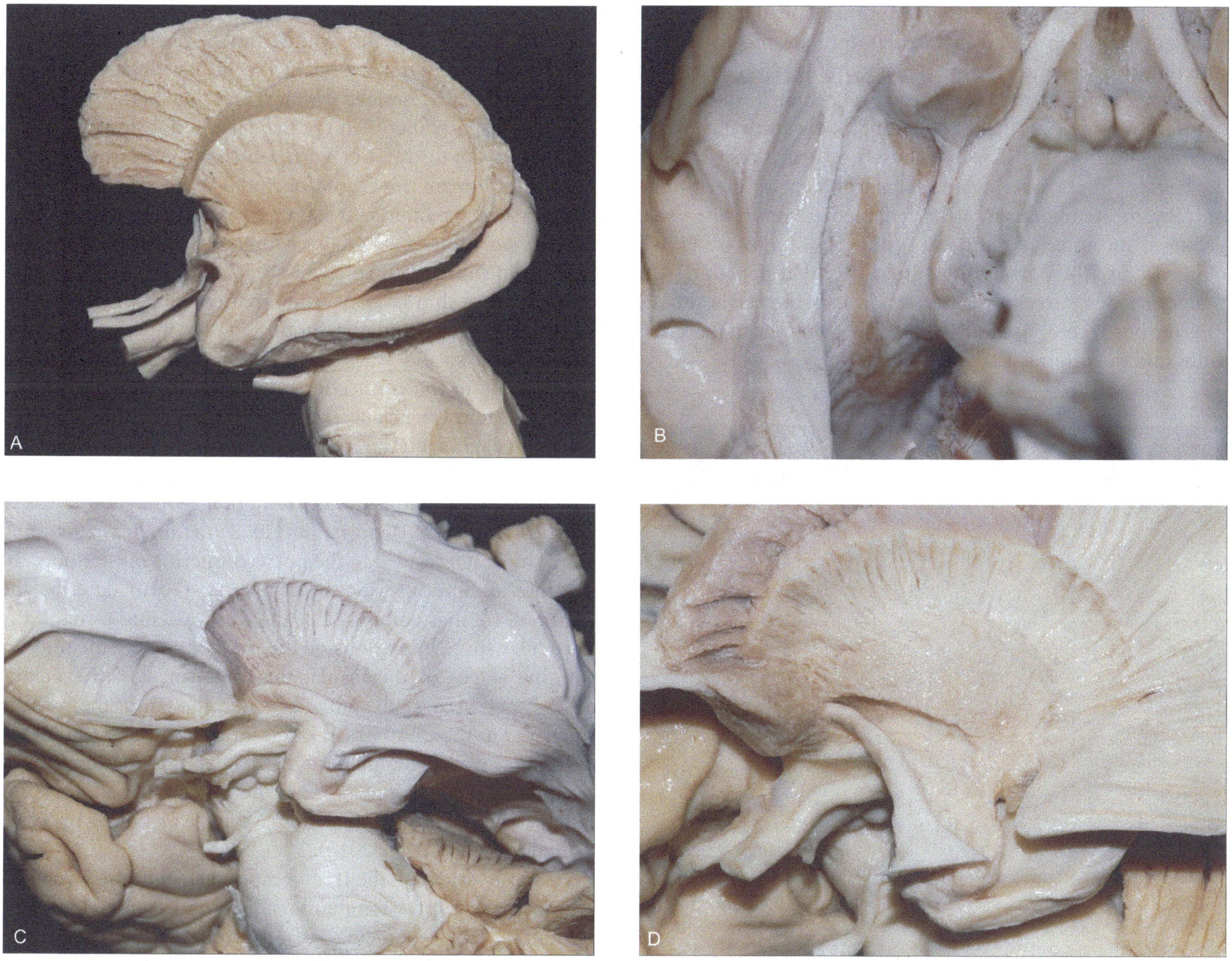

Figure 2.24 The amygdala and its relationships: (A) Lateral view showing that the amygdala is anterior and above the head of the hippocampus where it is contiguous with the tail of caudate; (B) View of the roof of the temporal horn showing the tail of the caudate reaching the amygdala with the stria terminalis running medially; (C) The ansa peduncularis (amygdalofugal fibers) runs inferiorly to the anterior commissure whose fibers laterally join the sagittal stratum; (D) Superiorly the amygdala is continuous with the globus pallidus, as seen after the removal of the anterior commissure from its groove at the base of the globus pallidus (channel of Gratiolet).

the inferior horn and atrium of the lateral ventricle, which are medially disposed along and underneath the inferior limiting sulcus of the insula, and that altogether are known as the sagittal stratum (Ludwig and Klinger, 1956; Türe *et al.*, 2000) (Figure 2.25).

The sagittal stratum lies under the subcortical white matter of the temporal lobe and under the temporal extension of the superior longitudinal fasciculus, and its fibers are organized in layers. From superior to inferior, it comprises the fibers of the inferior fronto-occipital fasciculus which ascend and vanish within the external capsule, the fibers of the anterior commissure which group more anteriorly and medially, the posterior and inferior thalamic peduncles which include the auditory and optic radiations with the visual fibers configuring Mayer's loop anteriorly, and the tapetum (Ludwig and Klinger, 1956; Türe *et al.*, 2000). The layer of splenial callosal fibers known as the tapetum lies under the optic radiation and then constitutes the most inferior layer of the sagittal stratum, being only separated from the ventricular cavity by the ependyma. The tapetum connects both posterior temporal areas (Catani and Schotten, 2012).

Anteriorly, the anterior commissure fibers leave the sagittal stratum and group together to join the anterior and mesial temporal peduncle. The most anterior aspect of Mayer's loop arch reaches the anterior temporal peduncle but does not group with its fibers, staying lateral to it. Any dorsal temporal surgical approach to the inferior horn or to the ventricular atrium will then divide the sagittal stratum, including the optic radiation fibers, to some extent (Figure 2.26).

With reference to the controversial concept of the temporal stem itself, initially authors such as Horel and associates (Horel, 1978; Horel and Misantone, 1974; Horel and Misantone, 1976) and Cirillo *et al.* (1989) described it generically as the combination of connections between the temporal cortex, the amygdala, the orbital cortex, the striatum, and the thalamus (Yasargil *et al.*, 2004; Choi *et al.*, 2011).

The further divergent understandings and definitions of the temporal stem found in the literature are mostly due to different considerations about understanding it as constituted only by the anterior and mesial temporal peduncle, only by the sagittal stratum fibers that lie along and underneath the insular inferior limiting sulcus, or by both sets of structures.

Regarding considering the temporal stem as constituted only by the temporal anterior and medial connections that group as an anterior temporal peduncle, Türe *et al.* (1999) defined it as "the portion of white matter that penetrates the temporal lobe between the anterior border of the insula and the inferior horn, composed of the inferior fronto-occipital fasciculus and the inferior thalamic peduncle."

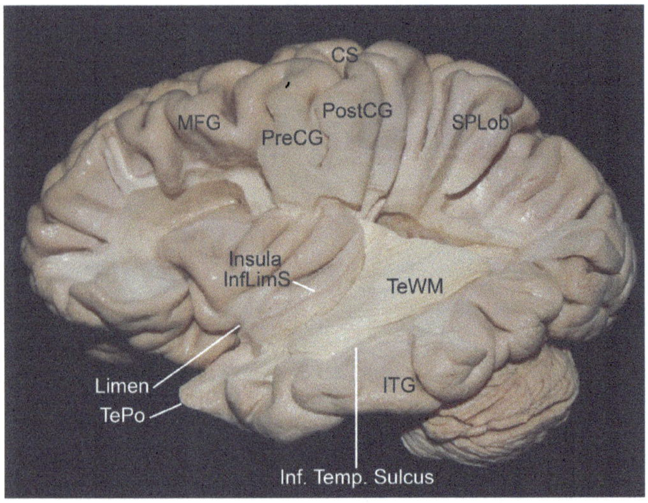

Figure 2.25 The removal of the inferior frontal gyrus, of the basal aspects of the pre- and postcentral gyri, and of the supramarginal, angular, superior, and middle temporal gyri exposes the insula surface and the temporal lobe subcortical white matter.

CS: central sulcus; Inf Temp Sulcus: inferior temporal sulcus; InfLimS: inferior limiting sulcus; ITG: inferior temporal gyrus; MFG: middle frontal gyrus; PostCG: postcentral gyrus; PreCG: precentral gyrus; SPLob: superior parietal lobule; TePo: temporal pole; TeWM: subcortical temporal white matter over sagittal stratum.

Among the authors that consider the temporal stem as constituted only by the white matter fibers anatomically related to the inferior aspect of the insula, Ebeling and von Cramon (1992a) described the temporal stem as the thin group of fibers disposed between the insular inferior limiting sulcus and the roof of the inferior horn, which includes "the uncinate fasciculus, the inferior fronto-occipital fasciculus, the anterior commissure, the inferior thalamic fibers with the Mayer's loop optical radiation fibers." Duvernoy (1998) described it more briefly but similarly, mentioning that "the temporal stem consists of only a thin layer of white matter situated between the ventricular cavity and the fundus of the superior temporal sulcus," and so did Wen *et al.* (1999) stating that the term refers "only to the connections between the mesial temporal structures and the insula, excluding the superior extension of the amygdala in the direction of the globus pallidus and the limen insulae."

Other authors consider the temporal stem as composed of both components. Wang *et al.* (2008) define it as extending from the limen insulae to the postero-inferior insular point of the inferior limiting sulcus. Choi *et al.* (2010) describe the temporal stem as composed of the fibers passing through the particular space located inside the line connecting the inferior limiting sulcus of the insula, the limen insulae, the medial Sylvian groove over the amygdala, and the tail of the caudate nucleus. For these authors, the temporal stem then includes the extreme capsule, the uncinate fasciculus, the inferior fronto-occipital fasciculus, the anterior commissure, the ansa peduncularis, and the inferior thalamic peduncle including the optic radiations (Choi *et al.*, 2010).

Yasargil criticizes the term temporal stem in the sense that "it causes the impression that this is the only connection of the temporal lobe, reducing its multidimensional activities (Yasargil, 2005; Yasargil *et al.*, 2004)." Nevertheless, he considers the term "anterior temporal stem (Cirillo *et al.*, 1989) seemingly correct" but still emphasizing that it should not establish a precedent with regard to its use for other lobar connections (Yasargil *et al.*, 2004), which is in accordance

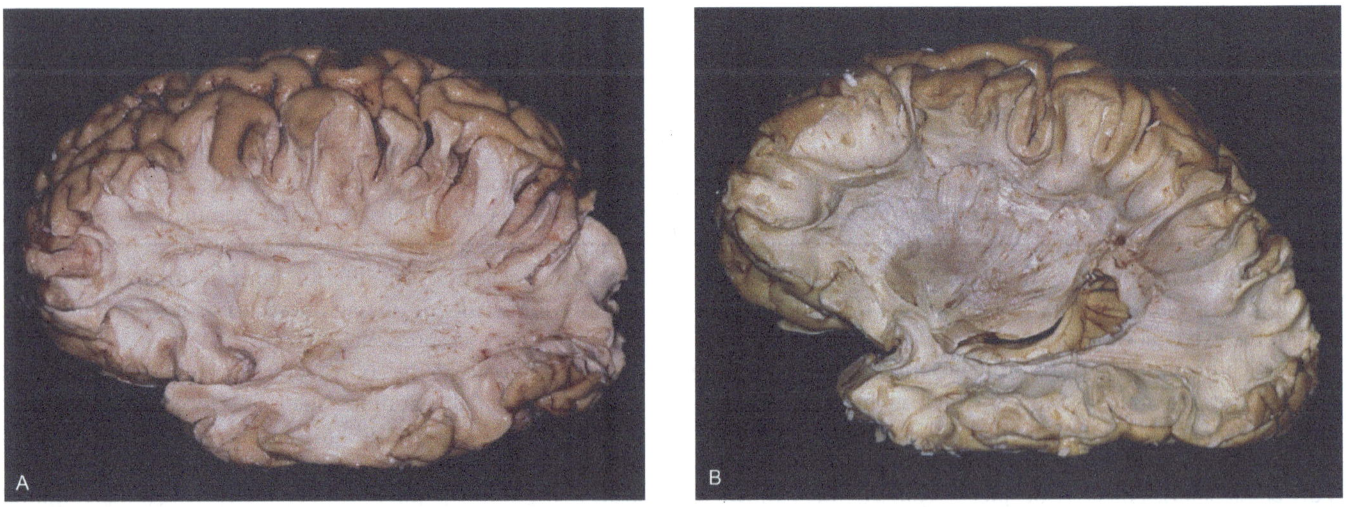

Figure 2.26 Bundles of fibers related to the temporal stem: (A) View of all white matter fibers which run underneath the inferior limiting sulcus of the insula, and (B) View of the anterior and mesial temporal peduncle after the removal of the bundles of fibers that comprise the sagittal stratum. See text for details.

with their previous comment that the temporal stem corresponds to "the portion of white matter that penetrates the temporal lobe between the anterior border of the insula and the inferior horn" (Türe *et al.*, 1999).

The morphological uniqueness of the anterior peduncular part of the medial temporal connection within the whole brain then justifies the distinction of calling this component the temporal stem. The fact that its deeper structures are evolutionarily much older than the further connections of the temporal lobe might explain its peculiar morphology, in contrast to the usual continuity of white matter in all lobes including the temporal lobe with the sagittal stratum itself.

The terms temporal stem and sagittal stratum refer then to two distinct arrangements of fibers at two different topographies, that are, in part, composed of the same bundles since they run along both topographies. While the temporal stem itself is situated anteriorly to the inferior horn connecting the anteromedial temporal structures to the basolateral frontal portion of the hemisphere, the sagittal stratum corresponds to the set of fibers disposed along the inferior limiting sulcus of the insula and that constitute the roof and lateral walls of the inferior horn and of the ventricular atrium.

Some MRI studies report the relationships of the temporal stem structures with social cognition and behavior, and even with the occurrence of autism (Lee *et al.*, 2007; Neeley *et al.*, 2007). Nevertheless, since its fibers intermingle and course in various directions forming a dense 3D network, accurate MRI tractographies are difficult to obtain for proper radiological evaluation (Peltier *et al.*, 2010).

2.2.3.6.3 The Basal Forebrain: the Anterior Perforated Substance, the Ventral-Striato-Pallidal and Septal Regions

The area known as the anterior perforated substance constitutes a particularly important topographical region of the basal forebrain. Macroscopically, this area is delineated anteriorly by the olfactory trigone and the lateral and medial olfactory striae, posteriorly by the edges of the optic tracts, medially by the interhemispheric fissure, and laterally by the uncus of the parahippocampal gyrus and by the limen insulae (Figure 2.22).

Topographically, the anterior perforated substance is situated just above the bifurcation of the internal carotid artery, thus forming the roof of the space that harbors the most distal portion of this artery and the proximal segments of the anterior and middle cerebral arteries. The perforating branches that emerge from those arterial segments constitute the lenticulostriate arteries that penetrate the anterior perforated substance through its multiple orifices, the reason for its name. This aspect is very easily seen in fixed anatomical specimens from which the arachnoid and blood vessels have been removed.

Laterally, the anterior perforated substance continues to the limen insulae, where it extends along the prepiriform cortex (the cortical area that lies lateral to the lateral olfactory stria and that is also occasionally referred to as the lateral olfactory gyrus). More posteriorly, it extends to the periamygdaloid area (the semilunar gyrus, where the lateral olfactory stria terminates and which harbors the cortical amygdaloid nuclei of the amygdaloid complex). The most posterior portion of the anterior perforated substance is traversed by the diagonal band of Broca, a particularly smooth bundle of fibers immediately facing the optic tract, which carry the amygdaloseptal fugal fibers.

Posteriorly, the anterior perforated substance extends along the cell aggregates and fibers that compose the so-called ventral-striato-pallidal region (Heimer, 1995; Heimer, 2003; Heimer *et al.*, 1982; Heimer *et al.*, 2008; Waldron and Lawton, 2009; Chang *et al.*, 2011). This region corresponds roughly to the basal forebrain region situated between the anterior perforated substance and the anterior commissure of each cerebral hemisphere. Superiorly, it is closely related to the most anterobasal portion of the anterior limb of the internal capsule, laterally it is continuous with the peduncle of the temporal stem, and medially it is continuous and particularly related to the septal region and the hypothalamus.

The ventral-striato-pallidal region, previously known as the innominata substance (Heimer, 1995), includes the fundus striati with the nucleus accumbens, which morphologically corresponds to the basal connection of the most anterior and inferior portions of the head of the caudate and the putamen (hence the name ventral striatum). It also includes the ventral part of the globus pallidus, the magnocellular nucleus of the basal forebrain (nucleus basalis of Meynert), and the fibers that constitute the amygdalofugal fibers of the ansa peduncularis together with the ventral extension of the amygdala which are, respectively directed toward the septal region, the hypothalamus, the thalamus, and to the bed nucleus of the stria terminalis located under the head of the caudate nucleus. Posteriorly to the ansa peduncularis lies the ansa lenticularis connecting the globus pallidus and the thalamus (Peuskens *et al.*, 2004).

The ventral-striato-pallidal region is superiorly covered by the anterior limb of the internal capsule (Figure 2.22C), which carries the projections of its structures to the prefrontal and anterior cingulate cortices (Heimer *et al.*, 1982; McGinty, 1999). Posteriorly, it is roughly delimited by the anterior commissure, which passes along a very evident anterior incisure of the globus pallidus, known as the channel of Gratiolet (Peuskens *et al.*, 2004; Déjérine, 1895) (Figure 2.22D). Because of its topography, the ventral-striato-pallidal region is crisscrossed by the perforating lenticulostriate arteries which penetrate the brain through the anterior perforated substance. Functionally, its structures are closely correlated with behavior and with neuropsychiatric dysfunctions (Heimer, 2003; Heimer and Van Hoesen, 2006; Heimer *et al.*, 2008; Ribas, 2007b).

The mediobasal frontal cortical area of each cerebral hemisphere, composed of the small and vertical paraolfactory gyri and the paraterminal gyrus, is also considered to be a limbic cortical area.

The anterior and posterior paraolfactory gyri are located anterior to the paraterminal gyrus, are separated by the anterior paraolfactory sulcus, and their cortical area is also known as the subcallosal area (Duvernoy, 1991). Anterior to the subcallosal area, there is always a fold that connects the basal-most portion of the cingulate gyrus with the gyrus rectus, encircling the posterior end of the superior rostral sulcus, and which is called the cingulate pole (Yasargil, 1994).

The paraterminal gyrus is situated on the medial wall of each cerebral hemisphere posteriorly to the paraolfactory gyri, immediately facing and quasi-continuous with the lamina terminalis, and is delineated anteriorly by a short and vertical sulcus known as the posterior olfactory sulcus. The small anterior curvature of the paraterminal gyrus is called the prehippocampal rudiment and extends superiorly along the previously described indusium griseum. Inferiorly, the paraterminal gyrus extends along the diagonal band of Broca and the lateral olfactory stria.

The paraterminal gyrus harbors the septal nuclei (Williams and Warwick, 1980) and constitutes the septal area, which corresponds to the so-called para-olfactory area of Broca (Lockard, 1977) (Figure 2.22B). This region is also known as the septum verum ("true septum"), or precommissural septum (Brodal, 1981; Heimer, 1995; Williams and Warwick, 1980), in counterpart to the septum pellucidum which does not contain neuronal cells and is situated posterior and above the anterior commissure, morphologically constituting the medial walls of the anterior horns and ventricular bodies. Functionally, the septal nuclei are responsible for connecting limbic structures with the hypothalamus and the brainstem, principally via the hippocampal formation and the medial prosencephalic fasciculus. The so-called septal syndrome is clinically characterized by exaggerated reactions to environmental stimuli and behavioral alterations principally related to eating and drinking habits, as well as by episodes of rage and disorders in the sexual sphere.

Topographically, it is interesting to note that the mediobasal frontal cortical areas (subcallosal area and paraterminal gyrus), the olfactory cortical areas (anterior perforated substance and components of the piriform lobe), and the ventral-striato-pallidal region with its subjacent nuclei and fibers, constitute a corticosubcortical continuum running along the ventral surface of the brain from the medial portion of the temporal lobe to the posterior mediobasal portion of the frontal lobe, underneath the anterior part of the cerebral central core, and with its posterior border being roughly delineated by the anterior commissure.

The ventral-striato-pallidal, or anterior perforated substance region, is then laterally continuous with the peduncle of the temporal stem and with the amygdaloid complex, and medially is continuous with the septal region.

Since these basal structures extend along the medial cerebral surface via the cingulate gyrus, and along the basal surface via the parahippocampal gyrus, with these two gyri being posteriorly continuous, the limbic lobe together with the basal forebrain of each hemisphere look like a slightly tilted circle, with its superior portion medial and its inferior portion lateral, encircling the diencephalic structures.

In parallel with these observations, Mesulam (1987) proposed that, because of their predominantly superficial presentation, the most medial portions of the amygdaloid complex, the substantia innominata (which corresponds to the ventral-striato-pallidal region), and the septal nuclei (within the paraterminal gyri), should be considered constituents of the cerebral mantle.

Table 2.6 Main limbic system structures

Main limbic system structures
Amygdala
Cingulate gyrus
Parahippocampal gyrus
Hippocampal formation
Hippocampus (Ammon's horn)
Subicular complex
Dentate gyrus
Entorhinal cortex
Prehippocampal rudiment/indusium griseum, gyrus fasciolaris
Frontal mediobasal cortical area
Paraterminal gyrus
Paraolfactory gyri or subcallosal area
Olfactory cortical areas

2.2.3.6.4 The Limbic System

Parallel to the strict concept of a limbic lobe (Federative Committee on Anatomical Terminology, 1998) which includes basically the cingulate and the parahippocampal gyri, the concept of the limbic system as a functional unit also involves the participation of deep structures and is controversial in terms of its conception and composition (Heimer, 1995; Heimer, 2003; Heimer and Van Hoesen, 2006).

The limbic system, in its entirety, is composed of cortical, subcortical, and nuclear structures that are interconnected and have connections with other areas of the CNS via a complex network of tracts. However, the main elements of the limbic system are the hippocampal formation and the amygdala, which participate in distinct circuits with the rest of the brain. The hippocampal formation is principally related to telencephalic and diencephalic structures via circuits whose basic purpose is to convert short-term memory into long-term memory, whereas the circuits that include the amygdala are more strictly related to the emotions and ultimately influence the effector systems (autonomic, neuroendocrine, and motor), primarily via the hypothalamus (Table 2.6).

The generic term olfactory cortical areas refers to the olfactory nerves, bulb, tract, trigone, lateral, and medial striae, as well as the anterior perforated substance, the diagonal band of Broca, and the piriform lobe, in each cerebral hemisphere. The piriform lobe comprises: 1) the prepiriform cortical area; 2) the lateral olfactory stria which extends to the gyrus semilunaris; 3) the uncus of the parahippocampal gyrus and its small gyri (uncinate gyrus, caudal portion of the dentate gyrus or band of Giacomini, and intralimbic gyrus); and 4) the entorhinal area.

From a functional point of view, one of the basic principles of the concept of the limbic system is that its structures project to the hypothalamus and not to the basal ganglia as occurs with the remainder of the cerebral cortex (Heimer, 1995, 2003; Heimer *et al.*, 2008).

However, since it has been shown that the portion most anterior and basal to the striatum (nucleus accumbens and striatal areas of the olfactory tubercle) receives projections not only from the olfactory cortex, hippocampus, entorhinal cortices, cingulate gyrus, and temporal pole, but also from the orbitomedial and insular cortices, and that the nucleus accumbens projects to the anterior-most portions of the globus pallidus, which in turn gives rise to anterior thalamocortical projections, Heimer and colleagues (Heimer and Van Hoesen, 2006; Heimer *et al.*, 1982) proposed to include within the concept of the "greater limbic lobe" the posterior regions of the orbital cortex and the insula.

These findings led to the conclusion that the ventral corticostriatopallidal system works distinctly from the classic dorsal corticostriatopallidal system which is related to motor activities, and that this ventral system is particularly related to neuropsychiatric abnormalities (Heimer, 2003; Heimer and Van Hoesen, 2006; Heimer *et al.*, 2008; Mello and Villares, 1997). While the dorsal system is related to neocortical connections (neocortex–dorsal striatum–dorsal pallidum–ventrolateral thalamic nuclei–motor cortex), the ventral system is related to allocortical and mesocortical connections (greater limbic lobe–ventral striatum–ventral pallidum–dorsomedial thalamic nuclei–prefrontal cortex/cortex of the anterior part of the cingulate gyrus) (Heimer, 1995).

From a morphological perspective, the structures that make up the limbic system present as a series of C-shaped curves centered around the thalamus and hypothalamus in each cerebral hemisphere. Nieuwenhuys *et al.* (1988) outlines five main circular circuits (medial to lateral): 1) stria medullaris thalami, habenular nuclei, and habenulointerpeduncular tract; 2) amygdala, posterior extension of the amygdala (stria terminalis), and anterior extension of the amygdala which also project to the bed nucleus of the stria terminalis, and that together constitute the so-called extended amygdala (de Olmos, 1972 apud Heimer, 2003; de Olmos and Heimer, 1999); 3) fimbria, crura, body, and column of fornix, which connect the hippocampus to the mammillary body; 4) hippocampus and indusium griseum, which connect the hippocampus with the paraterminal gyrus; and 5) cingulate gyrus and parahippocampal gyrus.

The amygdala (amygdaloid nuclear complex) consists of lateral, centromedial, and basal nuclei which are located mainly within the anterior half of the uncus, underneath the gyrus semilunaris, gyrus ambiens, and uncinate gyrus which lie along the medial aspect of the uncal surface. The amygdala is then mostly anterior to the head of the hippocampus comprising the anterior wall of the temporal horn, but it also extends posteriorly covering the head of the hippocampus close to the most anterior aspect of the tail of the caudate nucleus within the roof of the temporal horn. Superiorly, the amygdala is practically continuous with the globus pallidus (Figure 2.24).

Among its heterogeneous structure containing many different cell groups, a distinction can be made between a cortical or olfactory amygdala (related to olfactory structures), a basolateral amygdala (more closely related to many cortical areas), and a larger centromedial amygdala (more related to behavior and emotions).

In 1923, Johnston (Johnston, 1923 apud de Olmos and Heimer, 1999) described the stria terminalis as a dorsal extension of the centromedial portion of the amygdala, which dorsally wraps the thalamus ending in the bed nucleus of the stria terminalis close to the base of the head of the caudate nucleus, and in 1972, de Olmos (de Olmos, 1972 apud Heimer, 2003; de Olmos and Heimer, 1999) described its ventral extension, which runs underneath the lenticulate within the ventral-striato-pallidal or substantia innominata region and which also ends within the bed nucleus of the stria terminalis (Heimer, 2003; Heimer, 1995; de Olmos, 1972 apud Heimer, 2003; de Olmos and Heimer, 1999; Mc Ginty, 1999). Given its continuous circular extensions composed of fibers and cell columns, de Olmos and Heimer (1999) proposed the concept of extended amygdala for its centromedial part (Heimer, 1995; Heimer and Van Hoesen, 2006; de Olmos and Heimer, 1999).

The organization of the extensive subcortical and cortical connections of the amygdala is consistent with a role in emotional behavior. It receives highly processed unimodal and multimodal sensory information from the thalamus, sensory, and association cortices, olfactory information from the olfactory bulb and piriform cortex, and visceral and gustatory information relayed via brainstem structures and the thalamus. Its projections are widely distributed throughout the brain, including the endocrine and the autonomic domains of the hypothalamus and brainstem (Williams and Warwick, 1980).

2.2.4 The White Matter of the Cerebral Hemispheres

The white matter bulk of the cerebral hemispheres is composed of myelinated bundles of fibers, denominated fiber tracts or fasciculi, and they are categorized on the basis of their course and connections, as classically proposed by Theodor Meynert (1833–1891) in 1872 (Meynert, 1872 apud Türe *et al.*, 2000): association fibers, which link different cortical areas in the same hemisphere; commissural fibers, which link corresponding cortical areas of the two hemispheres; and projection fibers, which connect the cerebral cortex with the corpus striatum, diencephalon, brainstem, and the spinal cord.

The main fasciculi are described separately below, and some of them are also discussed within other related items (see also Section 2.2.3.5.2: The Insula and the Cerebral Central Core; Section 2.2.3.6.2: The Temporal Stem and the Sagittal Stratum; and Section 2.2.3.6.3: The Basal Forebrain).

2.2.4.1 Association Fibers

Association fibers may be either short association (arcuate or "U") fibers which connect adjacent gyri, or long association fibers which connect more widely separated gyri within the same hemisphere and which are grouped into bundles: cingulum, superior longitudinal fasciculus, inferior longitudinal fasciculus, uncinate fasciculus, and inferior fronto-occipital fasciculus.

2.2.4.2 Superior Longitudinal Fasciculus

The superior longitudinal fasciculus was initially identified by Reil in 1809 and by Aurenrieth in 1812 (Martino and Brogna, 2011) as a group of fibers disposed around the Sylvian fissure, and was more properly described by Burdach in 1819 (Burdach, 1819–1822–1826 apud Catani and Schotten, 2012; Burdach, 1844 apud Türe *et al.*, 2000) and later by Déjérine in 1895(Déjérine, 1895; Martino and Brogna, 2011).

Nevertheless, recent anatomical and neuroimaging studies (Catani *et al.*, 2005; Fernández-Miranda *et al.*, 2008; Martino and Brogna, 2011) have shown that the superior longitudinal fasciculus is indeed a complex association system composed of different subsets of fibers, with the arcuate fasciculus being one of them. Currently it is considered to be composed of three portions: a fronto-parietal or horizontal segment, a temporo-parietal or vertical segment, and a temporo-frontal segment or arcuate fasciculus (Figures 2.27, 2.28, 2.32, 2.33).

The fronto-parietal or horizontal segment runs deeply underneath the fronto-parietal operculum connecting the posterior aspect of the inferior frontal gyrus (Broca's area) with the inferior parietal lobule (supramarginal and angular gyri). More recent studies (Makris *et al.*, 2005; Martino and Brogna, 2011) suggest that this fronto-parietal portion of the superior longitudinal fasciculus (SLF) is actually composed of three dorsal to ventral components: SLF I, which connects the superior parietal lobule and the precuneus with the premotor and

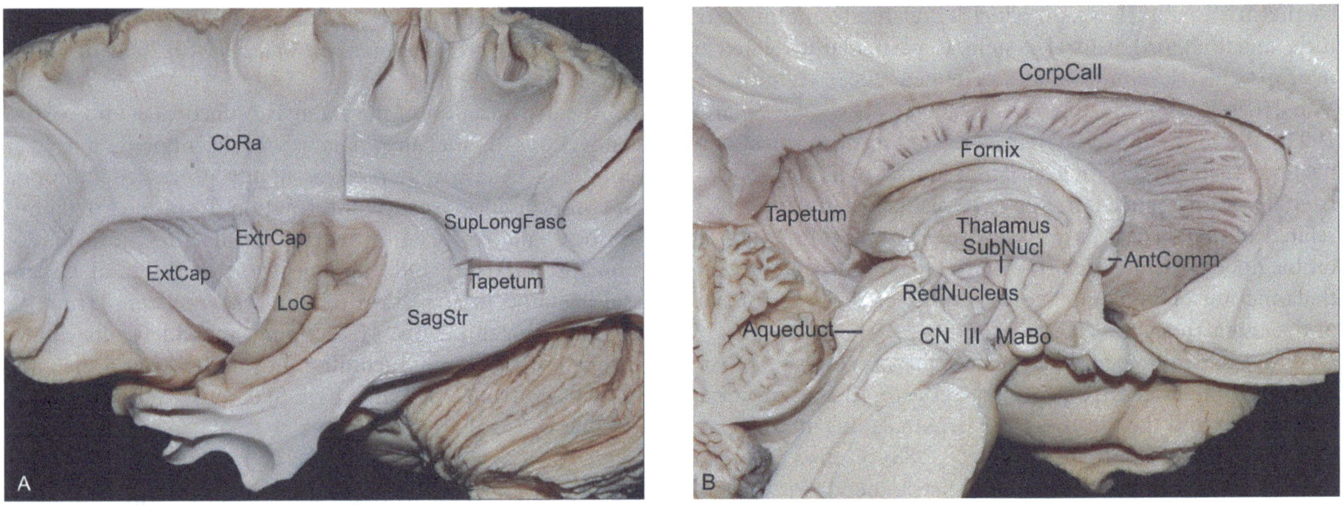

Figure 2.27 Cerebral white matter layers.
(A) Lateral view of the left hemisphere: the vertical segment of the superior longitudinal fasciculus (SupLongFasc) was removed, and a window was made in the sagittal stratum (SagStr) to expose the tapetum.
(B) Medial view of the left hemisphere: the ependyma of the lateral ventricle was removed, to show that the tapetum lies underneath the optic radiation along the lateral wall of the atrium.
CoRa: corona radiata; ExtCap: external capsule; ExtrCap: extreme capsule; LoG: long gyri of insula. AntComm: anterior commissure; CN III: cranial nerve III; CorpCall: corpus callosum; MaBo: mammillary body; SubNucl: subthalamic nucleus. (Adapted from Párraga *et al.* (2012).)

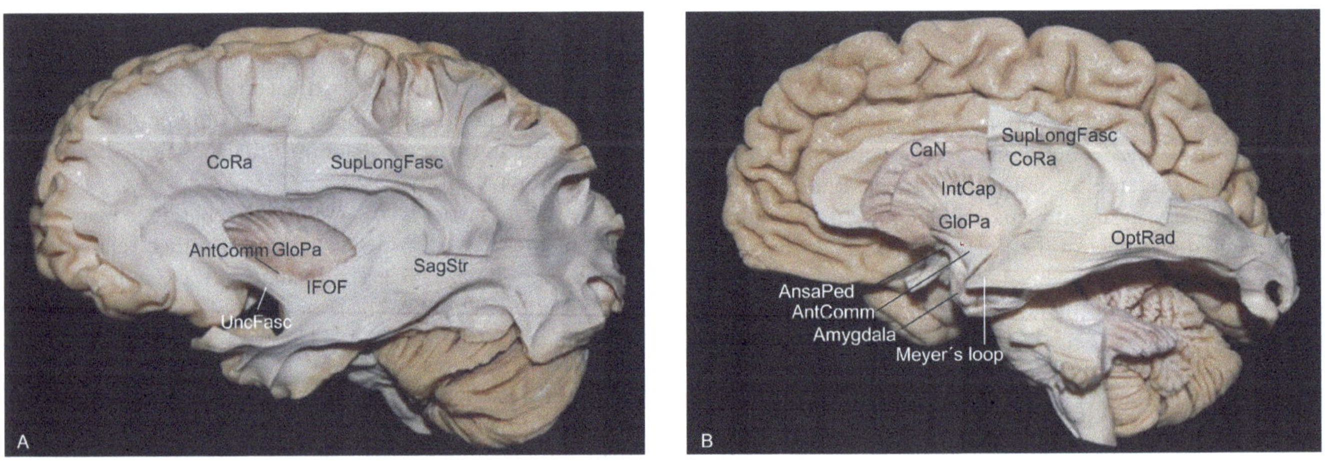

Figure 2.28 Progressive fiber dissection of lateral aspect of the left cerebral hemisphere:
(A) Parts of the superior longitudinal fasciculus (SupLongFasc) were removed to expose the corona radiata. The sagittal stratum (SagStr), inferior fronto-occipital fascicle (IFOF), and uncinate fasciculus (UncFasc) can be identified passing along the basal portion of the insular cortex.
(B) The removal of the uncinate fasciculus allows better exposure of the anterior commissure (AntComm), and the removal of the lateral fibers of the anterior commissure exposes the optic radiation fibers (OptRad).
AntComm: anterior commissure; CoRa: corona radiata; GloPa: globus pallidus; IFOF: inferior fronto-occipital fascicle; SagStr: sagittal stratum; SupLongFasc: superior longitudinal fasciculus; UncFasc: uncinate fasciculus. AnsaPed: Ansa peduncularis; AntComm: anterior commissure; CaN: caudate nucleus; CoRa: corona radiata; GloPa: globus pallidus; IntCap: internal capsule fibers; OptRad: optic radiation fibers; SupLongFasc: superior longitudinal fasciculus. (Adapted from Párraga *et al.* (2012).)

prefrontal cortex (areas 6, 8, and 9, and the supplementary motor area), SLF II, which runs above the superior limiting sulcus of the insula connecting the angular gyrus also with the dorsal premotor and prefrontal areas, and SLF III, which connects the supramarginal gyrus with the ventral premotor and prefrontal cortex (Broca's area) and which corresponds to the horizontal segment itself.

The temporal-parietal or vertical segment of the superior longitudinal fasciculus connects the posterior portions of the superior and middle temporal gyri (Wernicke's area) with the inferior parietal lobule (Catani *et al.*, 2005; Fernández-Miranda *et al.*, 2008; Martino and Brogna, 2011).

The temporal-frontal segment connects more diffuse areas of the posterior aspect of the temporal lobe with the posterior aspect of the frontal lobe, and corresponds to the arcuate fasciculus. This longer portion of the superior longitudinal fasciculus is anatomically more defined posteriorly where it arches around the distal aspect of the Sylvian fissure, and it runs parallel but medially to the vertical and horizontal segments, hence deeper within the fronto-parietal operculum (Bernal and Altman, 2010; Bernal and Ardila, 2009; Glasser and Rilling, 2008; Martino and Brogna, 2011).

The superior longitudinal fasciculus is then composed of an indirect pathway that links the Broca area with Wernicke's area through the inferior parietal lobule along its horizontal and vertical segments, and by a direct and deeper pathway which corresponds to the arcuate fasciculus, with both of them being related more particularly with language functions.

2.2.4.3 Inferior Fronto-Occipital Fasciculus

The inferior fronto-occipital fascicle was originally described by Curran in 1909 (Curran, 1909 apud Catani and Schotten, 2012), and is an associative bundle that runs mostly along the temporal lobe connecting the dorsolateral aspects of the frontal and occipital lobes (Figures 2.28, 2.32).

Anteriorly, the inferior fronto-occipital fasciculus is intermingled with other association fasciculi and with the most anterior fibers of the external capsule, and its frontal terminations are more particularly related to the dorsolateral prefrontal and orbitofrontal cortices (Catani and Thiebaut de Schotten, 2008; Catani *et al.*, 2002; Martino and Brogna, 2011; Forkel *et al.*, 2014). The claustrum, which is disposed above the external capsule, is particularly thinner anteriorly and approximates the fibers of the inferior fronto-occipital fasciculus, the extreme capsule, and the anterior aspect of the insular cortex. The external capsule itself is constituted mainly by claustrocortical fibers (Martino and Brogna, 2011) (see Section 2.2.3.5.2: The Insula and the Cerebral Central Core).

Inferiorly, the fibers of the inferior fronto-occipital fascicle converge crossing the anteroinferior portion of the external capsule and claustrum to join the temporal stem, underneath the anterior aspect of the inferior limiting sulcus of the insula and just behind the limen insulae and the uncinate fasciculus. While the uncinate fasciculus corresponds to the anterior one-third of the temporal stem, the inferior fronto-occipital fascicle corresponds to its posterior two-thirds reaching the level of the lateral geniculate body underneath the inferior limiting sulcus (Martino *et al.*, 2010).

Within the temporal lobe, the inferior fronto-occipital fasciculus joins the sagittal stratum covering the temporal horn and the atrium superiorly and laterally, running just superiorly to the optic radiation fibers (Türe *et al.*, 2000) (see Section 2.2.3.6.2: The Temporal Stem and the Sagittal Stratum) and inferiorly to the auditory radiation fibers (Martino *et al.*, 2010; Martino and Brogna, 2011).

According to the findings of studies based on subcortical brain mapping by electrical stimulation during awake neurosurgery, while the superior longitudinal fasciculus is more particularly related to phonological aspects of language, the inferior fronto-occipital fasciculus is more related to its semantic aspect (Duffau, 2011a).

2.2.4.4 Uncinate Fasciculus

The uncinate fasciculus is a hook-shaped associative bundle which connects the anteromedial temporal lobe (superior, middle, and inferior temporal gyri, cortical nuclei of amygdala) with the orbitofrontal region (medial and posterior orbital cortex, gyrus rectus, and subcallosal area) (Ebeling *et al.*, 1992a). Its fibers constitute a well-defined tract along the temporal stem, where it occupies its anterior one-third immediately posterior to the limen insulae and anterior to the inferior fronto-occipital fasciculus, underneath the most anterior aspect of the inferior limiting sulcus of the insula. Both the uncinate and the inferior fronto-occipital fasciculi intermingle with the most ventral fibers of the extreme and external capsules (Fernández-Miranda *et al.*, 2008; Ebeling *et al.*, 1992a).

2.2.4.5 Inferior Longitudinal Fasciculus

The inferior longitudinal fasciculus connects the anterior aspect of the temporal lobe with the posterior aspect of the occipital lobe along the cerebral basal aspect, reaching the cuneus, the lingual gyrus, and the convex surface of the occipital pole (Catani *et al.*, 2003; Martino and Brogna, 2011; Standring, 2008; Carpenter, 1991). It runs predominantly along and within the depth of the fusiform gyrus.

2.2.4.6 Cingulum

The cingulum lies within the depth of the cingulate and parahippocampal gyri. It starts below the rostrum of the corpus callosum within the paraolfactory gyri (paraolfactory area of Broca), and along its curved course, it receives fibers from the anterior thalamic nuclei, superior frontal gyrus, paracentral lobule, and precuneus which enlarge it significantly. It ends within the presubiculum and entorhinal cortex of the parahippocampal gyrus (Carpenter and Sutin, 1983; Martino and Brogna, 2011) (Figure 2.29).

2.2.5 Commissural Fibers

Commissural fibers cross the midline connecting corresponding areas in the two cerebral hemispheres: the corpus callosum, the anterior commissure, the hippocampal commissure, the posterior commissure, and the habenular commissure.

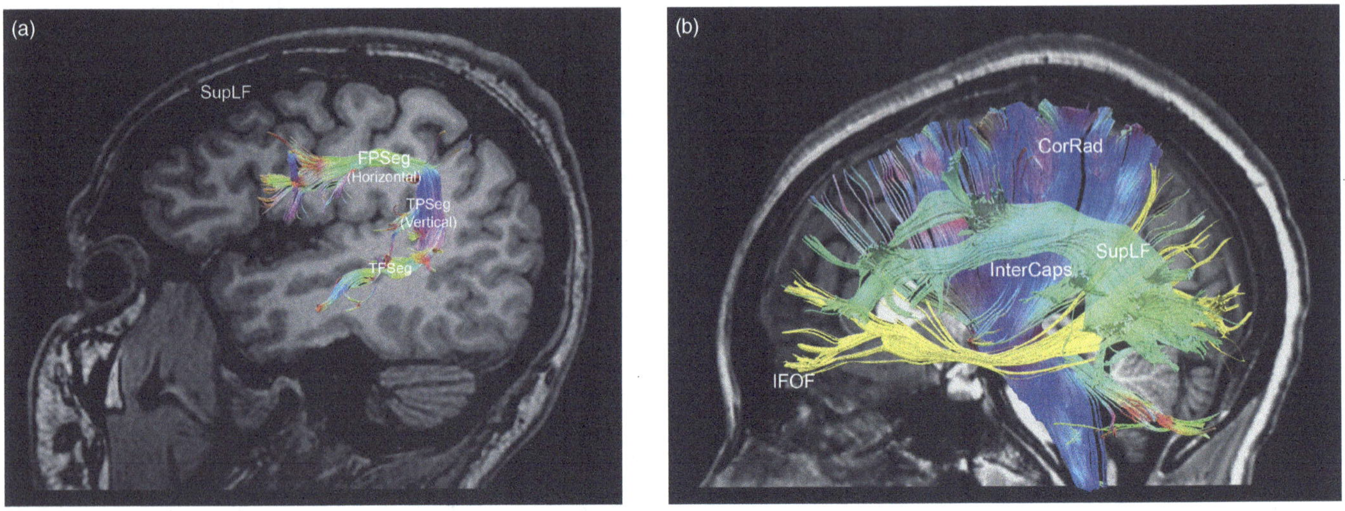

Figure 2.29 Diffuse tensor imaging (DTI): (A) of the superior longitudinal fascicle (SupLF), with its fronto-parietal or horizontal segment (FPSeg), temporo-parietal or vertical segment (TPSeg), and temporal-frontal segment (TFSeg), and (B) of the corona radiata (CorRad) which is continuous with the internal capsule (InterCaps), superior longitudinal fascicle (SupLF), and inferior fronto-occipital fascicle (IFOF). (Courtesy of E. Amaro, Department of Radiology, University of São Paulo Medical School.)

2.2.5.1 Corpus Callosum

The corpus callosum contains about 150 to 200 million fibers (Forkel *et al.*, 2014; Heimer, 1995) and constitutes the largest fiber pathway in the brain. The corpus callosum is compact and anatomically very well defined along the midline where it forms an arch approximately 10 cm long, classically divided into four portions: rostrum, genu, trunk, and splenium, and from where its fibers open widely to link the corresponding areas of the cerebral cortex in both hemispheres (Figure 2.30 A and B).

The genu is the most anterior portion of the corpus callosum, and is located approximately 4 cm from the frontal poles. The genu recurves posteroinferiorly in front of the septum pellucidum decreasing in thickness and extends to the upper end of the lamina terminalis as the rostrum (Williams and Warwick, 1980). While the genu corresponds to the anterior wall of the frontal horn of the lateral ventricle, the rostrum corresponds to its floor.

Posteriorly to the genu, the trunk of the corpus callosum arches back and is convex above, and ends posteriorly in the expanded splenium, which is the thickest part of the corpus callosum and is located approximately 6 cm from the occipital poles.

Superiorly, the median region of the trunk of the corpus callosum forms the floor of the great longitudinal fissure (interhemispheric fissure), supporting the anterior cerebral arteries and lying underneath the lower border of the falx cerebri, which may contact it behind. On each side, the trunk is overlapped by the cingulate gyrus, from which it is separated by the callosal sulcus.

The inferior surface of the corpus callosum is concave in its long axis, and is attached to the septum pellucidum along the trunk, genu, and rostrum, and fused with the crura of the fornix and with its commissure underneath the splenium. While the inferior surface of the trunk corresponds to the roof of both frontal horns and ventricular bodies, with the septum pellucidum as their medial walls, the inferior surface of the splenium overhangs the posterior part of the pulvinars of each thalamus and already covers the pineal region.

Since both layers of the septum pellucidum correspond to adjacent midline structures which are superiorly attached to the callosal trunk, anteriorly to the genu, and inferiorly to the rostrum anteriorly and to the bodies of the fornices posteriorly, both septum pellucidum layers correspond to the medial walls of the frontal horns and the walls of the lateral ventricular bodies. At the level where the bodies of the fornices turn into their crura which become attached to the inferior surface of the splenium, both layers of the septum pellucidum end establishing the anatomical limit between the lateral ventricular body and the atrium within each hemisphere (Rhoton, 2003; Timurkaynak *et al.*, 1986). While the frontal horns and ventricular bodies are located along the midline, the atria are already lateral cavities located posterior to both thalami and hence not related to the midline.

The superior surface is covered along each side by a thin layer of gray matter named the indusium griseum and which contains the medial and longitudinal striae. While anteriorly the indusium griseum extends into the paraterminal gyrus below the rostrum, posteriorly it is continuous with the dentate gyrus and hippocampus through the gyrus fasciolaris around the splenium.

A superior and an inferior layer of the tela choroidea advances below the splenium through the transverse fissure forming the velum interpositum cistern within the roof of the third ventricle and between both thalami, containing the distal branches of the medial posterior choroidal arteries and the internal cerebral veins, just below both bodies of the fornices (Yamamoto *et al.*, 1981; Wen *et al.*, 1988).

Both internal cerebral veins join together distally giving rise to the great cerebral vein of Galen, which runs upwards around the posterior aspect of the splenium toward the straight sinus placed along the falx-tentorium junction.

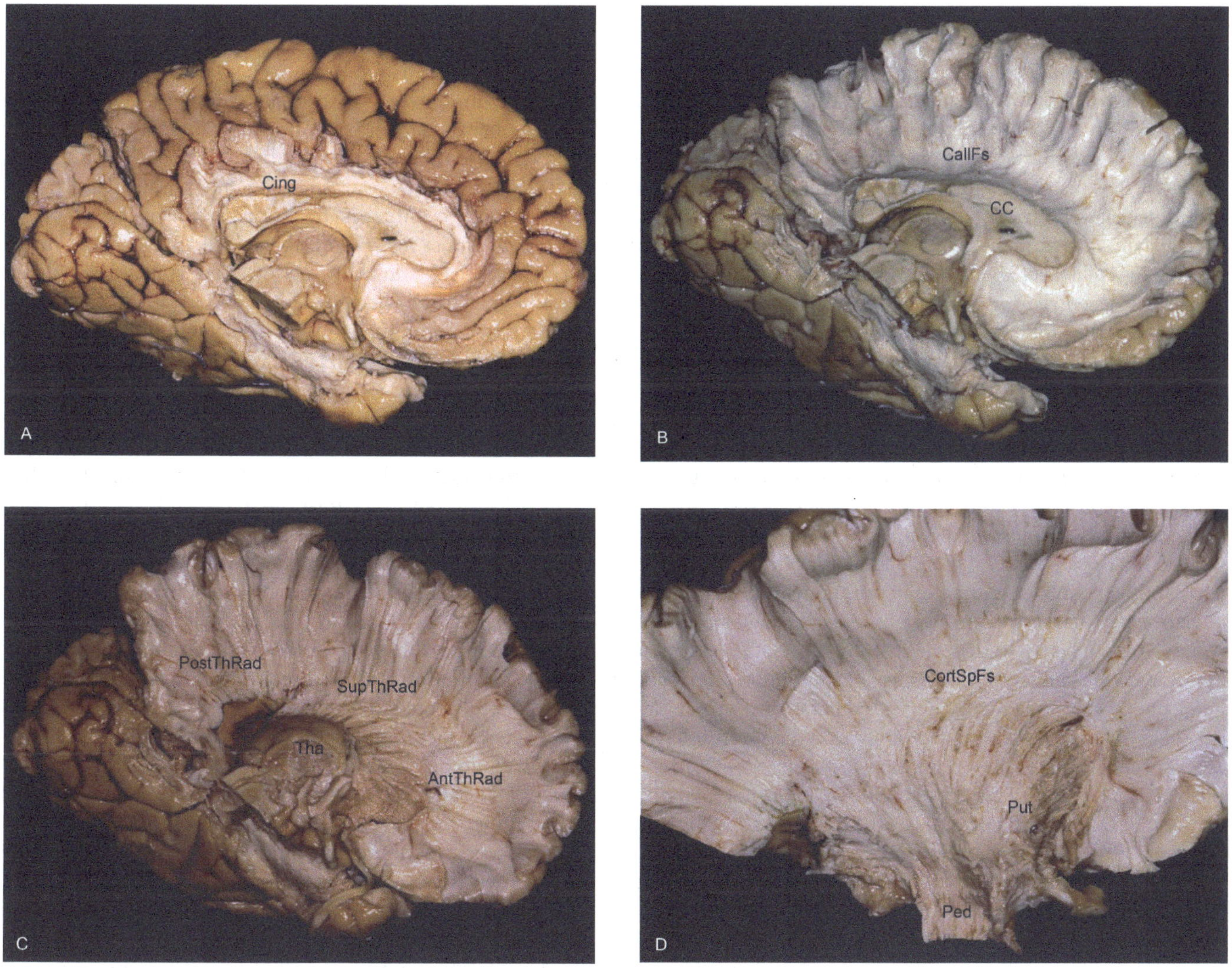

Figure 2.30 Progressive fiber dissections from the medial surface of the cerebral hemisphere disclosing (A) the cingulum within the cingulate and the parahippocampal gyri, (B) the callosal fibers, (C) the thalamus and the thalamic radiations, and (D) the corticospinal fibers within the most lateral aspect of the internal capsule, medially to the putamen.

AntThRad: anterior thalamic radiation; CallFs: callosal fibers; CC: corpus callosum; Cing: cingulum; CortSpFs: corticospinal fibers; Ped: cerebral peduncle; PostThRad: posterior thalamic radiation; Put: putamen; SupThRad: superior thalamic radiation (inferior thalamic radiation not shown); Tha: thalamus.

Callosal fibers of the rostrum connect the orbital surfaces of the frontal lobes, fibers of the genu constitute the forceps minor and connect the lateral and medial surfaces of the frontal lobes, and fibers of the trunk pass laterally, intersecting with the projection fibers of the corona radiata, and connect corresponding areas of the cerebral hemispheres. Fibers of the trunk and of the splenium, which form the roof and lateral wall of the atrium and the lateral wall of the inferior horn, constitute the tapetum which runs underneath the optic radiation fibers within the sagittal stratum (Ludwig and Klinger, 1956; Türe *et al.*, 2000). The remaining posterior fibers of the splenium curve back into the occipital lobes as the forceps major (Williams and Warwick, 1980).

It is interesting that cortical areas related to a clear representation of a contralateral sensorium have only their midline representation connected by callosal fibers. While the trunk representation is linked, the peripheral limb areas are not, and the same applies to the visual areas where only the cortices containing the representation of both midline retinal zones are linked (Williams and Warwick, 1980).

2.2.5.2 Anterior Commissure

The anterior commissure is a compact bundle of myelinated fibers which runs within the basal forebrain and which laterally fans out within both temporal lobes, predominantly connecting the medial temporal, olfactory, and anterior perforated substance structures in both hemispheres (Standring, 2008), which are not interconnected by the corpus callosum.

It has an average diameter of 4 mm (Peltier *et al.*, 2011) and it harbors about 3.5 million fibers, but with an overall axon density 2.4 times that of the corpus callosum which has about 200 million fibers (Foxman *et al.*, 1986 apud Peltier *et al.*, 2011). The optic nerve, which has a similar diameter, harbors 1.2 million fibers (Williams and Warwick, 1980).

The anterior commissure has the shape of a bicycle handlebar, and crosses the midline just ventral to the supraoptic recess of the third ventricle, immediately anteriorly to the major components of the columns of the fornices that project onto the mammillary bodies, and posteriorly to the smaller components of both fornices that project onto the septal nuclei located within the paraterminal gyri (Williams and Warwick, 1980). At this point, the anterior commissure bulges inside the third ventricle, within the upper aspect of this anterior wall and just underneath both interventricular foramina (of Monro).

The lamina terminalis, which is a thin sheet of gray matter covered by a pial layer and that corresponds to the anterior wall of the third ventricle, is attached superiorly to the midline segment of the anterior commissure and inferiorly to the upper surface of the optic chiasm. The cleft between the lamina terminalis and the midportion of the superior surface of the chiasm constitutes the optic recess of the third ventricle. Since the lamina terminalis embryologically corresponds to the upper closure site of the neural tube (the reason for its name), it is considered to be a telencephalic structure.

Each side of the anterior commissure is composed of a very well-defined posterolateral bundle known as the hemispheric part, and by a smaller and anterior component known as the olfactory part (Déjérine, 1895). While each smaller anterior component curves forward and vertically through the anterior perforated substance toward each olfactory tubercle, each hemispheric component curves posterolaterally with a handlebar shape, passing through a deep groove on the anteroinferior aspect of the globus pallidus known as the channel of Gratiolet (Debierre, 1907 apud Peltier *et al.*, 2011; De Ribet, 1957 apud Peltier *et al.*, 2011) (Figure 2.24C, 2.24D), and subsequently fans out mostly into the anterior part of the temporal lobe, including the parahippocampal gyrus (Standring, 2008), but also reaching the occipital lobe posteriorly (Déjérine, 1895) (Figure 2.31).

When passing underneath the inferior limiting sulcus of the insula superiorly to the temporal horn of the lateral ventricle, the fibers of the anterior commissure anteriorly join the temporal stem merging with the fibers of the uncinate and of the inferior fronto-occipital fascicle. They then proceed posteriorly more widely spaced constituting the sagittal stratum together with the inferior fronto-occipital fascicle and the optic radiation fibers (Ludwig and Klinger, 1956; Türe *et al.*, 2000) over the lateral aspect of the temporal horn and ventricular atrium. Within the temporal stem, the fibers of the anterior commissure are mostly medial to the fibers of the uncinate fascicle, and both sets of fibers run inferior to the fibers of the fronto-occipital fasciculus. Within the sagittal stratum, they intermingle but run predominantly underneath the inferior fronto-occipital fascicle and superiorly to the optic radiation fibers.

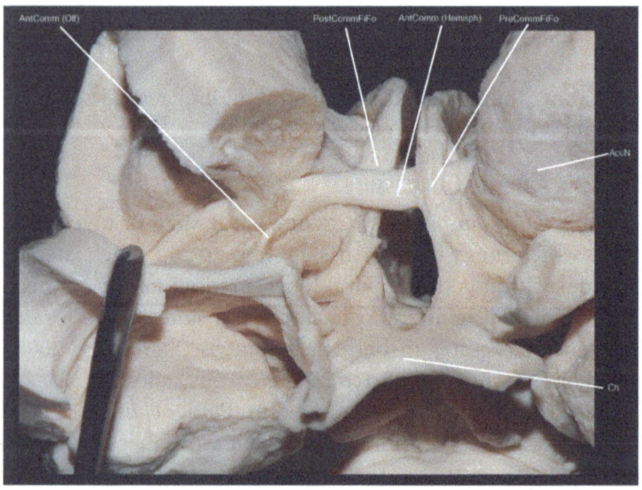

Figure 2.31 The anterior commissure with its hemispheric and olfactory parts.
AccN: accumbens nucleus; AntComm(Hemisph): anterior commissure hemispheric part; AntComm(Olf): anterior commissure olfactory part; Ch: optic chiasm; PostCommFiFo: postcommissural fibers of the fornix; PreCommFiFo: precommissural fibers of the fornix.

The anterior commissure was the main commissure in ancient reptiles and regressed together with the olfactory pathways throughout phylogeny. It is interesting to mention that, when reaching both olfactory tubercles, both olfactory parts can characterize an olfactory chiasm, as described by Theodor Meynert (Déjérine, 1895). With the emergence of the neocortex of the temporal lobes in primates, the fibers of the anterior commissure ended reaching the more inferior, lateral, and posterior temporal areas, constituting then the major component of the anterior commissure (Peltier *et al.*, 2011).

Supposedly, the anterior commissure connects the olfactory related structures, the anterior perforated substance, the nucleus accumbens part of the amygdaloid complex, the bed nucleus of the stria terminalis, and parts of the medial aspect of the parahippocampal gyrus (Williams and Warwick, 1980).

In humans, the anterior commissure seems to be related to the interhemispheric transfer of olfactory, gustative, visual, and auditory information (Peltier *et al.*, 2011; De Ribet, 1957 apud Peltier *et al.*, 2011).

The anterior commissure–posterior commissure line (AC–PC line) is a very important landmark in stereotactic atlases, for the proper localization of neuroanatomical targets utilized in stereotactic neurosurgical procedures.

2.2.5.3 Hippocampal Commissure

The hippocampal commissure or commissure of the fornix, also known as the lyre of David, psalterium (an instrument resembling a harp), and transverse fornix of Forel (Déjérine, 1895), is a thin triangular sheet of transverse fibers that lie between the two crura of the fornices, connecting functionally both hippocampi. As with the crura, the hippocampal commissure is situated underneath and intimately attached to the splenium, overhanging the pineal region.

2.2.5.4 Posterior Commissure

The posterior commissure lies below the pineal recess of the third ventricle, crossing the midline along the caudal lamina of the pineal stalk, and corresponds to the upper aspect of the aqueduct opening within the third ventricle.

It is a complex bundle that contains both decussating (e.g., medial longitudinal fasciculus) and commissural fibers that connect diencephalic and mesencephalic nuclei (interstitial and dorsal nuclei of the posterior commissure located within the periventricular gray matter, nucleus of Darkschewitsch of the periaqueductal gray matter, interstitial nucleus of Cajal located at the rostral end of the oculomotor nucleus and closely linked with the medial longitudinal fasciculus, and posterior thalamic, pretectal, tectal, and habenular nuclei), mostly still anatomically and functionally incompletely understood (Williams and Warwick, 1980).

2.2.5.5 Habenular Commissure

The habenular commissure lies between both habenula, which are small protuberances of both thalami located at the distal ends of both striae medullaris that course across the superior part of the medial surface of both thalami, within the posterior aspect of the lateral wall of the third ventricle.

Since the pineal gland is superiorly attached to the habenular commissure, and inferiorly attached to the posterior commissure, the pineal recess of the third ventricle is located between their two commissures.

As with the posterior commissure, the habenular commissure contains both decussating fibers (e.g., tectohabenular) and commissural fibers (predominantly connecting the habenular nuclei (Williams and Warwick, 1980; Heimer, 1995).

The habenular nuclei receive olfactory inputs from the septal nuclei, and transmit them mainly to the interpeduncular nucleus of the mesencephalon and to the rostral salivatory nucleus in the floor of the fourth ventricle to activate reflex salivation (Peltier *et al.*, 2011).

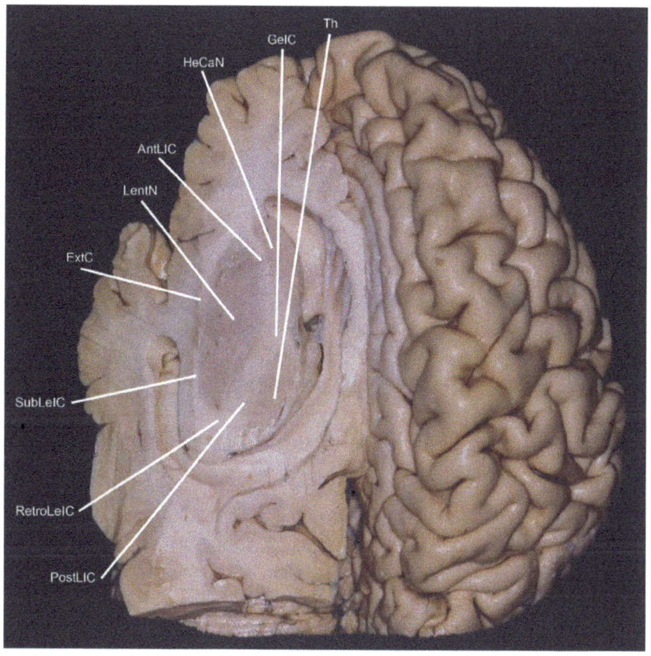

Figure 2.32 The internal and external capsules of the lenticular nucleus. AntLIC: anterior limb of internal capsule; ExtC: external capsule; GeIC: genu of internal capsule; HeCaN: head of caudate nucleus; LentN: lenticular nucleus (putamen); PostLIC: posterior limb of internal capsule: RetroLeIC: retrolenticular part of the internal capsule; SubLeIC: sublenticular part of the internal capsule; Th: thalamus.

2.2.6 Projection Fibers

The projection fibers comprise the corticofugal and corticopetal fibers that connect the cerebral cortex with the corpus striatum, the thalamus, cerebellum, brainstem, and spinal cord. Underneath the cerebral cortex, all of these fibers converge to form the corona radiata which intersects the commissural fibers and which is continuous with the internal capsule.

2.2.6.1 Internal Capsule

Since the internal capsule of Reil (Déjérine, 1895) corresponds to the caudal continuity of the corona radiata, this whole set of corticofugal and corticopetal fibers has the shape of a fan which opens upward and which covers the medial aspect of the lenticular nucleus (Figure 2.29B and Figure 2.30). The arbitrary limits of the internal capsule are then the superior and inferior aspects of the lenticular nucleus.

Given the round conformations of the head of the caudate nucleus anteriorly and of the thalamus posteriorly, the internal capsule, which is disposed laterally to these structures, has the shape of a V in horizontal cerebral sections (axial images), with its vertex oriented medially between these two structures and angled toward the interventricular foramen (of Monro). Therefore, based on the topography of its fibers, the internal capsule is divided into five parts: 1) the anterior limb, located between the putamen and the head of the caudate nucleus, 2) the genu, located within its vertex between the head of the caudate nucleus, putamen, and thalamus, therefore lateral and adjacent to the interventricular foramen, 3) the posterior limb, located between the putamen and the thalamus, upon which lies the body of the caudate nucleus, 4) the retrolenticular or retrolentiform portion, located posterior to the putamen, and 5) the sublenticular (or sublentiform) portion, located inferior to the putamen (Figure 2.32).

Cortical efferent fibers of the internal capsule continue to converge as they descend. Many, but not all, corticofugal fibers pass into the crus cerebri of the ventral midbrain. Here, corticospinal and corticobulbar fibers are located in the middle half of the crus. Frontopontine fibers are located medially, whereas corticopontine fibers from temporal, parietal, and occipital cortices are found laterally.

The anterior limb of the internal capsule contains frontopontine fibers which enter the opposite cerebellar hemisphere through the middle cerebellar peduncle, and anterior thalamic radiations which interconnect the medial and anterior thalamic nuclei and various hypothalamic nuclei and limbic structures with the frontal cortex (Table 2.7).

The genu of the internal capsule contains the corticobulbar fibers, which end mostly in the contralateral motor nuclei of cranial nerves, and some of the anterior fibers, of the superior thalamic radiation.

The posterior limb of the internal capsule includes the corticospinal or pyramidal tract. While the fibers concerned with the upper limb are anterior, the fibers pertinent to the trunk and lower limbs are located posterior.

The corticospinal or pyramidal tract provides direct control by the cerebral cortex over motor centers of the spinal cord. A homologous pathway to the brainstem, the corticobulbar projection, fulfils a similar function in relation to motor nuclei of the brainstem. The corticospinal tract does not

Table 2.7 Principal fibers of the internal capsule

Anterior limb	Frontopontine fibers Anterior thalamic radiation (frontal cortex, cingulum)
Genu	Corticonuclear fibers Anterior part of the superior thalamic radiation
Posterior limb	Frontopontine fibers Corticospinal fibers Corticoreticular fibers Corticorubral fibers Pallidothalamic fibers Superior thalamic radiation (premotor, motor and somato-sensitive cortex)
Retrolenticular portion	Parietopontine fibers Occipitopontine fibers Posterior thalamic radiation (parietal, occipital and temporal cortex, including optical radiations) Intraparietal and occipital pulvinar connections
Sublenticular part	Temporopontine fibers parietopontine fibers Inferior thalamic radiation (temporal cortex, amygdaloid nucleus, auditory radiation)

Adapted from Brodal (Brodal, 1981), Standring (Standring, 2008), Williams and Warwick (Williams and Warwick, 1980), and Yasargil (Yasargil, 1994).

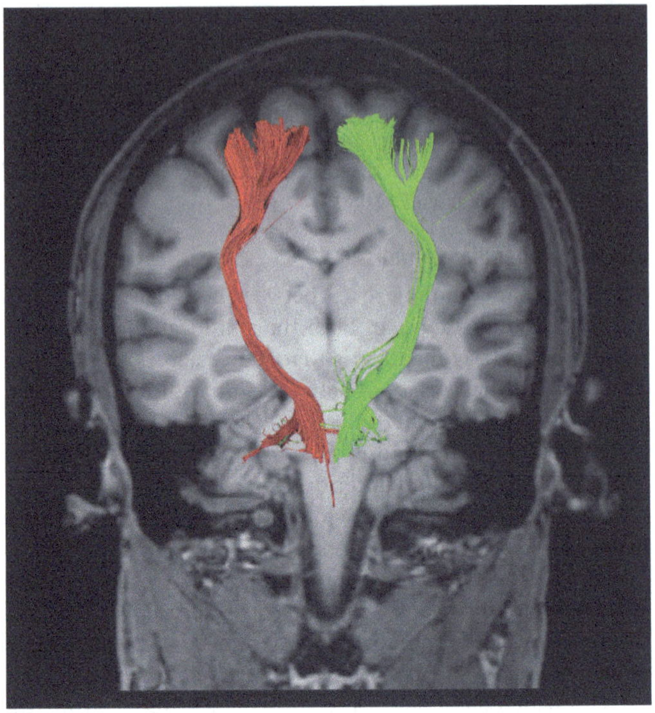

Figure 2.33 Diffuse tensor imaging (DTI) of the right (red) and left (green) cerebral hemispheres. (Courtesy of E. Amaro, Department of Radiology, University of São Paulo Medical School.)

originate solely from the motor cortex, but is conveniently considered in conjunction with it.

The percentage of corticospinal fibers that arise from the primary motor cortex may actually be quite small, probably in the region of 20 to 30 percent. They arise from pyramidal cells in layer V and give rise to the largest diameter corticospinal axons. There is also a widespread origin from other parts of the frontal lobe, including the premotor cortex and the supplementary motor area, and between 40 and 60 percent of pyramidal tract axons arise from parietal areas (Standring, 2008; Williams and Warwick, 1980).

The pyramidal tract fibers are disposed as a fan throughout the corona radiata and converge toward the genu of the internal capsule and posterior limb (Figure 2.30, 2.32, 2.33). The transition of pyramidal fibers between the corona radiata and the internal capsule is defined medially by the superior aspect of the body of the caudate nucleus, and by the fibers of the splenium, that together constitute the lateral upper edge of the lateral ventricle body. The transition is defined laterally by the superior aspect of the putamen and by the superior insular sulcus, since the most lateral pyramidal fibers run like a bow above and around these structures (Ebeling and Reulen, 1992b). To join the internal capsule, other than converging, the pyramidal tract fibers suffer an internal rotation of approximately 90 degrees, since the main axis of the precentral gyrus and of the genu of the internal capsule and posterior limb are almost perpendicular. Throughout their convergence and rotation, the fibers retain their somatopic motor arrangement according to the homuncular cortical representation (Penfield and Baldwin, 1952 apud Hansebout, 1977; Penfield and Boldrey apud Brodal, 1981), and end having an anterior-cranial to a posterior-caudal arrangement along the genu and the anterior portion of the posterior limb of the internal capsule (Brodal, 1981; Ebeling and Reulen, 1992b). Radiologically and surgically, this important portion of the internal capsule can have its topography estimated from the position of the interventricular foramen (of Monro) that lies medially and adjacent to the genu of the internal capsule, which contains the corticonuclear bundle (Brodal, 1981; Ebeling and Reulen, 1992b).

The posterior limb also harbors frontopontine fibers, corticorubral fibers, and fibers of the superior thalamic radiation (the somesthetic radiation) ascending to the postcentral gyrus (Standring, 2008; Williams and Warwick, 1980).

The retrolenticular part of the internal capsule contains parietopontine, occipitopontine, and occipitotectal fibers, and the posterior thalamic radiation including part of the optic radiation (Standring, 2008; Williams and Warwick, 1980).

The sublenticular part of the internal capsule carries the temporopontine fibers, most of the optic radiation, and the inferior thalamic radiation including the auditory radiation (Standring, 2008; Williams and Warwick, 1980).

The fibers of the optic radiation arise at the lateral geniculate body and its adjacencies within the pulvinar, join the retro and the sublenticular parts of the internal capsule, run within the sagittal stratum over the inferior horn and ventricular atrium, and project posteriorly passing superiorly and inferiorly to the posterior horn as part of the posterior thalamic peduncle to reach both the superior and inferior lips of the calcarine fissure (Párraga *et al.*, 2012; Ebeling and Reulen, 1988; Peltier *et al.*, 2006; Rasmussen, 1943; Sincoff *et al.*, 2004; Mahaney and Abdulrauf, 2008) (Figure 2.28B).

Within the temporal lobe, the optic radiation fibers are located along the depths of the superior and middle temporal gyri about 2 cm from the brain surface, inferiorly to the vertical segment of the superior longitudinal fasciculus, and always superiorly to the inferior temporal sulcus (Párraga *et al.*, 2012). Within the sagittal stratum, the optic radiation fibers intermingle with the other tracts but they run predominantly underneath the inferior fronto-occipital fasciculus and the anterior commissure fibers, and above the tapetum (see Section 2.2.3.6.2: The Temporal Stem and the Sagittal Stratum).

In coronal sections, while anteriorly, the optic radiation fibers appear predominantly flat, posteriorly, they have the shape of a comma (Martino *et al.*, 2010 apud Duffau, 2011b). The optic radiation fibers are classically divided into three portions: anterior, central, and posterior bundles (Ebeling and Reulen, 1988).

The fibers of the anterior bundle initially follow an anterolateral direction along the roof of the inferior horn until approximately 5 mm anteriorly to its tip and 3 cm from the temporal pole, and then shift backward constituting Meyer's loop and assuming a posterolateral course laterally to the inferior horn and to the atrium, to end predominantly along the inferior lip of the calcarine fissure within the lingual gyrus. The anterior bundle carries visual fibers related to the superior quadrant of the corresponding visual field (Walsh and Hoy, 1969).

The central bundle initially follows a lateral direction superiorly to the roof of the inferior horn, and turns sharply following a posterior course laterally to the atrium and posterior horn to end predominantly over the lateral aspect of the occipital pole (Párraga *et al.*, 2012). Its fibers are related to macular (central part of the retina) visual inputs (Walsh and Hoy, 1969).

The posterior bundle runs posteriorly as the lateral wall and part of the roof of the atrium and posterior horn, to reach the superior lip of the calcarine fissure within the cuneus, carrying fibers related to the inferior quadrant of the corresponding visual field (Walsh and Hoy, 1969).

Chapter

3 Cranial-Cerebral Relationships Applied to Microneurosurgery

The determination of the exact relations of the primary fissures and convolutions of the brain to the surface of the cranium is of importance to the physician and surgeon, as a guide to the localization and estimation of the effects of diseases and injuries of the brain and its coverings . . .
David Ferrier, 1843–1928 (Ferrier, 1876 apud Greenblatt, 1997)

3.1 Microneurosurgical Anatomy – General Remarks

Although evident, it is interesting to point out that the neuroimaging and intraoperative identification of intracranial structures, as with other body organs, are done from and based on the initial recognition of their surrounding natural spaces. Intracranially, this is constituted by the cerebrospinal fluid (CSF) filled spaces, and surgery is always preferably done through the same natural spaces, hence also preferably through CSF spaces for intracranial surgery.

This ideal practice became possible only with the advent of microneurosurgery. This was led particularly by the contributions of Yasargil (1999), evolved through the progressive development of initial transfissural and transcisternal approaches, particularly for the removal of extrinsic lesions (Yasargil *et al.*, 1976), to posterior transsulcal approaches for intrinsic lesions (Harkey *et al.*, 1989; Pia, 1986; Yasargil, 1994; Yasargil, 1996; Yasargil *et al.*, 1988a), and with the consequent establishment of the sulci as fundamental anatomical landmarks for its practice.

The brain sulci can be used as microsurgical corridors for the removal of cortical and subcortical lesions, to reach the ventricular cavities, or to serve as landmarks and limiting surgical boundaries for subpial or transgyral approaches (Figure 3.1).

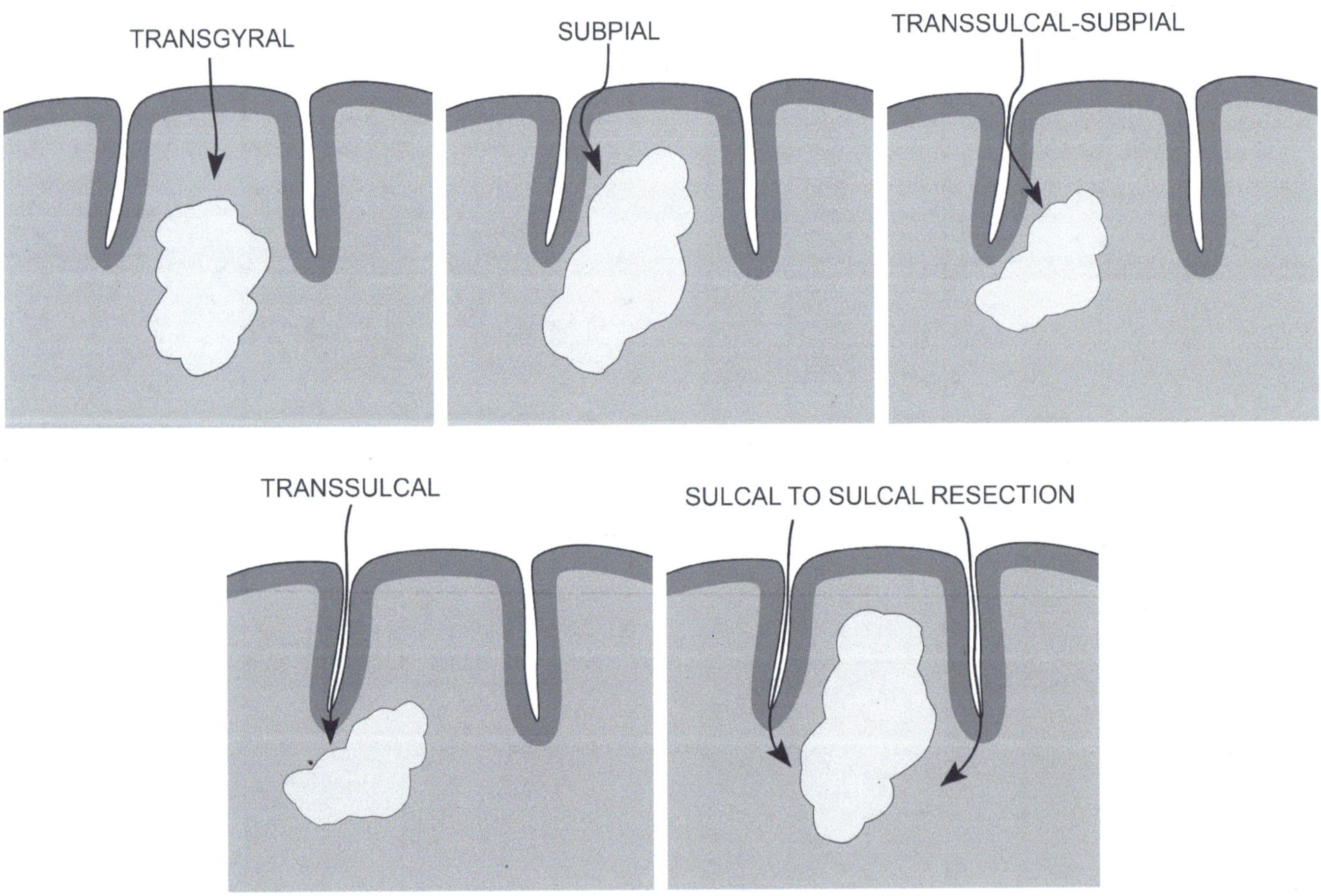

Figure 3.1 Possible transcerebral microneurosurgical routes.

Given the actual brain anatomy with the gyri constituting a real continuum throughout their multiple, and to some extent also variable, superficial, and deep connections that, respectively interrupt and limit the depth of their related sulci, it is important to emphasize that, despite being distinctively named, the gyri should be understood as arbitrary circumscribed regions of the brain surface. They are delimited by sulci that correspond to extensions of the subarachnoid space and that should also be understood as arbitrary circumscribed spaces of the brain surface which can be constituted by single or multiple segments, and with a variable morphology to some extent.

When compared to the subpial and transgyral approaches, besides the obvious advantage of providing a natural closer proximity to deep spaces and lesions, the transsulcal approaches are naturally oriented toward the nearest part of the ventricular cavity, which can be very helpful when dealing with peri- and intraventricular lesions. This unique feature of the radial orientation of sulci in relation to the nearest ventricular space, which is well seen in MRI coronal cuts, is due to the evolutionary fact that the sulci of the superolateral surface of the brain are a product of an infolding process of the cerebral surface. This took place mainly throughout the evolution of mammals in order to increase the cortical surface, and it occurred concomitant to the C-shaped bending of the telencephalon in relation to a center constituted by the thalami, which together carried the morphological modifications of the primitive prosencephalic vesicle that gave rise to the lateral ventricles through the same C-shaped bending process (Sarnat and Netsky, 1981; Squire *et al.*, 2003; Williams and Warwick, 1980). Despite their anatomical variations, the main sulci have then constant topographical relationships with their related ventricular cavities and hence with the deep neural structures (Harkey *et al.*, 1989; Ono *et al.*, 1990; Rhoton, 2003; Seeger, 1978; Ribas *et al.*, 2006).

Once the cortex is thicker over the crest of a convolution and thinner in the depth of a sulcus (Carpenter and Sutin, 1983), theoretically, while the actual transgyral approaches sacrifice a larger number of neurons and of projection fibers, the transsulcal approaches sacrifice a larger number of U fibers (Carpenter and Sutin, 1983; Harkey *et al.*, 1989) (Figure 3.2).

The subpial approaches can be started either through a transcortical opening just next to a sulcus or be initiated through a more limited sulcal opening.

The major disadvantage of the transsulcal approach is that the surgeon has to deal with intrasulcal vessels with diameters proportional to the dimensions of the sulci, and with occasional cortical veins that can run along the sulci surface (Figure 3.3).

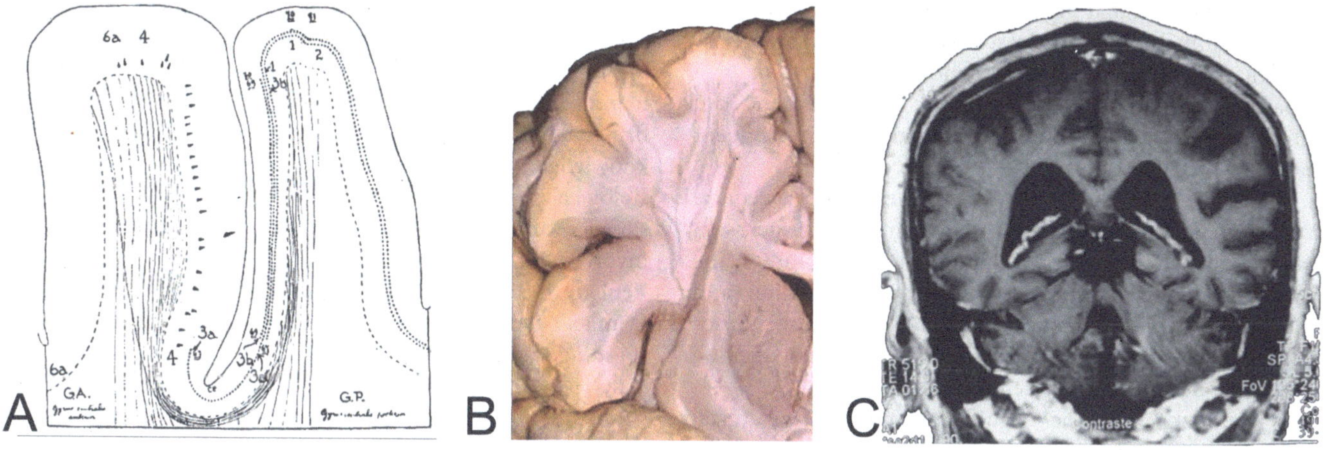

Figure 3.2 (A) Classic sketch by Vogt C, Vogt O, 1919, 1928, (B) cadaveric specimen, and (C) MRI coronal image, showing 1) that while the projection fibers arise from the crest of the gyri, the bottom of the sulci are related mainly to U-fibers, and 2) that while the main sulci of the superolateral and basal brain surfaces point to the nearest ventricular cavity, the sulci of the medial surface are parallel to the corpus callosum, and their organization depends on its normal development.

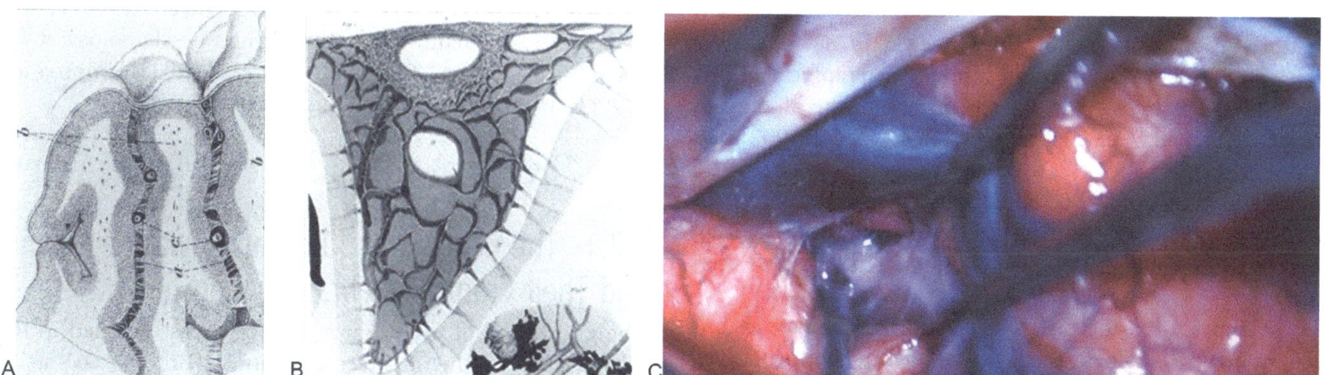

Figure 3.3 (A) Classic sketch by Key and Reteius (Key and Reteius, 1875 apud Yasargil, 1984a), 1875, and (B) Microneurosurgical opening of the Sylvian fissure, showing that, while the arteries are loosely attached to arachnoid bands within the intrasulcal spaces, the veins are more firmly attached to the pia mater and brain surface. (C) Microneurosurgical opening of the Sylvian fissure showing the arachnoid space (Arach), artery (Art) and vein (Vein).

Besides the respective vascular impairments, damage to these vessels can cause bleeding that spreads through the adjacent subarachnoid space and that can obliterate the clear microsurgical view. Even small vessels can be critical in eloquent areas of the brain.

In order to avoid stretching and tearing these vessels, and to optimize opening of the sulci, the arachnoid should be divided preferably with sharp instruments and the sulci should be progressively opened along their entire required extent. The running arteries should be freed and protected toward one side after the coagulation and division of their tiny contralateral perforating branches. The coagulation and division of larger veins are dependent on their location, and small intrasulcal veins should usually be coagulated to prevent their posterior bleeding during subsequent maneuvers. Vessels at the sulci depth can be avoided if necessary by entering the white matter before reaching them in order to proceed subpially. Larger sulcal opening extents provide less traction of the sulcal related vessels and walls, easing the transsulcal work by decreasing the need for Stille retractors.

For removal of hemispheric intrinsic lesions, the transsulcal approach can be useful to reach lesions that can then be removed piecemeal or en bloc, and also to delimit the removal of a gyral region that encloses the lesion. In particular, for the infiltrative gliomas that are so common and that frequently remain confined within their site of origin for some time (Yasargil, 1994), the anatomical removal of a gyral or of a lobular sector that encloses the tumor is justified and can facilitate and enhance its radical resection in non-eloquent areas.

In similitude to the brain extrinsic lesions that require complete dissection and exposure for their correct microsurgical treatment, as with the clipping of aneurysms or the removal of benign tumors, the strategy of isolation and removal of a gyral sector that contains an infiltrative tumor provided by its delimiting sulci identification and opening should then be considered when feasible.

In parallel with the significant microneurosurgical (Yasargil, 1999) and intracranial microanatomic knowledge (Rhoton, 2003; Yasargil, 1984a; Yasargil, 1994) gained over the last decades, the current localization of the brain sulci and gyri on the external cranial surface for the correct positioning of supratentorial craniotomies and for general transoperatory orientation (Rhoton, 1999; Seeger, 1978; Uematsu *et al.*, 1992) is still mostly based on cranial-topographic anatomy studies done particularly in the second half of the nineteenth century (Gusmão *et al.*, 2000; Finger, 1994; Kocher, 1907 apud Krause, 1912; Krause, 1912; Krönlein, 1898 apud Krause, 1912; Taylor and Haughton, 1900 apud Uematsu *et al.*, 1992; Testut and Jacob, 1932; Uematsu *et al.*, 1992) or done with the aid of stereotactic (Chin *et al.*, 1999) or sophisticated frameless imaging devices (Watanabe *et al.*, 1987).

The appraisal of the surface projection of intrinsic lesions seen in neuroradiological images frequently performed by neurosurgeons is difficult and error-prone due to the irregular oval shape of the skull and of the brain, and to the obliqueness and variable levels, particularly of axial and coronal images. Special techniques developed for this aim may require specific devices and are based on calculations that are also not free from error (von Economo, 1987; Fernández-Miranda *et al.*, 2008; Hinck and Clifton, 1981; King and Walker, 1980; Krol *et al.*, 1988; O'Leary and Lavyne, 1978; Penning, 1987).

The intraoperative frameless imaging devices developed during the last decade (Watanabe *et al.*, 1987), when available, obviously should not replace the cranial-cerebral anatomic knowledge that every neurosurgeon has to have and has to improve throughout his practice. Moreover, transoperatory brain displacement can affect the accuracy of these navigation systems (Dorward *et al.*, 1999; Roberts *et al.*, 1998; Sure *et al.*, 2000) and, although real-time corrections can nowadays be eventually made by the fusion of ultrasound images with the neuronavigation (Unsgaard *et al.*, 2002) and using intraoperative MRI (Black and Pikul, 1997; Black *et al.*, 1997; Wirtz *et al.*, 1997), correct transoperatory anatomical orientation is of course mandatory for the interpretation and for checking of all these imaging data. The same argument can be made about any new neurosurgical instrument or imaging technique, since the planning, practice, and evaluation of any surgical procedure intrinsically require accurate anatomical knowledge and can be particularly enhanced by a tridimensional understanding.

Regarding the functional reliability of utilizing anatomical sulcal and gyral landmarks for microneurosurgical orientation, it is mandatory to consider that any transoperatory anatomical identification of any eloquent cortical area, even when confirmed by a localizing imaging system, cannot safely replace the knowledge given by transoperatory functional or neurophysiological testing. This is because of common anatomical functional variations, their possible displacements and/or involvement by the underlying pathology (Ebeling and Reulen, 1992b; Ojemann *et al.*, 1989; Simos *et al.*, 1999; Uematsu *et al.*, 1992), or the plasticity more common in long standing lesions (Duffau, 2011b).

On the other hand, it is meaningful to bear in mind that studies on functional neuroimaging and intraoperative cortical stimulation denote findings that, in general, corroborate the expected relationships between elicited functional responses and their respective eloquent anatomical sites (Berger *et al.*, 1990; Boling *et al.*, 1999; Brannen *et al.*, 2001; Ebeling *et al.*, 1992a; Ebeling and Reulen, 1992b; Fitzgerald *et al.*, 1997; Lobel *et al.*, 2001; Ojemann *et al.*, 1989; Quiñones-Hinojosa *et al.*, 2003; Rutten *et al.*, 2002; Schiffbauer *et al.*, 2002; Simos *et al.*, 1999; Uematsu *et al.*, 1992; Yousry *et al.*, 1995).

3.2 The Sulcal, Gyral, and Cranial Key Points

3.2.1 The Concept of Sulcal and Gyral Key Points and Their Cranial-Cerebral Relationships

The knowledge of the primary cortical areas obtained in the second half of the nineteenth century (Broca, 1861 apud Finger, 1994; Ferrier, 1873 apud Finger, 1994; Fritsch and Hitzig, 1960 apud Finger, 1994; Jackson, 1863 apud Finger, 1994) generated the need to relate the brain sulci and gyri to the skull surface in order to properly expose and operate on intracranial lesions diagnosed only through neurological focal findings. This gave rise to several methods to establish the main cranial-cerebral relationships (Bischoff, 1868 apud Broca, 1876; Broca, 1876a apud Stone, 1991; Broca, 1876b; Horsley apud Ebeling *et al.*, 1987; Kocher, 1907; Krause, 1912; Krönlein, 1898 apud Krause, 1912; Taylor and Haughton, 1900 apud Uematsu *et al.*, 1992; Testut and Jacob, 1932). These descriptions were led particularly by Broca in France (Broca, 1876a apud Stone, 1991; Broca, 1876b; Broca, 1861 apud Finger, 1994), and related the brain sulci and gyri mostly to cranial sutures and to craniometric points (Broca, 1861 apud Finger, 1994), and many of these methods are still utilized at the present time.

As already stressed, the development of microneurosurgery established the sulci as the fundamental landmarks of the brain surface and made the subpial and transsulcal microneurosurgical approaches possible (Harkey *et al.*, 1989; Pia, 1986; Yasargil *et al.*, 1988b; Yasargil, 1999; Yasargil, 1994); however, in parallel with the fact that the main sulci and gyri of the brain are currently easily identified in standard magnetic resonance images, their accurate visual transoperative recognition is notoriously difficult because of their common anatomic interruptions and variations, and their arachnoid, cerebrospinal fluid, and frequent vessel coverings.

Upon the exposure of their sites eased by the knowledge of basic cranial-cerebral relationships, the identification of the main sulci may be facilitated by the initial identification of some more remarkable sulci and gyri points constituted by the main sulci extremities and/or intersections, and by the cortical sites that underlie the most prominent cranial points. This identification can then be completed from these starting points through recognition of the exposed sulci and gyri according to previous knowledge of their usual orientations, shapes, and more frequent anatomical variations. Currently, 3D rendering reconstructions of MR images can be very helpful for their preoperative appraisal.

On the superolateral surface of the brain, besides the always evident lateral or Sylvian fissure, the central sulcus, the precentral sulcus, and the postcentral sulcus, the other main sulci are the superior frontal sulcus, the inferior frontal sulcus, the superior temporal sulcus, and the intraparietal sulcus. The essential microneurosurgical sulcal and cortical key points are naturally those constituted by these main sulci extremities and/or intersections, and by the gyral sites that underlie the most prominent cranial points. Besides being anatomically more constant, the sulcal key points constituted by an intersection of two important sulci can be identified usually as a site with a variable enlargement of the subarachnoid space (Ribas *et al.*, 2006).

In order to project a cortical or a subcortical lesion seen on MR images onto the cranial surface for planning of a craniotomy, similar to navigation systems that localize any given point according to its position in relation to points with previously known coordinates, with the aid of these key points, any intrinsic cerebral lesion can be initially understood with regard to the structure and/or the intracranial space that contains the lesion. Then through the known relationships of this site with its most related cortical and sulcal key points, the lesion can have its external cranial projection estimated considering the position of the corresponding cranial points for these key points.

In addition to determining the external projection of the lesion, its most related sulcal key points will also serve as natural references pertinent to the best transsulcal, subpial, or transgyral approach for the target lesion, and hence contribute particularly to the correct placement of the planned craniotomy.

The sulcal and gyral key points described later are divided into fronto-opercular, superior frontal, and central, parietal, posterior temporal, occipital, and basal supratentorial key points which delineate the cerebral base. They are related to their respective cranial points within intervals smaller than 2 cm (Ribas *et al.*, 2006), which is acceptable for the surgical purposes of placement of craniotomies and intraoperative visual identification of sulcal key points.

Altogether, they constitute a cranial-cerebral anatomic framework which can aid the understanding of the location of any intrinsic brain lesion, orient the placement of craniotomies, and ease the identification of brain sulci and gyri.

Since their locations are particularly related to cranial sutures and the most prominent cranial points (Broca, 1861 apud Finger, 1994), the precise initial identification of these cranial landmarks is mandatory (Figure 3.4).

While the coronal sutures are usually palpable laterally and above the superior temporal lines, distances from the nasion to the bregma, and from the bregma to the lambda vary roughly from 12 to 14 cm in adults (Ribas *et al.*, 2006). This knowledge is very helpful for the localization of these two important craniometric points along the midline.

3.2.2 Fronto-Opercular Key Points

The frontoparietal operculum generally covers the superior half of the insular surface, with the triangular and opercular parts of the inferior frontal gyrus covering its anterior aspect and with the basal parts of the pre- and postcentral gyri covering its posterior aspect. The fronto-opercular sulcal key points are: 1) the Anterior Sylvian Point, 2) the Inferior Rolandic Point, and 3) the Inferior Frontal and Precentral Sulci Meeting Point.

3.2.2.1 The Anterior Sylvian Point

The lateral or Sylvian fissure (SyF) is definitely the most identifiable feature of the superolateral face of the brain, and constitutes the main microneurosurgical corridor to the base of the brain (Yasargil *et al.*, 1976; Yasargil, 1984a; Yasargil, 1994; Yasargil *et al.*, 1988a; Yasargil *et al.*, 1975; Yasargil *et al.*, 2002a).

The SyF is divided into a proximal segment (stem, sphenoidal, anterior ramus) and a distal segment (lateral, posterior ramus) by the Anterior Sylvian Point (ASyP) (Türe *et al.*, 1999; Yasargil *et al.*, 2002a; Ribas *et al.*, 2005a). This corresponds with a variable but anatomically constant enlargement of the Sylvian fissure located inferior to the triangular part and

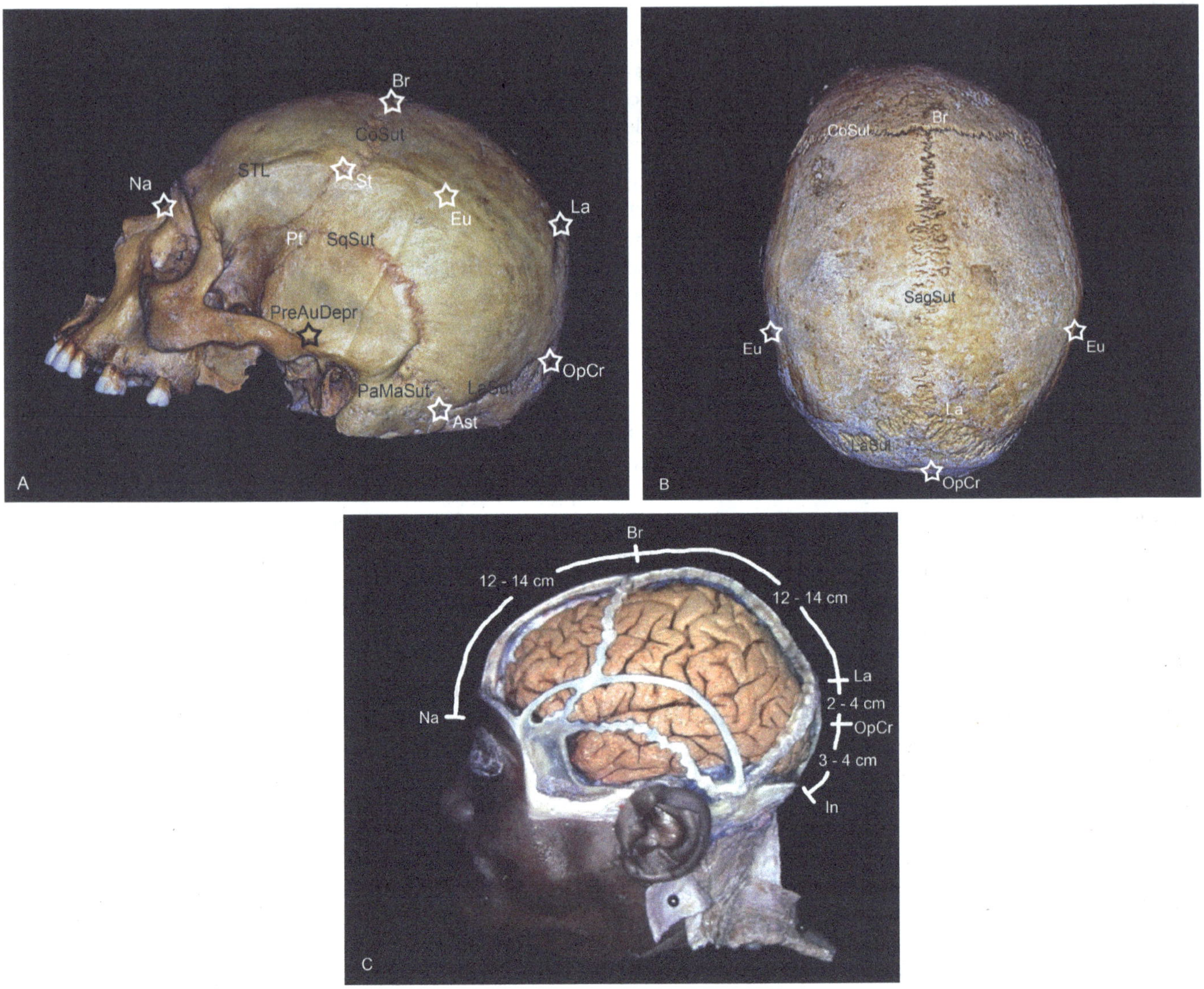

Figure 3.4 Average cranial suture and main midline measurements. (A) and (B), Adult skull with its main sutures and most prominent points; (C), their average distances and their relationships with the sulci and gyri of the brain. Average measurements are from Ribas *et al.* (2006).

Ast: asterion (meeting point of the lambdoid occipitomastoid and parietomastoid sutures); Br: bregma (meeting point of the sagittal and coronal sutures); CoSut: coronal suture; Eu: euryon (most prominent point of the parietal bossa or tuberosity); In: inion (prominence given by the external occipital protuberance); La: lambda (meeting point of the sagittal and lambdoid sutures); LaSut: lambdoid suture; Na: nasion (intersection of the nasion bones with the frontal bone); OpCr: opisthocranion (most prominent point of the occipital bossa); PaMaSut: parietomastoid suture; PreAuDepr: preauricular depression (upper aspect of the most posterior aspect of the zygomatic arch, anterior to the tragus); Pt: pterion (region where the frontal, parietal, temporal and sphenoid bones join together); SagSut: sagittal suture; SqSut: squamous suture; St: stephanion (meeting point of the coronal suture and superior temporal line); STL: superior temporal line (from Ribas *et al.*, 2006).

anterior/inferior to the opercular part of the inferior frontal gyrus (IFG), and which is evident due to an usual retraction of the triangular part (Figure 3.5).

The horizontal and anterior ascending branches of the SyF originate from the ASyP and delineate the triangular part of the IFG, which always harbors a small descending segment of the inferior frontal sulcus (IFS). Anteriorly to it lies the more prominent orbital part of the IFG which is basally continuous with the most lateral orbital gyrus, and posteriorly to it lies the anatomically constant U-shaped opercular part of the IFG, always harboring the most inferior segment of the precentral sulcus (Ribas *et al.*, 2005a).

Given its constant location and striking cisternal appearance as already shown in old illustrations (Krause, 1912; Taylor and Haughton, 1900 apud Uematsu *et al.*, 1992) and in recent publications (Duvernoy, 1991; Krings *et al.*, 2001; Ono *et al.*, 1990; Pernkoff, 1980; Rhoton, 2003; Seeger, 1995; Seeger, 1978; Squire *et al.*, 2003; Tamraz and Comair, 2000; Türe *et al.*, 1999; Yasargil, 1984a; Yasargil, 1994; Yasargil *et al.*, 2002a), the ASyP can be used not only as a starting site to open the SyF but also as an initial landmark to identify intraoperatively other important neural and sulcal structures along the fissure. These structures are usually hidden by their arachnoidal and vascular coverings, features that characterize the ASyP as the prototype of a microneurosurgical sulcal key point.

Taylor and Haughton (1900 apud Uematsu *et al.*, 1992), in their study of the topography of the convolutions and fissures of the brain published in 1900, used the term Sylvian point,

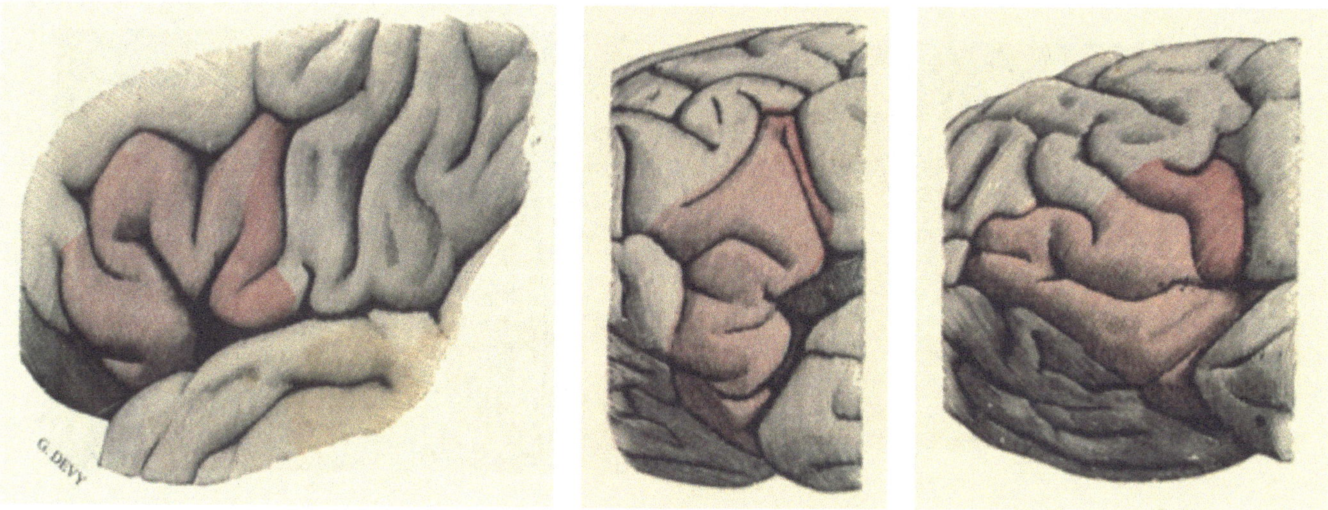

Figure 3.5 Variations of the IFG illustrated by Testut and Jacob, showing the typical enlargement of the SyF beneath its triangular part. (Reprinted from Testut and Jacob, 1932; Ribas *et al.*, 2005b.)

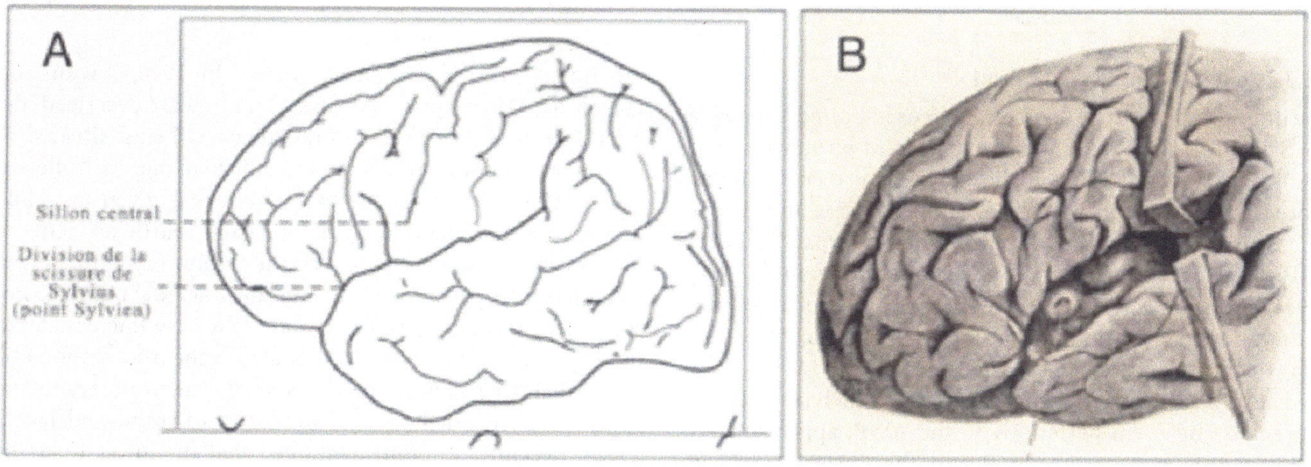

Figure 3.6 Reproduction of an old illustration of the Sylvian Point by August von Froriep (A), and opening of the Sylvian fissure by F. Krause (B). (Reprinted from Krause, 1912.)

defining it as "the point where the main stem of the fissure of Sylyius reaches the outer aspect of the hemisphere." In his textbook published in 1912, Krause (1912) reproduced illustrations by the German anatomist August von Froriep (1849–1917) (Lockard, 1977) with identification of the Sylvian point and also illustrated an anatomical opening of the SyF for exposure of a superficial insular lesion (Figure 3.6). Recently, Türe *et al.* (1999) stressed the use of the term Sylvian point.

Nevertheless, its designation as the Anterior Sylvian Point (ASyP) seems more appropriate, and in line with the term Posterior Sylvian Point (Ribas *et al.*, 2005a; Ribas *et al.*, 2005b; Yasargil and Abdulrauf, 2003), which corresponds to the distal extremity of the posterior ramus of the Sylvian fissure, and that is the starting point of the ascending terminal ramus and the occasional descending terminal ramus (Ono *et al.*, 1990).

The ASyP can also be identified intraoperatively as the SyF segment located just posteriorly to the IFG orbital part since this convolution frequently bulges significantly after dural opening, in contrast to its posterior adjacent triangular part (Figure 3.7).

Yasargil and colleagues emphasized that "the Sylvian point is located in the same plane of the IFG triangular part, and 10 to 15 mm anterior to the Sylvian venous confluence constituted by frontal and temporal tributaries veins," and advised "to begin opening the fissure immediately anterior to this vein confluence at a point where a temporal or frontal artery or where both arteries appear at the surface of the fissure" (Yasargil *et al.*, 2002b), hence at the ASyP area. Upon opening of the Sylvian fissure, the insular apex can be identified just below the ASyP.

Regarding its cranial relationship, the ASyP lies underneath the most anterior aspect of the squamosal suture, hence just posterior to the sphenoparietal suture that corresponds to the H central bar that characterizes the pterion, and just superior to the sphenotemporal suture (Ribas *et al.*, 2005b).

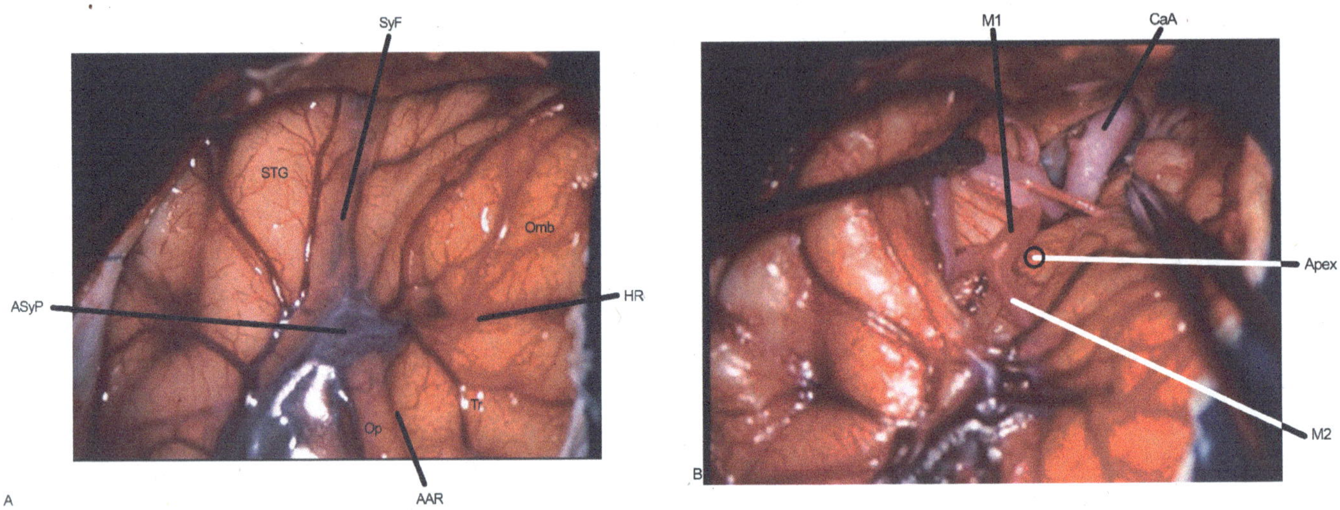

Figure 3.7 Surgical exposure of the stem of the Sylvian fissure (SyF), Anterior Sylvian Point (ASyP), of the Horizontal (HR) and Anterior Ascending Rami (AAR) of the Sylvian fissure which define the Triangular Part of the Inferior Frontal Gyrus (Tr), its posterior Opercular Part (Op), Superior Temporal Gyrus (STG), Carotid artery (CaA), branches of the middle cerebral artery (M1 and M2), and insular apex (Apex).

AAR: Anterior ascending ramus of SyF; Apex: insular apex; ASyP: anterior Sylvian point; CaA: Carotid artery; HR: horizontal ramus of SyF; M1 and M2: branches of the middle cerebral artery; Op: opercular part of the inferior frontal gyrus; STG: superior temporal gyrus; SyF: Sylvian fissure; Tr: Triangular part of the inferior frontal gyrus.

3.2.2.2 The Inferior Rolandic Point

The inferior extremity of the central sulcus is located just above the Sylvian fissure (SyF) in about 80 percent of humans, and inside the Sylvian fissure in the other 20 percent with the subcentral gyrus then completely hidden inside the fissure (Ribas *et al.*, 2006). The so-called Inferior Rolandic Point (IRP) (Taylor and Haughton, 1900 apud Uematsu *et al.*, 1992) corresponds to the projection of the inferior extremity of the central sulcus onto the lateral SyF, or to their intersection when the central sulcus reaches the fissure.

The IRP is located along the lateral (Sylvian) fissure between 2 and 3 cm posteriorly to the ASyP, approximately mid-distance between the ASyP and the Posterior Sylvian Point (PSyP) at the end of the lateral (Sylvian) fissure (Ribas *et al.*, 2005b).

Regarding its cranial relationships, in adults, the IRP lies underneath the point of intersection of the squamous suture with a 4 cm high vertical line originating in the preauricular depression which lies in front of the tragus, and which corresponds to the upper and most posterior aspect of the zygomatic root (Ribas *et al.*, 2006). This intersection point also corresponds to the highest segment of the concave squamous suture, which then indicates that the subcentral gyrus lies underneath the highest part of the squamous suture (Ribas *et al.*, 2005b; Ribas *et al.*, 2006).

It is interesting to note that the early authors also related the inferior extremity of the central sulcus (CS) to the same vertical line originating at the preauricular depression, but none of them studied the relationship of the projection of the inferior extremity of the CS over the Sylvian fissure with the squamous suture level. Poirier described the lower extremity of the central sulcus as being situated over a line perpendicular to the zygomatic arch and located immediately anterior to the tragus, 7 cm superior to the preauricular point which can be characterized as an evident small depression just anterior to the tragus (Testut and Jacob, 1932). In 1900, Taylor and Haughton (1900 apud Uematsu *et al.*, 1992) described the inferior extremity of the central sulcus as being situated at the intersection of this same perpendicular line with the so-called Sylvian line, that for these authors is given by a line drawn from the junction of the third and fourth segments of the Nasion-Inion curvature to the orbito-temporal angle. Championnière positioned the inferior Rolandic point 3.5 cm superiorly to the posterior extremity of a 7 cm line parallel to the zygomatic arch and which initiated at the frontozygomatic point that corresponds to the site of the frontozygomatic suture situated on the lateral orbital rim (Testut and Jacob, 1932). Recently, Rhoton mentioned that the lower Rolandic point is located approximately 2.5 cm posterior to the Pterion on the Sylvian fissure line, which corresponds to a line drawn between the frontozygomatic point and the three-quarter point of the Nasion-Inion distance (Rhoton, 2003).

In relation to the coronal suture, Passet found the inferior extremity of the central sulcus to be situated 25 mm (range: 0–65 mm) posteriorly to the coronal suture (Passet apud Ebeling *et al.*, 1987), Horsley between 20 and 30 mm (Horsley apud Ebeling *et al.*, 1987), and Lang 27.3 mm (range: 17–33 mm) (Lang, 1985 apud Ebeling *et al.*, 1987).

3.2.2.3 The Inferior Frontal and Precentral Sulci Meeting Point

The inferior frontal sulcus is always interrupted and can end in connection with the precentral sulcus or very close to this sulcus. Their connection point, or the point of connection of an inferior frontal sulcus prolongation line with the precentral sulcus when they do not actually connect, is designated as the inferior frontal and precentral sulci meeting point (IFS/PreCS). This is a practical neurosurgical key point that 1) delineates anteriorly the precentral gyrus at its inferior third level which corresponds to the face motor activation area (Penfield and Rasmussen, 1950b; Penfield and Boldrey apud

Brodal, 1981) and 2) indicates the posterior and superior limit of the opercular part of the inferior frontal gyrus.

The IFS/PreCS lies underneath the coronal suture and the superior temporal line meeting point, which corresponds to the craniometric point named the Stephanion (St) (Broca, 1876b; Ribas *et al.*, 2006). Its topographic relationship with the inferior frontal sulcus had already been shown by Broca (1876b), and more recently, Seeger (1995) clearly related the inferior aspect of the coronal suture to the inferior aspect of the precentral sulcus.

3.2.2.4 The Frontoparietal Operculum

Identification of the fronto-opercular key points ASyP, IRP, and IFS/PreCS can be helpful for the identification of all the main sulci and convolutions of the frontoparietal suprasylvian operculum both in preoperative radiologic images and intraoperatively (Ribas *et al.*, 2005a), and for the correct placement of craniotomies.

The superior and inferior margins of the SyF constitute, respectively, the cisternal borders of the frontoparietal and temporal operculi (*operculum*, from Latin: cover, curtain) which cover the superior and inferior aspects of the insula. Once by definition the frontoparietal operculum extends from the anterior to the posterior ascending branch of the SyF (Williams and Warwick, 1980), hence with the orbital part (Orb) of the inferior frontal gyrus (IFG) disposed anteriorly, the suprasylvian structures can be understood as a series of convolutions morphologically roughly arranged as a V-shaped convolution with its vertex constituted by the ASyP, followed by three U-shaped and one C-shaped convolution, all enclosing sulci terminal segments and extremities (Figures 3.8 and 3.9). The bottom of the three U-shaped convolutions and their related sulcal extremities can be situated either superiorly to the SyF or inside the fissure, then causing the false visual impression that their related sulci end at the SyF (Ribas *et al.*, 2005a).

The anterior V-shaped convolution is constituted by the triangular part (Tr) of the IFG, and is located just superiorly to the anterior Sylvian point (ASyP) where the horizontal (HR) and the anterior ascending (AAR) rami of the SyF originate, and delineate this convolution. Usually, the Tr contains a descending branch of the inferior frontal sulcus (IFS).

The most anterior U-shaped convolution is the opercular part (Op) of the IFG that encloses the inferior aspect of the precentral sulcus (PreCS) (Ono *et al.*, 1990; Ebeling *et al.*, 1989; Ribas *et al.*, 2005a; Ribas, 2005b). The PreCS ends superiorly or adjacent to the SyF (in 44 percent of humans) or inside the SyF (56 percent) (Ribas *et al.*, 2005a; Ribas, 2005b), always generating an anatomically constant U-shaped convolution which contains the inferior segment of the PreCS inside, and which corresponds anteriorly to the opercular part itself and posteriorly to its connection with the precentral gyrus (PreCG). Anteriorly, the Op is delimited by the anterior ascending ramus (AAR) of the SyF, and posteriorly by the anterior subcentral ramus (ASCR) of the SyF.

The middle U-shaped convolution is composed of the subcentral gyrus (SCG) that is constituted by the pre- (PreCG) and postcentral (PostCG) connection, also called the inferior

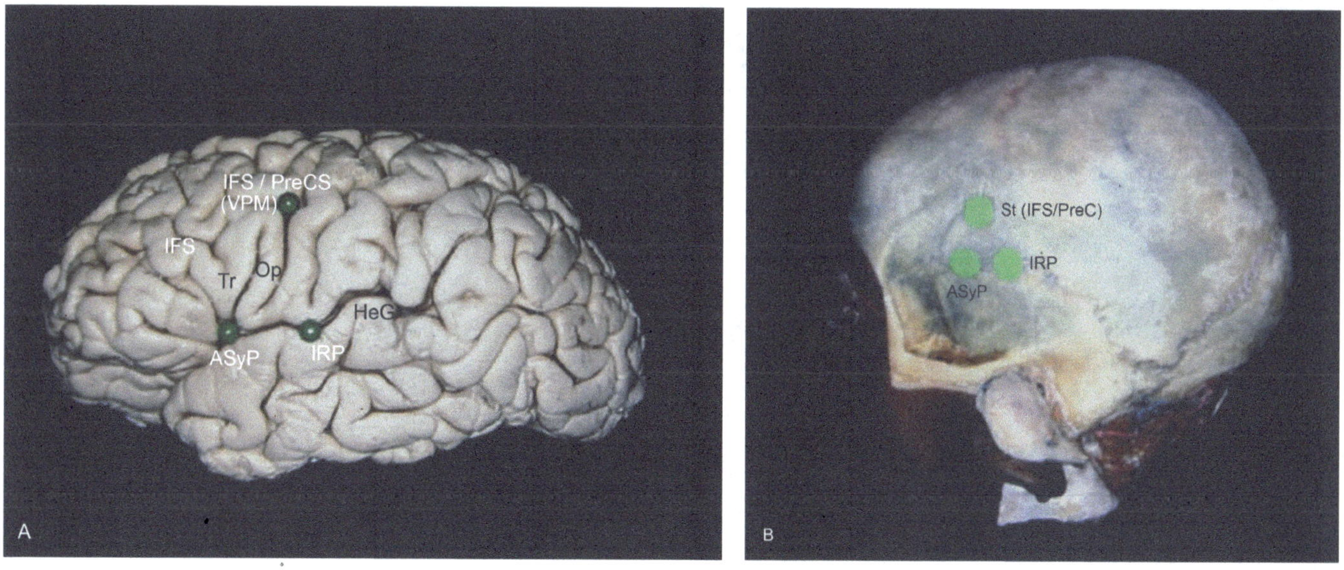

Figure 3.8 (A) Fronto-opercular key points and (B) their corresponding cranial sites: 1) the anterior Sylvian point (ASyP) is characterized by enlargement of the Sylvian fissure inferior to the triangular part (Tr) and anterior to the opercular part (Op) of the inferior frontal gyrus, and lies underneath the most anterior aspect of the squamous suture, just posterior to the pterion; 2) the inferior Rolandic point (IRP) is located along the Sylvian fissure 2 to 3 cm posteriorly to the ASyP, just anteriorly to Heschl's gyrus (HeG), and lies underneath the highest aspect of the squamous suture, which also corresponds with the intersection of this suture with a vertical line originating at the preauricular depression, about 4 cm high in adults; and 3) the inferior frontal and precentral sulci meeting point (IFS/PreCS), which indicates the superior aspect of the opercular part (Op) of the IFS (up to 3 cm above the Sylvian fissure), which corresponds to the face motor activation/ventral premotor area (VPM), and which lies underneath the craniometric point known as the stephanion (St) which corresponds to the site of intersection of the coronal suture with the superior temporal line (Ribas *et al.*, 2005b; Ribas *et al.*, 2006).

ASyP: anterior Sylvian point; HeG: Heschl's gyrus; IFG: inferior frontal gyrus; IFS/PreCS: inferior frontal and precentral sulci meeting point; IFS: inferior frontal sulcus; IRP: inferior Rolandic point; Op: opercular part; St: Stephanion (meeting point of the coronal suture and superior temporal line); Tr: triangular part of the inferior frontal gyrus; VPM: ventral premotor area.

frontoparietal "plis de passage" of Broca, and the Rolandic operculum that encircles the inferior part of the central sulcus (CS). The position of the base of the U-shaped convolution, here constituted by the SCG, in relation to the SyF varies in accordance with the position of the inferior Rolandic point (IRP) in relation to the SyF, and it can be found to be either superior to or adjacent to the SyF (in 83 percent of humans) or enclosed inside the SyF (17 percent) (Ribas *et al.*, 2005a; Ribas, 2005b). The SCG or Rolandic operculum is delimited by the anterior (ASCR) and posterior (PSCR) subcentral rami of the SyF.

The third U-shaped convolution is composed of the connecting arm between the postcentral gyrus (PostCG) and the supramarginal gyrus (SMG) that contains the inferior part of the postcentral sulcus (PostCS), and which is delimited anteriorly by the posterior subcentral ramus (PSCR) of the SyF, and posteriorly by the posterior ascending ramus (PAR) of the SyF. According to the position of the inferior extremity of the PostCS in relation to the SyF, the bottom of this third U-shaped convolution can be either superior to the SyF (in 61 percent of humans) or inside the SyF (39 percent) (Ribas *et al.*, 2005a; Ribas, 2005b).

The C-shaped convolution that completes the frontoparietal or suprasylvian operculum is constituted by the connecting arm between the postcentral (PostCG) and the superior temporal (STG) gyri, that encircle the posterior end of the SyF. The inferior margin of the SyF is related only to the STG that constitutes the temporal operculum.

The temporal operculum, which covers the inferior half of the insula, is solely comprised by the superior temporal gyrus (STG).

3.2.2.5 Frontotemporal Craniotomies and Exposures

Frontotemporal exposures are currently based on the pterional or fronto-temporo-sphenoidal craniotomy described by Yasargil (Yasargil, 1984a; Yasargil *et al.*, 1975), and probably constitute the most utilized and systematized neurosurgical procedure.

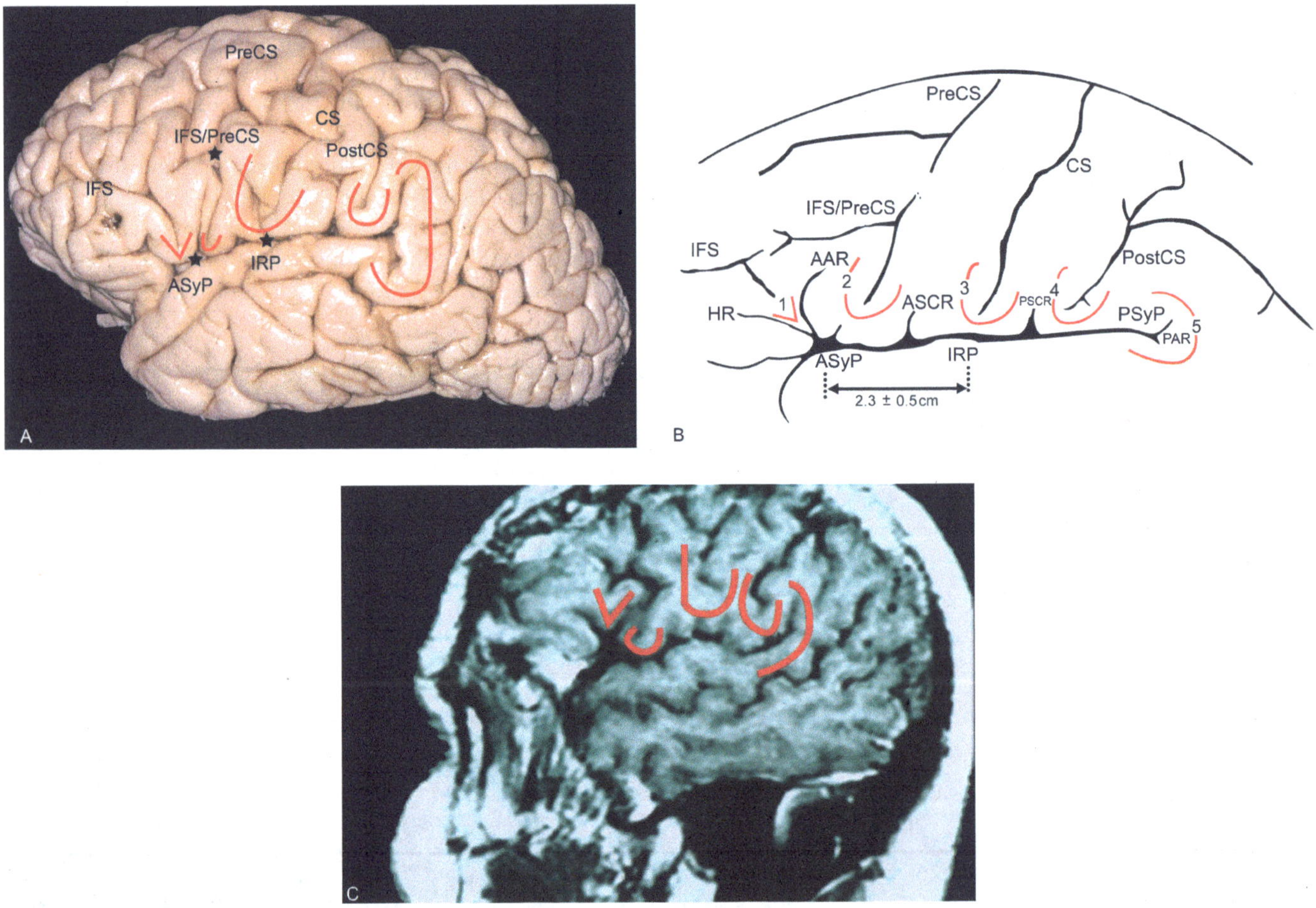

Figure 3.9 The frontoparietal operculum. (A) A cadaveric specimen, (B) a sketch of the neural and sulcal morphology, and (C) a MR sagittal image, disclosing the frontoparietal structures and the fronto-opercular key points, and with the identification of 1) the V-shaped convolution constituted by the triangular part of the IFG located just superiorly to the ASyP, and usually containing a descending branch of the IFS; and of its following three U-shaped convolutions, respectively comprised by 2) the opercular part of the IFG, which always harbors the inferior part of the precentral sulcus; 3) the subcentral gyrus or Rolandic operculum composed of the inferior connection of the pre- and postcentral gyri enclosing the inferior part of the central sulcus; 4) the connecting arm between the postcentral and the supramarginal gyri that contains the inferior part of the postcentral sulcus; followed 5) by the C-shaped convolution constituted by the connection of the supramarginal and superior temporal gyri that encircle the posterior end of the SyF. The bottoms of the U-shaped convolutions and their related sulcal extremities can be either superior to or inside the fissure.

AAR: anterior ascending ramus of SyF; ASCR: anterior subcentral ramus of Sylvian fissure; ASyP: anterior Sylvian point; CS: central sulcus; HR: horizontal ramus of SyF; IFS: inferior frontal sulcus; IFS/PreCS: inferior frontal and precentral sulci meeting point; IRP: inferior Rolandic point; PAR: posterior ascending ramus of SyF; PostCS: postcentral sulcus; PreCS: precentral sulcus; PSCR: posterior subcentral ramus of Sylvian fissure; PSyP: posterior Sylvian point. (Adapted from Ribas *et al.*, 2005a.)

The transsylvian approach (Yasargil *et al.*, 1976; Yasargil *et al.*, 2002b) provided by the pterional craniotomy is particularly useful for all sorts of anterior basal extrinsic lesions and for frontobasal, mesial temporal and insular intrinsic intracranial lesions (Yasargil, 1984a; Yasargil, 1994; Yasargil *et al.*, 2002c). The more recently proposed basal frontotemporal craniotomies derived from pterional and supraorbital (Jane *et al.*, 1967) craniotomies, such as the combined epi- and subdural approach with anterior clinoid removal (Dolenc, 1985; Dolenc, 1989), and the orbitozygomatic extension of pterional craniotomy (Fujitsu and Kuwabara, 1985; Hakuba *et al.*, 1986), enhance the basal approaches and minimize brain retraction but do not disregard the opening of the Sylvian fissure to optimize its ideal exposure.

Once having understood the location of any given lesion in relation to the fronto-opercular key points, their corresponding cranial sites can aid in the correct placement of frontotemporal craniotomies, particularly with regard to their posterior extent (Figure 3.8).

While the most anterior aspect of the squamosal suture covers the always evident ASyP, which allows identification of the triangular and opercular parts of the inferior frontal gyrus, with the U-shaped opercular part always harboring the inferior aspect of the precentral sulcus, the highest segment of the squamosal suture lies over the subcentral gyrus with its highest point corresponding to the IRP. Just posterior to the IRP, there is the prominence formed by Heschl's gyrus always underlying the postcentral gyrus (Figure 3.10).

With the cortical exposure, the ASyP can usually be easily recognized due to its cisternal aspect, and the IRP lies 2 to 3 cm posteriorly to the ASyP along the mid-third of the horizontal or posterior SyF segment (Ono *et al.*, 1990).

Since the opercular aspect of the postcentral gyrus (PostCG) always lies over Heschl's gyrus (HeG) (Wen *et al.*, 1999), the IRP also indicates the position of the anterior margin of HeG along the SyF, and hence the limit between the polar (PoPl) and the temporal planum (TePl) of the temporal opercular surface.

The posterior segment of the inferior frontal sulcus (IFS) and the IFS/PreCS key point can confine the superior limit of the opercular part of the IFG (about 3 cm above the Sylvian fissure in adults) (Ribas, 2005b), and indicate the face area of the PreCG, which roughly corresponds to the ventral premotor area (VPM) (Duffau, 2011b). Together with the ASyP and the IRP, they can then constitute important landmarks to estimate intraoperatively the so-called Broca's area in the dominant hemisphere, and guide restricted removal of the inferior portion of the motor strip, which is safer in the non-dominant hemisphere, and occasionally necessary in vascular, tumor, and in epilepsy surgery (Hansebout, 1982). The frontal or Broca's speech area occupies one or both frontal opercular convolutions anterior to the precentral gyrus of the dominant hemisphere (Hansebout, 1982; Rasmussen and Milner, 1975 apud Hansebout, 1982), and their removal is not justified. The pre- and postcentral face area can be removed, if pial barriers are respected, in order to preserve the blood supply to the upper Rolandic areas, and this may result in contralateral facial paresis that usually subsequently improves but that may leave some mild facial deficit (Hansebout, 1982; Rasmussen and Milner, 1975 apud Hansebout, 1982).

Considering that the IRP indicates the position of Heschl's gyrus (HeG), the removal of the superior and middle temporal gyri posteriorly to the IRP in the dominant hemisphere carries a greater risk of permanent dysphasia (Hansebout, 1982; Rasmussen and Milner, 1975 apud Hansebout, 1982).

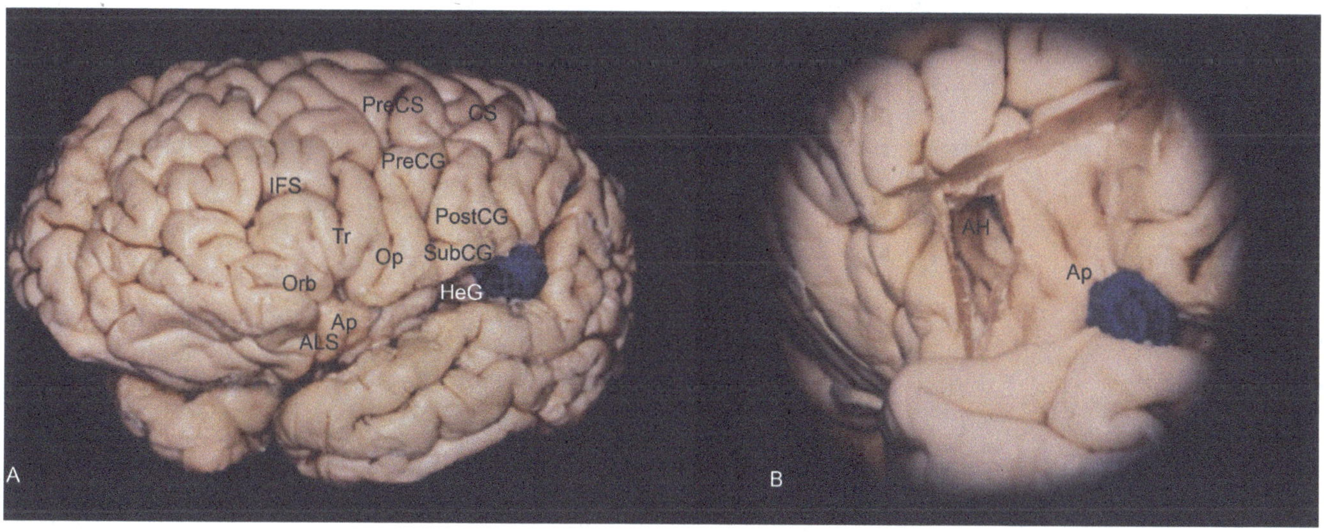

Figure 3.10 (A) The wide opening of the Sylvian fissure discloses the insular apex (Ap) located at the anterior Sylvian point coronal level, just posteriorly to the anterior limiting sulcus (ALS) of the insula. The opercular part (Op) of the postcentral gyrus (PostCG) lies over Heschl's gyrus (HeG), which separates the anterior polar plane from the posterior temporal plane of the temporo-opercular surface. (B) The depth of the anterior limiting sulcus of the insula, superior to the insular apex (Ap) level, is closely related to the most anterior aspect of the anterior horn of the lateral ventricle (AH), having in between mostly fibers of the anterior limb of the internal capsule.

AH: anterior horn of the lateral ventricle; ALS: anterior limiting sulcus; Ap: Sylvian fissure discloses the insular apex; CS: central sulcus; HeG: Heschl's gyrus; IFS: inferior frontal sulcus; Op: opercular part of inferior frontal gyrus; Orb, inferior frontal gyrus, orbital part; PreCS: precentral sulcus; PreCG, precentral gyrus; PostCG, postcentral gyrus; SubCG, subcentral gyrus (pre- and postcentral gyri inferior connection arm); Tr: triangular part of the inferior frontal gyrus.

The opening of the SyF at the ASyP level discloses the apex of the insula at its depth (Türe *et al.*, 1999), and the limen insula and the middle cerebral artery bifurcation are located a little deeper and anteriorly, 10 to 20 mm perpendicular to the ASyP itself (Yasargil *et al.*, 2002b).

Opening of the Sylvian fissure posteriorly to the ASyP exposes the lateral aspect of the insula, and opening of its stem anteriorly to the ASyP leads to the suprasellar cisterns. When both are opened in conjunction with opening of the Sylvian anterior ascending ramus (AAR), this enables exposure of its continuous insular anterior limiting sulcus (ALS) or anterior periinsular sulcus (Türe *et al.*, 1999), and thus of the anterior aspect of the insula situated behind the posterior orbital gyrus. The depth of the superior aspect of the anterior limiting sulcus (ALS) lies very close to the most anterior portion of the anterior horn, just in front of the head of the caudate nucleus, and is separated from the ventricle by local fibers, and by fibers of the anterior arm of the internal capsule (Türe *et al.*, 1999) (Figure 3.11).

3.2.2.6 Anatomical Remarks Pertinent to Common Frontotemporal Transcerebral Procedures

The frontotemporal approaches definitely constitute the most common and standard procedures in neurosurgical practice, given their frequently related extrinsic and intrinsic lesions and the very common use of the transsylvian route for Sylvian, insular, temporal mesial, subfrontal, and suprasellar lesions (Yasargil, 1984a; Yasargil *et al.*, 1985; Yasargil *et al.*, 2002a).

All of these approaches start with exposure of the frontoparietal and temporal opercula, and should have their temporal gyri recognized (Figure 3.9).

This section discusses the main anatomical issues related to the most standardized frontotemporal transcerebral procedures, with a particular focus on the procedures which require exposure of the temporal horn.

Approaches to the Temporal Horn of the Lateral Ventricle

Given the confinement of the temporal horn within the mesial portion of the temporal lobe, currently considered to belong to the limbic lobe (Federative Committee on Anatomical Terminology, 1998), this portion of the lateral ventricle can only be approached surgically through transcerebral routes and for their understanding, it is mandatory to have in mind some key anatomical features.

Although lying along the hippocampus, most of the temporal horn cavity itself lies mainly along the depth of the fusiform gyrus, about 3 cm deep from the temporal lobe lateral surface, and with its tip located also about 3 cm posterior to the temporal pole (Rasmussen and Jasper, 1958 apud Hansebout, 1977; Wiebe *et al.*, 2001; Wen *et al.*, 2006) (Figure 3.12).

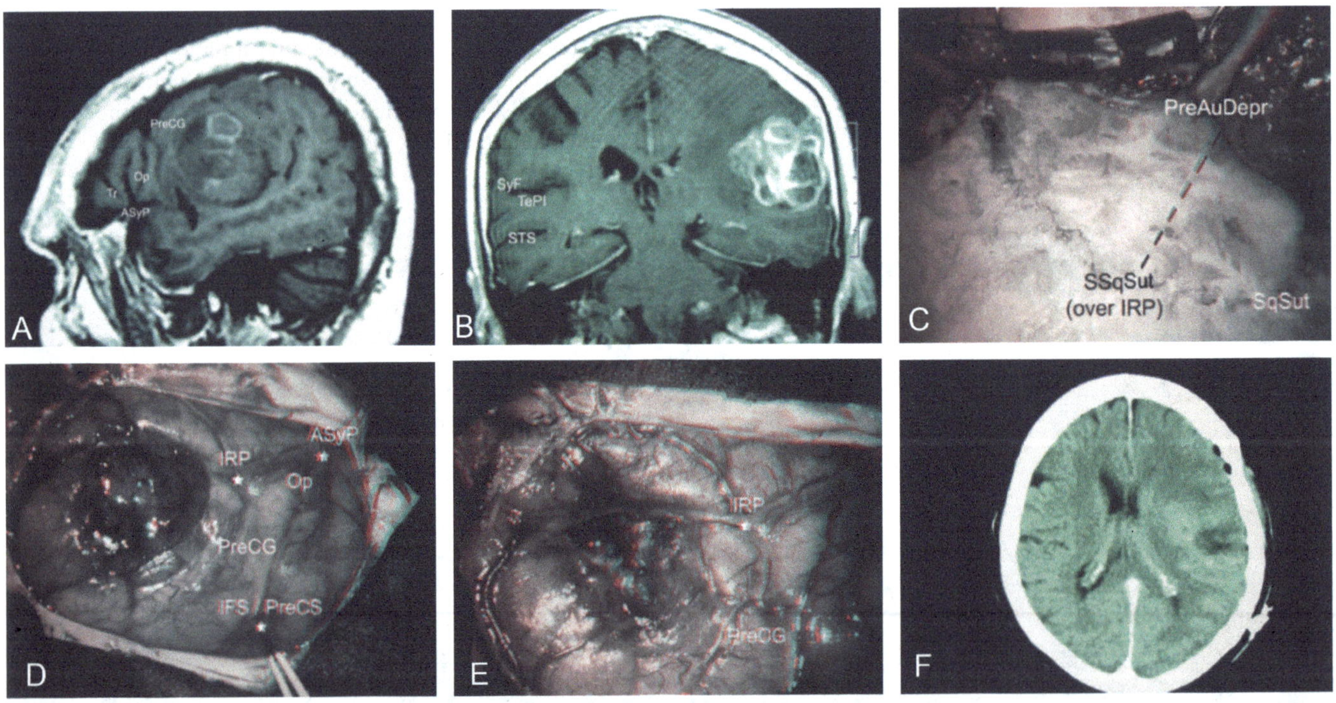

Figure 3.11 Frontotemporal craniotomy for exposure of the suprasylvian operculum and debulking of a glioblastoma multiforme within the inferior aspect of the left postcentral gyrus of a 75-year-old woman without focal deficits. (A) Sagittal MR image; and (B) coronal MR image showing the tumor over the flat aspect of the distal Sylvian fissure that corresponds to the temporal plane; (C) patient in the lateral position and intraoperative identification of the most superior aspect of the squamous suture, which corresponds to the intersection site between the squamous suture and a vertical line originating at the preauricular depression and which overlies the inferior Rolandic point (IRP); (D) exposure of the suprasylvian operculum through a frontotemporal craniotomy centered on the most superior segment of the squamous suture, and identification of the IRP, anterior Sylvian point, and the inferior frontal and precentral sulcus meeting point (IFS/PreCS), which enabled estimation of the topography of their related sulci and gyri; (E) surgical image and (F) CT scan image after the PostCG glioblastoma multiforme debulking.

ASyP: anterior Sylvian point; IFS/PreCS: inferior frontal and precentral sulci meeting point; IRP: inferior Rolandic point; Op: inferior frontal gyrus opercular part; PreAuDepr: preauricular depression; PreCG: precentral gyrus; SqSut: squamous suture; SSqSut: most superior aspect of the squamous suture, over IRP; STS: superior temporal sulcus; SyF: Sylvian fissure; TePl: temporal planum; Tr: inferior frontal gyrus triangular part.

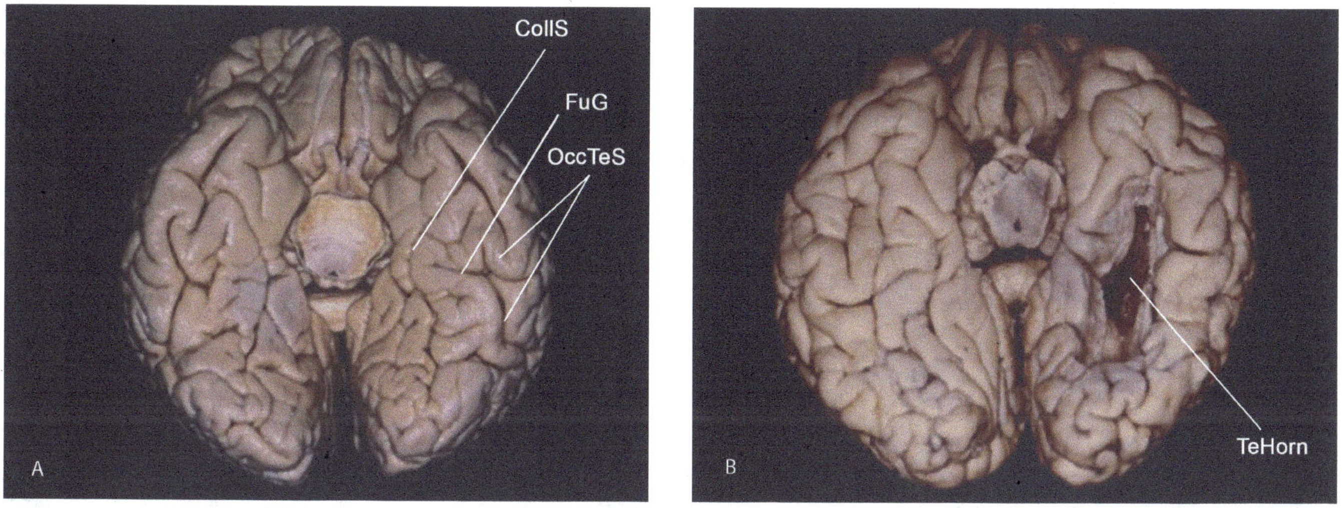

Figure 3.12 (A) The fusiform gyrus, between the collateral sulcus and the occipitotemporal sulcus, constitutes the floor of the temporal horn (B). CollS: collateral sulcus; FuG: fusiform gyrus; OccTeS: occipitotemporal sulcus; TeHorn: temporal horn with its choroid plexus.

Anteriorly to the tip of the temporal horn, while the bulk of the amygdala is enclosed within the anterior half of the uncus which can have its anterior and superior surfaces exposed through wide opening of the stem of the Sylvian fissure since its surfaces lie within the carotid cistern, the head of the hippocampus lies inside the posterior half of the uncus which cannot be exposed through any anterior and/or lateral cisternal approach. The posterior half of the uncus is incorporated in the most lateral aspect of the basal forebrain along a peduncular bundle of structures that pass between the limen insulae and the most anterior aspect of the temporal horn, and which includes the uncinated and the inferior fronto-occipital fascicles, fibers of the anterior commissure, and the upper extension of the amygdala toward the globus pallidus. Medially to them there is the ventral pallidal-striatum region located behind the anterior perforated substance and already within the basal forebrain, which is more medially continuous with the septal region. Posteriorly, this peduncular bundle of structures is continuous with the fibers that are running underneath the inferior limiting sulcus of the insula, which altogether correspond with the sublentiform part of the internal capsule and which spread laterally covering the temporal horn and the ventricular atrium.

While the different bundles of fibers that incorporate the temporal lobe into the rest of the cerebral hemisphere are collectively referred to as the temporal stem (Horel and Misantone, 1974; Cirillo *et al.*, 1989; Türe *et al.*, 1999; Ebeling *et al.*, 1992a; Duvernoy, 1998; Wang *et al.*, 2008; Choi *et al.*, 2010; Yasargil *et al.*, 2004), when passing underneath the inferior limiting sulcus of the insula, the continuous group of bundles of fibers that cover the temporal horn and the atrium more laterally are referred to as the sagittal stratum (Ludwig and Klinger, 1956; Türe *et al.*, 2000). In order to perform an anterior temporal lobectomy, both the temporal stem and the sagittal stratum should then be divided.

Within the temporal horn, the choroidal fissure starts at the inferior choroidal point, between the head and the body of the hippocampus, lies posteriorly along all its medial aspect, and its opening detaches the mesial temporal structures from the thalamus (Nagata *et al.*, 1988).

The approaches to the temporal horn are relatively standardized since they were developed mainly to remove the amygdala and the anterior portion of the hippocampus to treat patients with uncontrollable seizures due to mesial temporal sclerosis, and with good results.

Anterior Temporal Lobectomy and Lateral Approaches for Exposure of the Temporal Horn

Anterior temporal lobectomy for the surgical treatment of temporal lobe epilepsy was the first standardized procedure for the ventricular exposure and removal of deep and mesial temporal structures (Penfield and Flanigin, 1950a apud Maxwell and Tummala, 2004; Spencer *et al.*, 1984), and is still currently used with different modifications. Its rationale is to remove initially the lateral (neocortical) aspect of the temporal lobe in order to expose the temporal horn and ease the removal of the amygdala and hippocampus (allocortical structures) (Figure 3.13).

The most original descriptions of standard temporal lobectomies proposed that the subpial dissection should be started along the summit of the superior temporal gyrus, pulling away its gray matter in order to expose the white matter that should then be suctioned until exposure of the pia-arachnoid which covers the insula and the middle cerebral artery branches. Currently, there is a trend to spare at least the most superior aspect of the superior temporal gyrus, initiating the subpial removal along its inferior aspect or immediately next and inferiorly to the superior temporal sulcus (Maxwell *et al.*, 2004). Nevertheless, since the superior temporal gyrus constitutes the temporal operculum which covers the inferior half of the insula, its removal enhances the basal insular exposure and is still proposed by many authors (Wiebe *et al.*, 2001), particularly with awake surgeries when in the dominant hemisphere (Duffau, 2011b). Once the insula and its inferior limiting

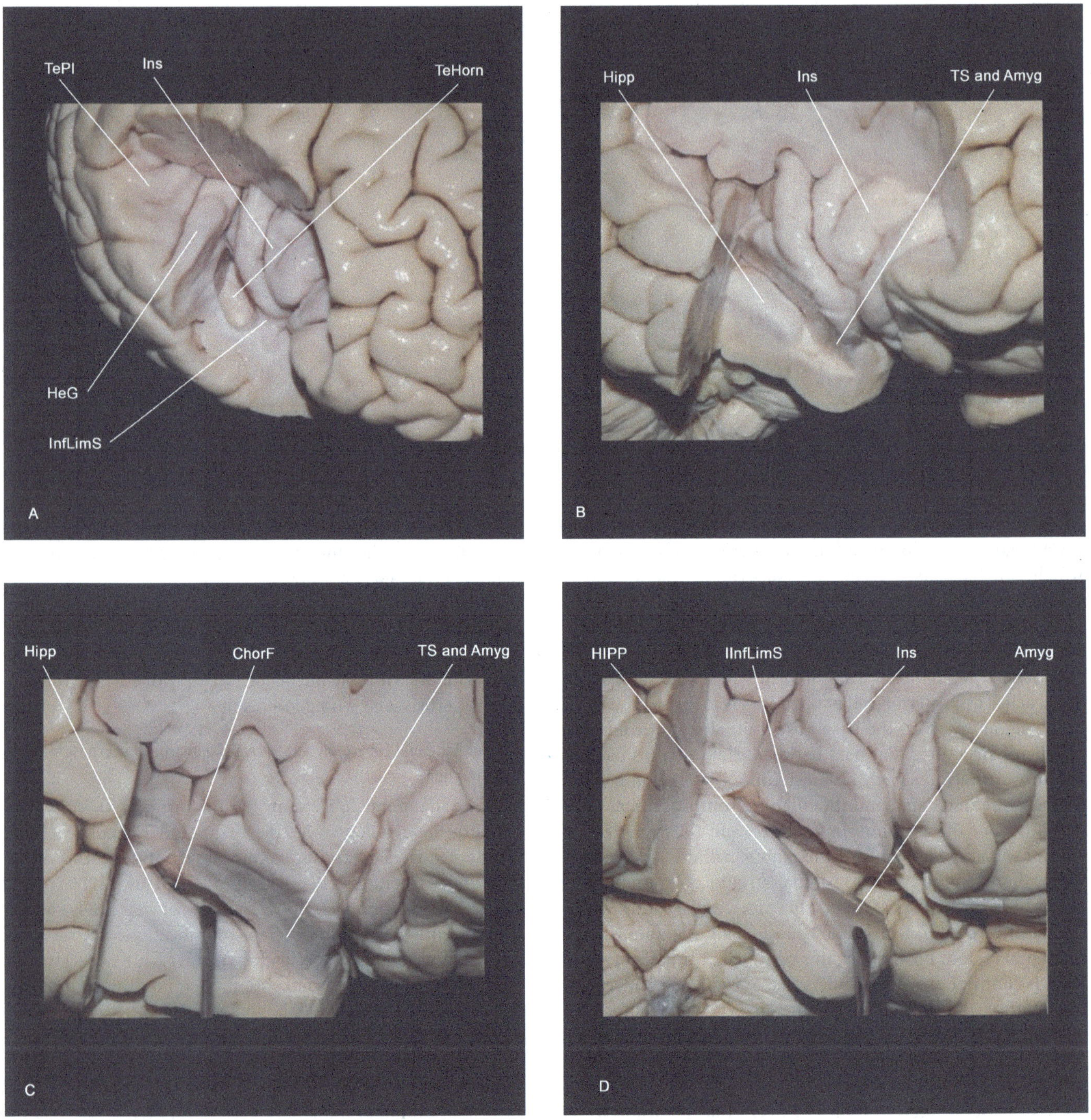

Figure 3.13 All techniques for temporal lobectomies are based on exposure of the temporal horn, which can be achieved through different routes. (A) View of the insula after removal of the frontoparietal operculum and of the superior temporal gyrus, and exposure of the temporal horn through an opening along the inferior limiting sulcus of the insula. (B) View of the hippocampus within the temporal horn and of the temporal stem, after removal of the neocortical structures of the temporal lobe (temporal gyri and temporal lobe). (C) View of the choroidal fissure medially to the hippocampus. (D) View of the allocortical structures (hippocampus and amygdala) after the division of the temporal stem.

Amyg: amygdala; ChorF: choroidal fissure; HeG: Heschl's gyrus; Hipp: hippocampus; InfLimS: inferior limiting sulcus; Ins: insula; TeHorn: temporal horn; TS: temporal stem; TePl: temporal planum.

sulcus are exposed, the suction should proceed through the temporal stem medially toward the middle fossa floor at an angle of 45°, and finally along the fusiform gyrus reaching the middle fossa skull base. The anterior incision should then be carried out anteroinferiorly until it meets the basal temporal incision (Hansebout, 1977).

After the coagulation and division of anterior and basal temporal veins, the whole disconnected anterior temporal lobe is lifted out, usually leaving some white matter overlying the temporal horn (Hansebout, 1977) which is then carefully removed by suction until the hippocampus is exposed.

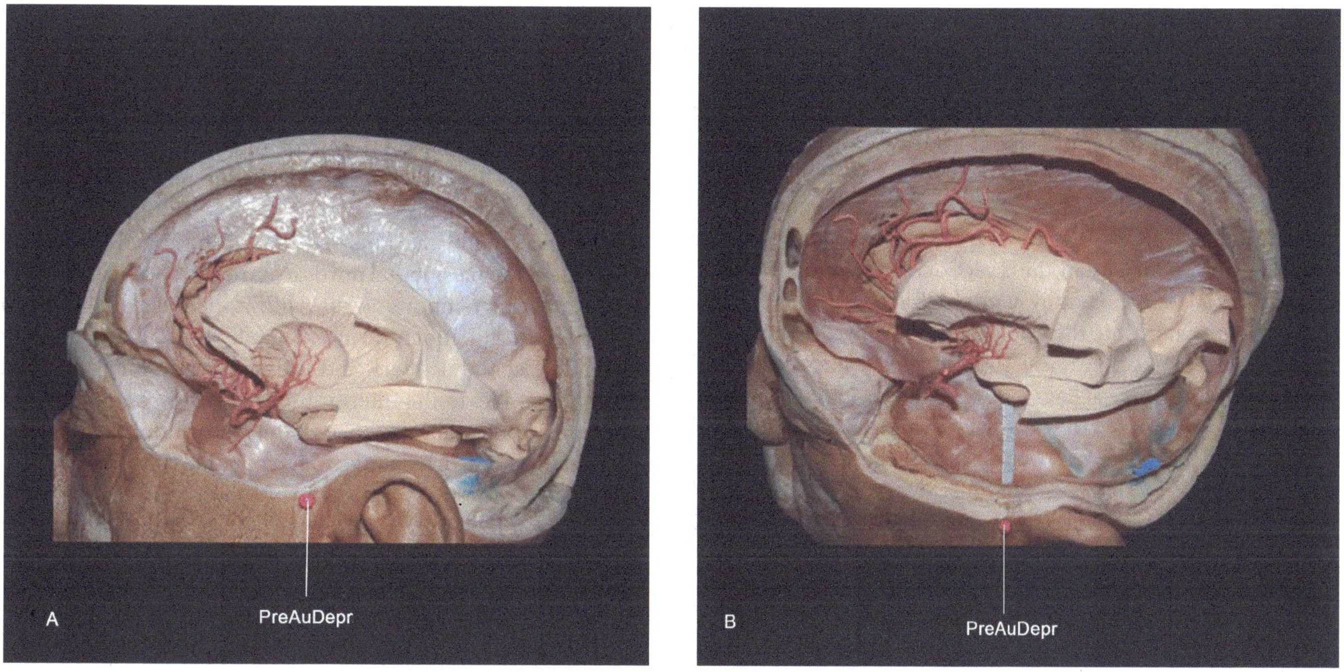

Figure 3.14 (A and B) The preauricular depression is related to the posterior aspect of the hippocampus along a coronal plane. PreAuDepr: preauricular depression.

Further dissection and exposure lead to the identification of the amygdala anteriorly, and of the head and body of the hippocampus within the temporal horn. The choroid plexus is seen as a fringe covering the head of the hippocampus, and its lifting allows the exposure and opening of the choroid fissure. En bloc removal of the amygdala and of the anterior part of the hippocampus within the parahippocampal gyrus can be done through further cutting of the medial temporal stem between the most anterior aspect of the choroidal fissure (anterior choroidal point) and the limen insulae, opening of the choroidal fissure leaving the choroid plexus superiorly attached to the thalamus, and division of the body of the hippocampus usually at the level of the lateral mesencephalic sulcus, which roughly corresponds to 2 cm of its length.

Regarding the posterior extent of the temporal lobectomy, it is interesting to point out that in 1952, Penfield and Baldwin (Penfield and Baldwin, 1952 apud Hansebout, 1977) and in 1955, Falconer and colleagues (Falconer *et al.*, 1955 apud Hansebout, 1977) had suggested that the dominant temporal lobe resection could be extended posteriorly as far as the vein of Labbé. In 1958, Rasmussen and Jasper suggested that this removal could comprise 5 to 6 cm of the dominant temporal lobe (Rasmussen and Jasper, 1958 apud Hansebout, 1977), and in 1975, Rasmussen considered that, due to the variable position of the vein of Labbé, the safest landmark pertinent to the posterior level of the dominant temporal lobe resection would be the junction of the Rolandic and Sylvian fissures (Rasmussen, 1975 apud Hansebout, 1977). This point corresponds to the inferior projection of the central sulcus into the Sylvian fissure, which is known as the Inferior Rolandic Point and which is located underneath the highest aspect of the cranial squamous suture, 4 cm vertically above the preauricular depression (upper surface of the most posterior aspect of the zygomatic root, just anteriorly to the tragus) (Ribas *et al.*, 2005a). The Inferior Rolandic Point is located along the Sylvian fissure about 2.0 to 2.5 cm posteriorly to the Anterior Sylvian Point (Ribas *et al.*, 2005a), and about 5 cm from the temporal pole. Since there might be some difficulty in obtaining intraoperative measurements from the temporal pole, the preauricular depression can then be considered an easier and fairly good landmark to establish the posterior limit of the resection (Figure 3.14).

Rasmussen also reported that visual field defects were rarely seen if this limit was respected (Rasmussen, 1975 apud Hansebout, 1977), and Rasmussen and Milner considered what they called the parietal speech zone as the cortical area extending along the superior and middle temporal gyri from 2 to 4 cm behind the postcentral sulcus, and superiorly 1 to 4 cm above the Sylvian fissure (Rasmussen and Milner, 1975 apud Hansebout, 1982).

More recently, Wiebe *et al.* suggested that posterior temporal resection in the dominant hemisphere can be extended for 4.0 to 4.5 cm, and 6.0 to 6.5 cm in the non-dominant side, and that the mesial resection should include the amygdala and a minimum of 1.0 to 3.0 cm of the hippocampus (Wiebe *et al.*, 2001).

Less extensive lateral temporal neocortical resections for exposure of the temporal horns, and more selective mesial temporal resections for the surgical treatment of mesial temporal sclerosis, were initiated by Niemeyer with the proposal to access the ventricle through the middle temporal gyrus (Niemeyer, 1958), followed by the proposal to access it through the superior temporal gyrus (Olivier, 1991), and more recently by the transsylvian approach by Yasargil (Wieser and Yasargil, 1982).

The average distances from the temporal pole to the temporal horn, and from the surface of the middle temporal gyrus to this ventricular cavity, are both about 3 cm (Rasmussen and Jasper, 1958 apud Hansebout, 1977; Wiebe *et al.*, 2001; Wen *et al.*, 2006). While accessing the temporal horn through the middle temporal gyrus constitutes a route with no defined anatomical landmarks, a progressive subpial dissection along the inferior margin of the superior temporal sulcus leads the surgeon more naturally in the direction of the temporal horn (Maxwell *et al.*, 2004; Harkey *et al.*, 1989).

In order to facilitate the exposure of the temporal horn and to follow the correct surgical route during transsylvian and lateral temporal approaches, Wen *et al.* suggest identifying the gray matter which overlies the rhinal and occipitotemporal sulci during the white matter resection toward the temporal base. This gray matter is located just lateral to the temporal horn and can be preoperatively analyzed in coronal MR images (Wen *et al.*, 2006).

This anatomical feature can also be of great help for a more posterior and straightforward approach to the temporal horn. For this purpose, a basal frontotemporal craniotomy should be performed after a question mark-shaped scalp incision which starts at the superior border of the zygomatic arch but which extends posteriorly to the ear, in order to allow a transcerebral vertical incision to be made through the middle and inferior temporal gyri at the level of the preauricular depression (upper surface of the most posterior aspect of the zygomatic root, just anteriorly to the tragus). The progressive and careful removal of brain parenchyma through the whole length of this incision will lead initially to a possible identification of the occipitotemporal sulcus and subsequently of the also vertical but more prominent collateral sulcus gray matter, and the temporal horn will be found 2 to 3 mm superiorly to the latter (Gwinn, 2015).

The transcerebral approach performed at the level of the preauricular depression will expose the posterior portion of the head of the hippocampus, and enlargement of the ventricular cavity exposure can then be achieved with further subpial removal of both the middle and inferior temporal gyri, and also of the superior temporal gyrus anteriorly, until the sphenoid wing and the transpial visualization of M1. In the case of performing an amygdalohippocampectomy, the amygdala can be removed anteriorly and medially within the uncus, and the hippocampus can be removed together with the mesiobasal temporal structures after the opening of the choroidal fissure, until the transpial visualization of the contents of the ambient cistern (Gwinn, 2015).

In relation to the superior aspect of the resection, Wen *et al.* proposed the carotid-choroidal line (from the internal carotid artery bifurcation or the proximal segment of M1, to the inferior choroidal point) as the superior extraventricular limit for the removal of the uncus that is mostly below this line, and the superior intraventricular limit for the removal of the superior extension of the amygdala which bulges on the roof of the temporal horn underneath the globus pallidus (Wen *et al.*, 1999). The lateral geniculate body is located superiorly to the body of the hippocampus.

Transsylvian Approaches to the Temporal Horn

The transsylvian approaches to the temporal horn, as proposed originally by Yasargil to perform a selective amygdalohippocampectomy (Wieser and Yasargil, 1982), require an initial wide opening of the stem and of the posterior part of the Sylvian fissure in order to expose the limen insulae and the inferior limiting sulcus of the insula.

A transcerebral incision of about 15 mm should then be made along the mesiobasal portion of the intraopercular aspect of the superior temporal gyrus, within the polar planum just posteriorly to the limen insulae, laterally to the bifurcation of the middle cerebral artery and to the M2 inferior trunk, just next and parallel to the inferior limiting sulcus, obliquely with an inclination toward the edge of the tentorium (Figure 3.15).

This incision corresponds to the opening of the most anterior aspect of the temporal stem, and the ventricular cavity is found only a few millimeters below. Once within the inferior horn, this incision can be split occipitally unroofing the ventricular cavity for a distance of 2.5 to 3.0 cm from its tip (Maxwell *et al.*, 2004; Wieser and Yasargil, 1982). The head and anterior aspect of the hippocampus, covered by the choroid plexus, can then be exposed, and the amygdala can be identified anteriorly by its more brownish color.

Within the temporal horn, the choroidal fissure can be explored by lifting up the choroid plexus toward the thalamus and can be opened along the taenia fimbria, exposing the subiculum already within the lateral wing of the transverse fissure, and the apex of the uncus more anteriorly. The anterior limit of the choroidal fissure corresponds to the inferior choroidal point, the point of entrance of the anterior choroidal artery. Hippocampal arteries originating along the P2 and P3 segments of the posterior cerebral artery can be seen entering along the choroidal fissure (Nagata *et al.*, 1988) and should be coagulated and divided if the temporomesial structures are to be removed.

A selective amygdalohippocampectomy can then be performed subpially with removal of the amygdala within the anterior part of the uncus, and of the hippocampus along its anterior axis, until the cisternal structures and the lateral aspect of the peduncle can be seen through the transparent pial and arachnoid membranes (Wieser and Yasargil, 1982), or it can be performed en bloc.

For an en bloc removal, the hippocampus and the parahippocampal gyrus can be medially transected along the ascending fimbria, posteriorly at the level of the hippocampal body and tail junction (the level of the lateral mesencephalic sulcus), laterally in between the hippocampus and the collateral eminence, inferiorly toward the collateral sulcus and the tentorium, and anteriorly including the bulk of the amygdala. Further medial resection of the parahippocampal gyrus should then be performed subpially exploring the posterior cerebral artery on the other side of the pia and arachnoid, facilitating then the lateral rotation of the hippocampus and its final removal. Anteriorly, the lateral limit for the removal of the amygdala is the rhinal sulcus, which separates the uncus from the rest of the temporal pole (Maxwell *et al.*, 2004; Wieser and Yasargil, 1982).

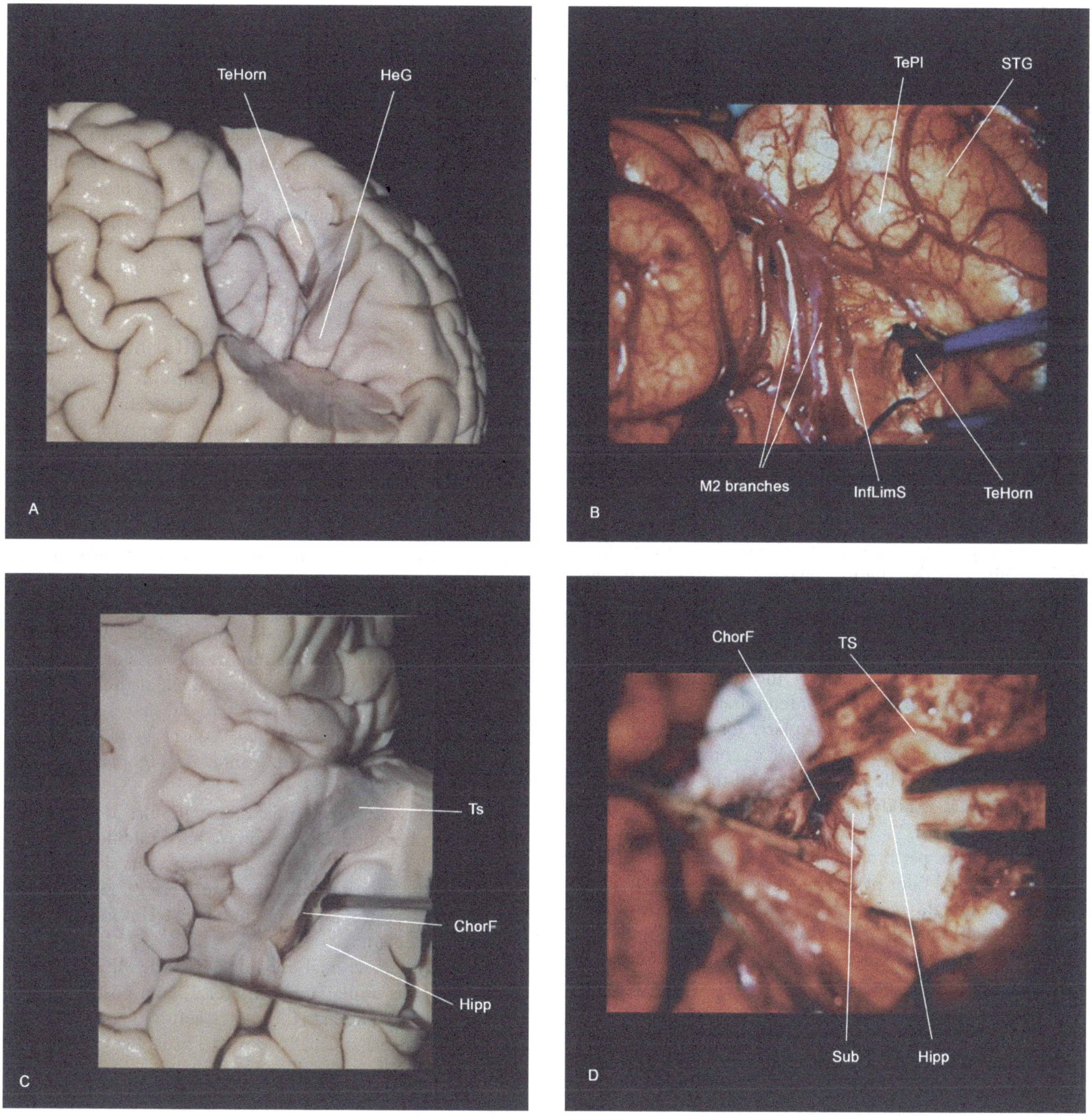

Figure 3.15 Exposure of the temporal horn through the transsylvian approach as seen from a pterional-transsylvian perspective (A) in an anatomical specimen after removal of the frontoparietal and temporal (superior temporal gyrus) operculi and (B) in an operative view after a wide opening of the Sylvian fissure: intraventricular exposure of the hippocampus and of the choroidal fissure medial to the subiculum (C) in an anatomical specimen after the removal of the neocortical structures (temporal gyri and temporal pole) and (D) in an transsylvian operative view.

ChorF: choroidal fissure; HeG: Heschl's gyrus; Hipp: hippocampus; InfLimS: inferior limiting sulcus; STG: superior temporal gyrus; Sub: subiculum; TeHorn: temporal horn; TePl: temporal plane; TS: temporal stem.

As a variation of the transsylvian route to the temporal horn, Vajkoczy *et al.* proposed a transsylvian transcisternal approach initiated by a wide opening of the Sylvian fissure, and with exposure and retraction of the temporal pole in order to reach the temporal horn through the rhinal sulcus. For these authors, the distance between the rhinal sulcus and the ventricular cavity was 17.9 ± 2.5 mm, and the amygdala and the hippocampus could be removed en bloc (Vajkoczy *et al.*, 1998).

The advantages of the transsylvian route to the temporal horn are its nearness to the ventricular cavity, and its possible navigation by more well-defined anatomical landmarks. Its disadvantages are having to open widely the Sylvian fissure, having to deal with vessels within the Sylvian fissure, and its limitation to expose the most posterior part of the temporal horn due to the natural limitations of the opening of the posterior aspect of the fissure.

More particularly, in cases of intrinsic tumors, if there is a need for more posterior resections of the hippocampus and parahippocampal gyrus, a complementary temporal lobectomy should be performed. Given the V-shaped format of the distal end of the Sylvian fissure, more posterior exposures require further removals along the superior temporal gyrus, and the extent of the temporal lobectomy depends mostly on the tumor extent.

A transsylvian temporal lobectomy with a variable posterior extent should be performed after exposure of the temporal horn and, preferably, before removal of the mesiobasal temporal structures since it significantly enhances their exposure. Once having the temporal horn unroofed and exposed, the dorsal (neocortical) temporal lobectomy can be started through an incision from the anterior aspect of the ventricular cavity toward the rhinal sulcus, followed by an incision along the lateral margin of the hippocampus vertically toward the middle fossa floor, and completed by a posterior and also vertical incision. The early temporal branch from the middle cerebral artery and the anterior and basal temporal veins should be coagulated and divided for the en bloc removal of the anterior portion of the temporal lobe. Once the temporal horn is fully exposed, the mesiobasal structures can be more easily removed as already described.

The wide opening of the Sylvian fissure exposes more particularly the inferior half of the insula and its inferior limiting sulcus which are covered by the temporal operculum, which corresponds to the superior temporal gyrus. It is important then to bear in mind, particularly for surgery involving intrinsic tumors, that the insular surface constitutes the external shield of the so-called central core of the brain and of its adjoining ventral pallidal-striatum or substantia innominata region (Figure 3.16).

The anterior perforated substance corresponds to the anterior wall and floor of the ventral pallidal-striatal or substantia innominata region, the anterior commissure to its posterior wall, and the fibers of the anterior limb of the internal capsule to its roof. The carotid artery bifurcation and the proximal segments of the anterior and middle cerebral arteries (A1 and M1 segments) lie underneath the anterior perforated substance and give rise to the lenticulostriate perforating arteries which run within the ventral pallidal-striatum region (Figure 3.17).

Basal Approaches

In order to spare the lateral aspect of the temporal lobe and avoid any damage to the optic radiations, some authors described subtemporal approaches to reach the temporal horn and the mesiobasal temporal structures. These approaches do avoid damage to the optic radiation but imply having to go round the base of the temporal lobe and are frequently limited by retraction of the vein of Labbé.

Park *et al.* proposed a subtemporal transparahippocampal exposure of the temporal horn retracting the anterior uncus superiorly, in order to perform a subsequent amygdalohippocampectomy (Park *et al.*, 1996). With the same aim but with the intent of avoiding the more voluminous and steep basal inclination of the anterior aspect of the temporal lobe into the middle fossa, Hori *et al.* proposed a more posterolateral subtemporal approach to the temporal horn, to be performed anteriorly to the vein of Labbé and through a 1.5 cm corticotomy of the fusiform gyrus (Hori *et al.*, 1993).

A more complex but ingenious basal approach to the mesiobasal temporal region, and hence to the temporal horn, is through the supracerebellar transtentorial route. This access was initially used by Voigt and Yasargil (1976), first described by Yonekawa *et al.* (2001), and more recently reviewed with further details (de Oliveira *et al.*, 2012; Türe *et al.*, 2012; Quesada, 2015).

3.2.3 Superior Frontal and Central Key Points

The superior frontal and central key points are, respectively 1) the Superior Frontal and Precentral Sulci Meeting Point (SFS/PreCS) and 2) the Superior Rolandic Point (SRP) (Ribas, 2005b; Ribas *et al.*, 2006).

3.2.3.1 The Superior Frontal and Precentral Sulci Meeting Point

Given its usual constancy, straightness, depth, and its reliable relationship with the underlying ventricular frontal horn, the superior frontal sulcus constitutes an important microneurosurgical corridor (Harkey *et al.*, 1989). Its posterior extremity, which usually joins or lies very close to the precentral sulcus, is an important key point which 1) delineates anteriorly the precentral gyrus at the level of the omega region which corresponds to the hand motor activation area (Boling *et al.*, 1999; Yousry *et al.*, 1995) and which 2) limits the superior frontal sulcus opening posteriorly (Figure 3.18A).

The Superior Frontal and Precentral Sulci Meeting Point (SFS/PreCS) lies about 2.5 to 3 cm from the midline (Harkey *et al.*, 1989; Ribas *et al.*, 2006) and anteriorly to its site, the SFS is parallel to the interhemispheric fissure (IHF) and is usually characterized as a continuous or almost continuous sulcus (Ribas *et al.*, 2006).

Regarding its cranial relationships, the SFS/PreCS lies underneath the cranial area centered 1.5 cm posterior to the bregma and 3 cm lateral to the sagittal suture (Figure 3.18B). In adults, the bregma is usually located 12 to 14 cm posterior to the nasion (Ribas, 2005b; Ribas *et al.*, 2006).

Considering its relationships along the level of the coronal plane, the SFS/PreCS constitutes an important microsurgical landmark both for the superior frontal transsulcal and for the interhemispheric transcallosal approaches to the ventricular cavity, once the SFS/PreCS key point was found to be always related coronally to the superior surface of the thalamus (Ribas, 2005b; Ribas *et al.*, 2006), hence with the floor of the lateral ventricle body (Rhoton, 2003), just behind the foramen of Monro (Figure 3.18C).

These findings are in accordance with text books and atlases (Krause, 1912; Pernkoff, 1980; Rhoton, 2003; Rhoton, 1999; Seeger, 1978; Seeger, 1995; Testut and Jacob, 1932; Yasargil *et al.*, 1988b); with previous studies (Ebeling *et al.*, 1987; Gusmão *et al.*, 2000; Rowland and Mettler, 1948; Yousry *et al.*, 1995) that relate the coronal suture with the precentral

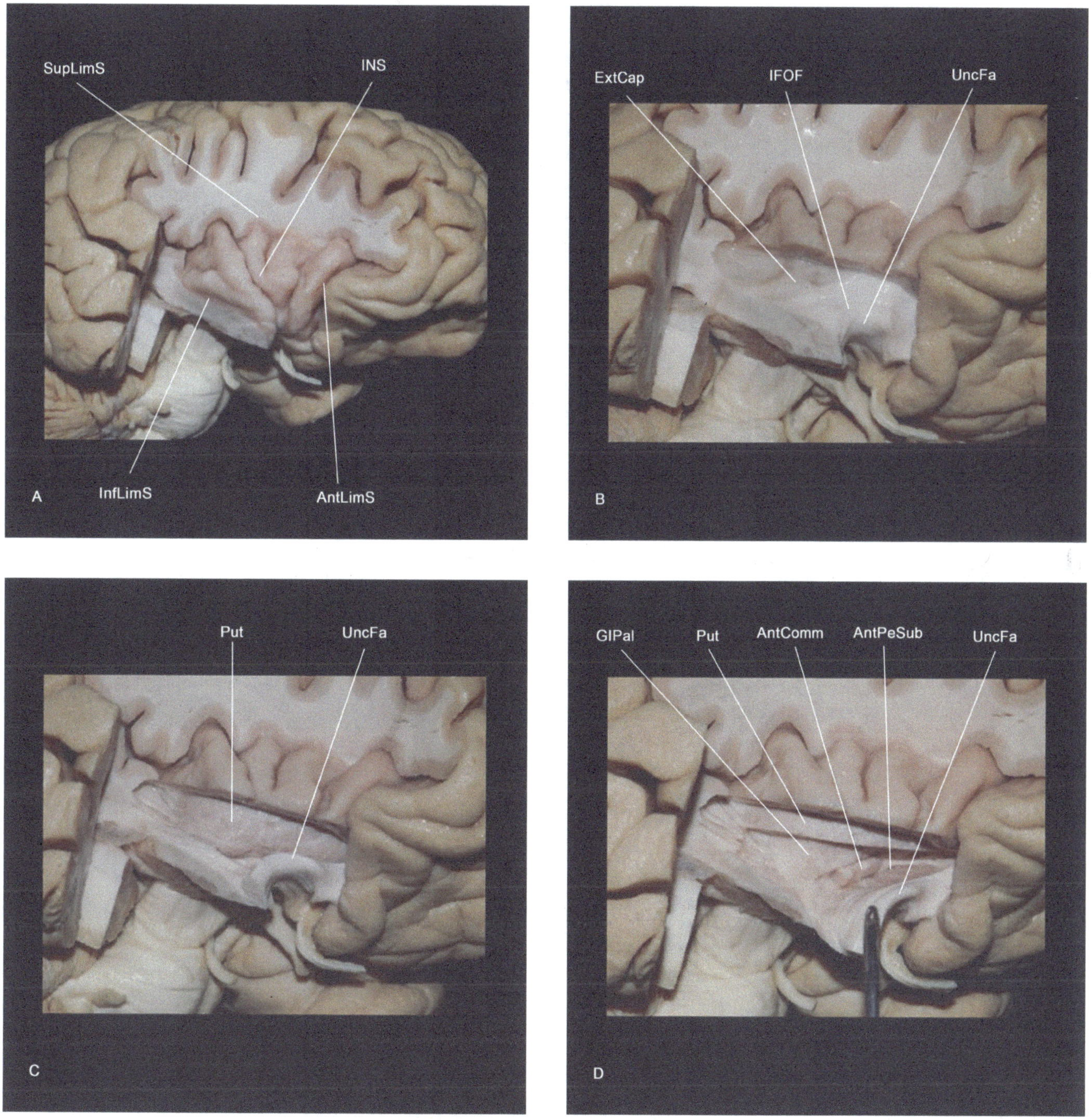

Figure 3.16 The sub-insular structures. (A) View of the lateral insular surface and of its superior, inferior and anterior limiting sulci, after the removal of the frontoparietal operculum, with the orbital part of the inferior frontal gyrus left, and of the whole temporal lobe; (B) view of the fibers of the inferior fronto-occipital fascicle, and of their contiguous fibers of the external capsule which cover the putamen, after the removal of the insular cortex and of the extreme capsule which corresponds to the insular surface white matter; (C) view of the putamen after the removal of the external capsule; (D) view of the globus pallidus underneath the putamen, and of the anterior commissure which runs along the channel of Gratiolet; (E) view of the fibers of the internal capsule after further removal of the putamen; and (F) with the removal of the internal capsule fibers, view of the head of the caudate and the accumbens nucleus within the ventral striatum region.

Acc: accumbens nucleus; AntComm: anterior commissure; AntLimS: anterior limiting sulcus of insula; AntPeSub: anterior perforated substance; ExtCap: external capsule fibers; GlPal: globus pallidus; HeCa: head of caudate nucleus; IFOF: inferior fronto-occipital (or occipito-frontal) fascicle fibers; InfLimS: inferior limiting sulcus; INS: insula; IntCap: internal capsule fibers; Put: putamen; SupLimS: superior limiting sulcus of insula; UncFa: uncinate fascicle fibers; VeStr(Acc): accumbens nucleus within the ventral striatum.

sulcus on the brain surface, and with the foramen of Monro along its coronal level (Apuzzo and Amar, 1988; Ehni and Ehni, 1988; Lavyne and Patterson, 1988; McComb, 1988; Pernkoff, 1980; Seeger, 1978; Shucart, 1988; Yasargil *et al.*, 1988b), and also with the studies of the topography of the hand motor activation area, done with both positron emission tomography (PET) and functional magnetic resonance imaging (fMRI) (Boling *et al.*, 1999; Yousry *et al.*, 1995).

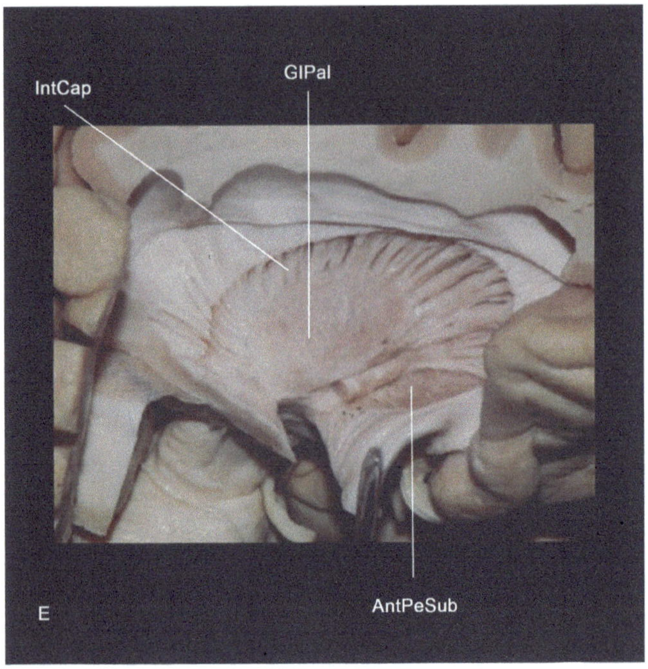

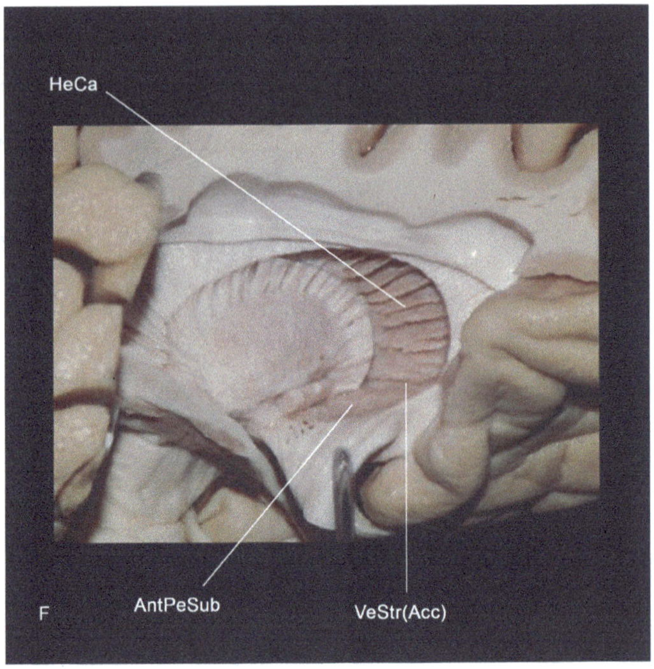

Figure 3.16 (Cont.)

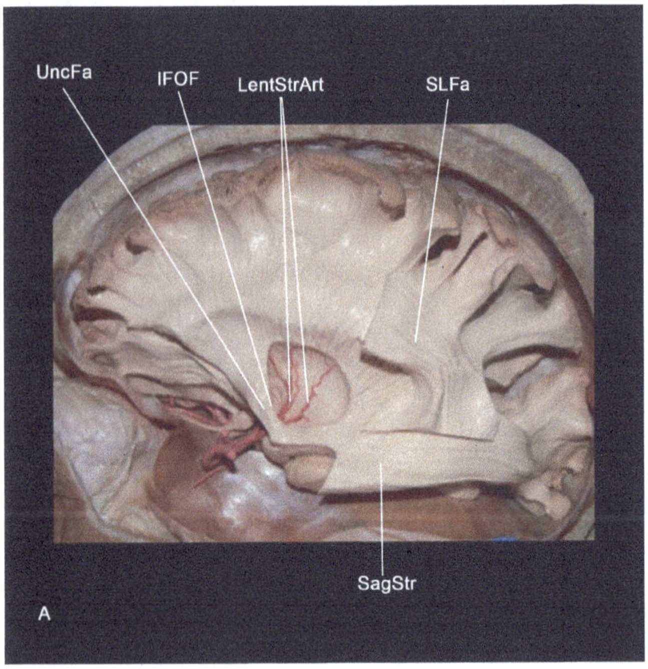

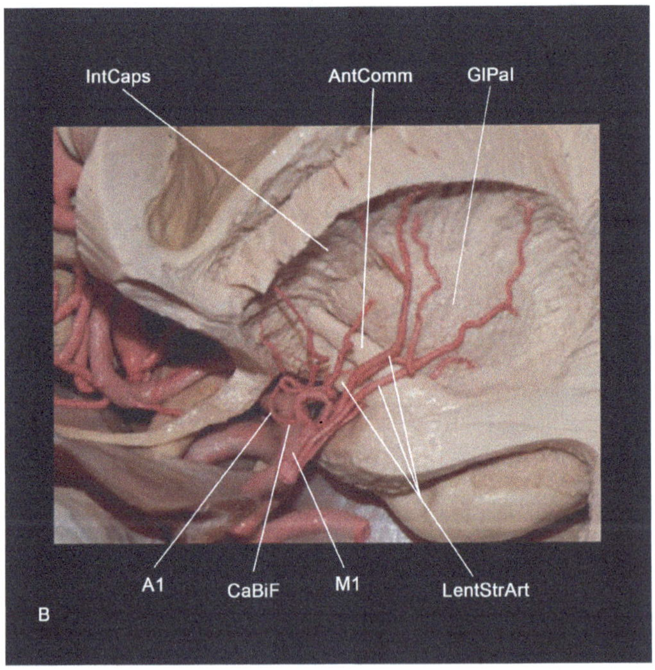

Figure 3.17 (A) and (B) Arteries within the ventral pallidal-striatum region.
A1: A1 segment of the anterior cerebral artery; AntComm: anterior commissure; CaBiF: carotid bifurcation; GlPal: globus pallidus; IFOF: inferior fronto-occipital (or occipito-frontal) fascicle fibers; IntCaps: internal capsule; LentStrArt: lenticulostriate arteries; M1: M1 segment of the middle cerebral artery; SagStr: sagittal stratum; SLFa: superior longitudinal fascicle; UncFa: uncinate fascicle fibers.

3.2.3.2 The Superior Rolandic Point

The superior extremity of the central sulcus (CS) is always located on the medial surface of each cerebral hemisphere, and its projection on the superior margin of the cerebral hemisphere, which corresponds to the intersection of the CS with the superior margin of the interhemispheric fissure (IHF), is usually designated as the Superior Rolandic point (SRP) (Taylor and Haughton, 1900 apud Uematsu *et al.*, 1992) (Figure 3.19A).

In relation to the skull surface, the SRP is located roughly 5 cm behind the bregma (Ribas *et al.*, 2006), in accordance with the classic studies of the nineteenth century done originally by

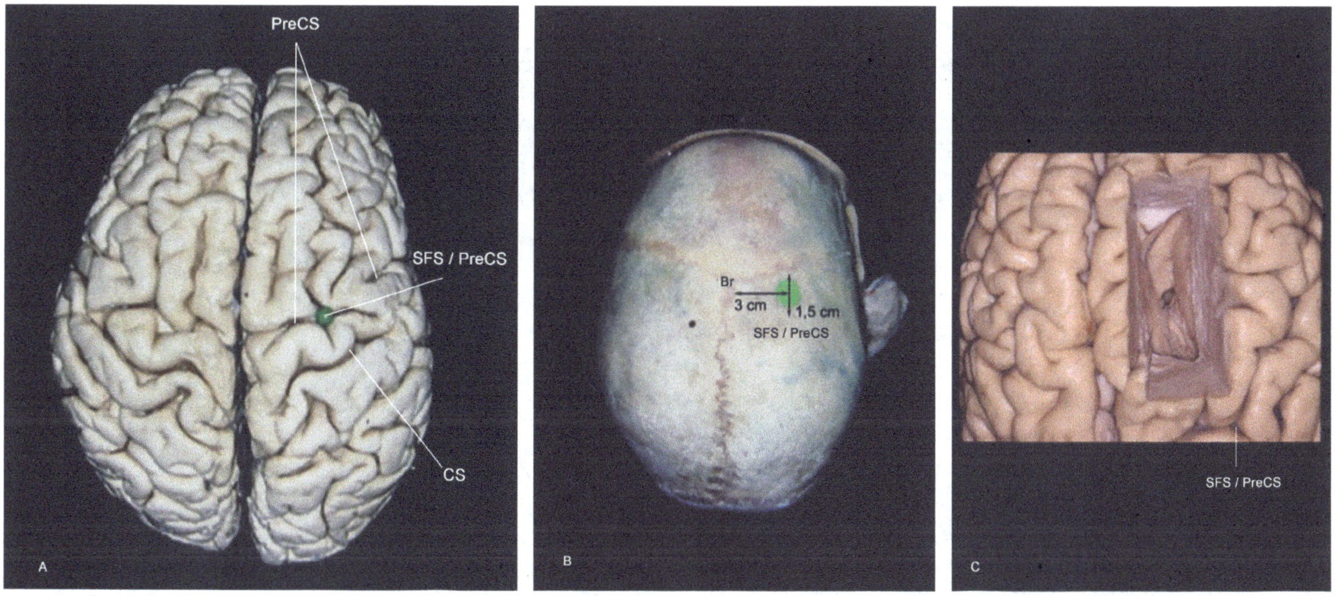

Figure 3.18 (A) Superior frontal and precentral sulci meeting point; (B) its corresponding cranial site: the superior frontal and precentral sulci meeting point (SFS/PreCS) is located underneath the cranial site situated 1.5 cm posterior to the coronal suture and 3 cm lateral to the sagittal suture, and (C) relationship of the superior frontal sulcus with the anterior horn and body of the lateral ventricle.
Br: bregma; CS: central sulcus; PreCS: precentral sulcus; SFS/PreCS: superior frontal and precentral sulci meeting point.

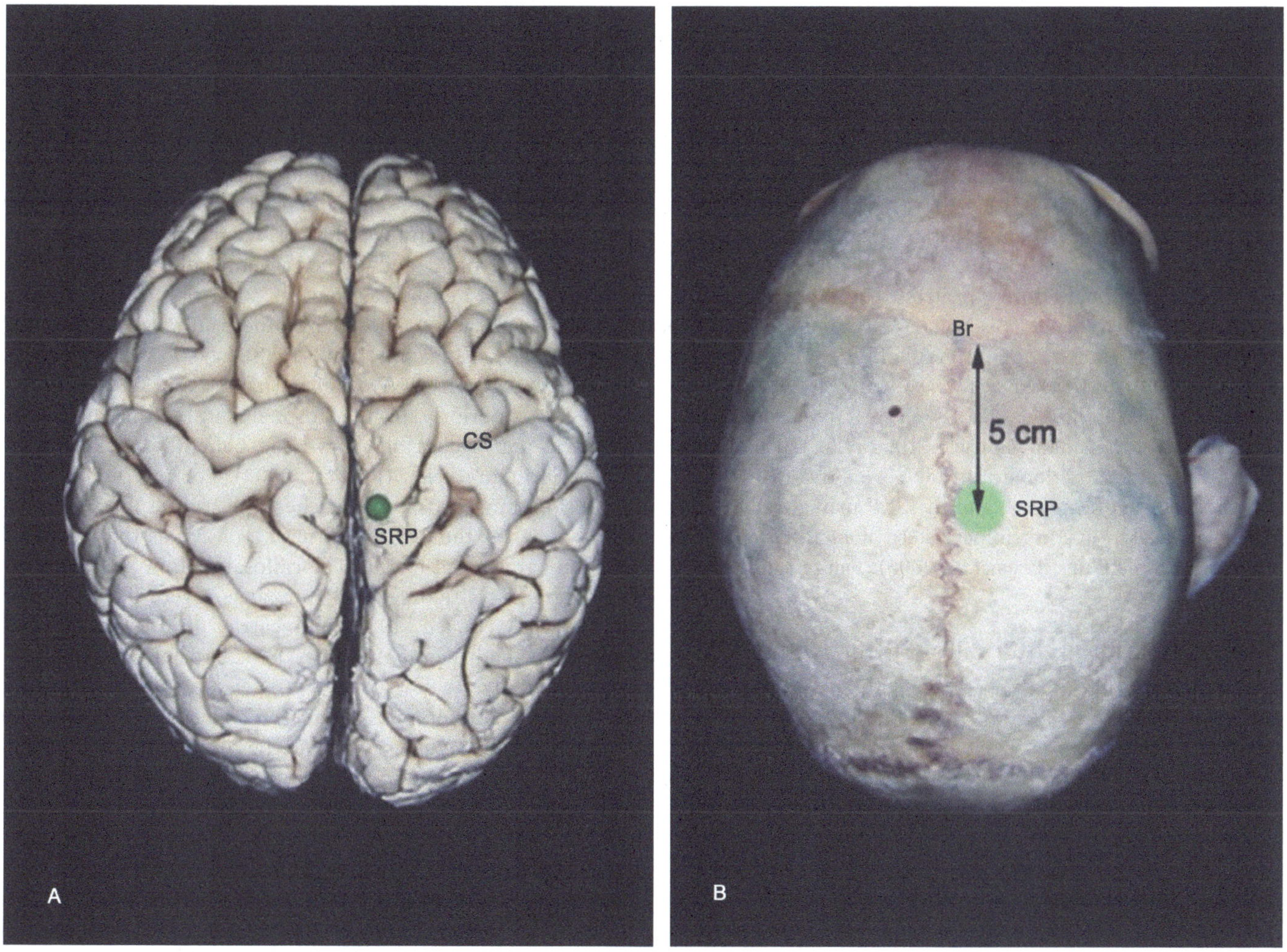

Figure 3.19 (A) The superior Rolandic point and (B) its corresponding cranial site: the superior Rolandic point corresponds to the intersection of the central sulcus (CS) and the interhemispheric fissure, and is located underneath the cranial site 5 cm posterior to the bregma.
Br: bregma; CS: central sulcus; SRP: superior Rolandic point.

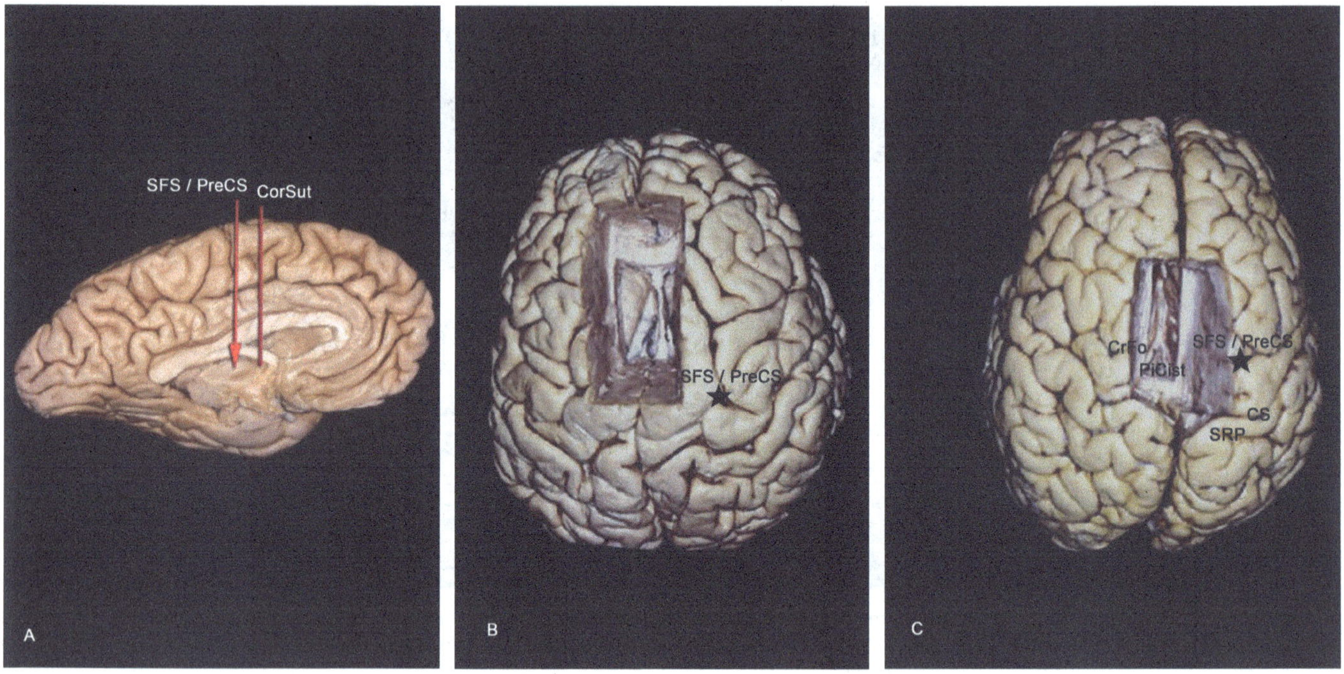

Figure 3.20 The superior frontal, the superior Rolandic point and the lateral ventricles. (A, B) While the coronal suture is related to the foramen of Monro and the coronal level of the superior frontal and precentral sulci meeting point is related to the body of the lateral ventricle; (C) the opening of the corpus callosum at the level of the superior Rolandic point may already lead to the subsplenial pineal or quadrigeminal cistern, posterior to the junction of both fornices.
CorSut: coronal suture; CrFo: crura of the fornix; CS: central sulcus; PiCist: pineal or quadrigeminal cistern; SFS/PreCS: superior frontal and precentral sulci meeting point; SRP: superior Rolandic point.

Broca (Gusmão *et al.*, 2000), Championnière (Testut and Jacob, 1932), Poirier (Testut and Jacob, 1932), Passet (Passet apud Ebeling *et al.*, 1987), Horsley (Horsley apud Ebeling *et al.*, 1987), and more recently Lang (Lang, 1985 apud Ebeling *et al.*, 1987) and Ebeling *et al.* (Ebeling *et al.*, 1987) (Figure 3.19B).

While the coronal suture is related to the foramen of Monro along its coronal plane (Bischoff, 1868 apud Broca, 1876; Ebeling and Steinmetz, 1995b; Pernkoff, 1980; Seeger, 1978; Shucart, 1988), and the SFS/PreCS is vertically related to the superior surface of the thalamus, which corresponds to the floor of the body of the lateral ventricle (Ribas *et al.*, 2006; Rhoton, 2003), the paracentral lobule already covers the atrium of the lateral ventricle off midline, and the SRP may already project over the pineal or quadrigeminal cistern along its coronal plan, through the splenium (Ribas *et al.*, 2006) (Figure 3.20).

3.2.4 Superior Frontal and Central Craniotomies

Given their relationships particularly with important eloquent motor cortical areas and also with the anterior ventricular cavities, both the superior frontal and precentral sulci meeting point (SFS/PreCS) and the superior Rolandic point (SRP) are landmarks that can be helpful for exposure of frontal lobar and anterior ventricular lesions.

In the cortical surface, the SFS/PreCS lies immediately anteriorly to the hand motor activation area (Boling *et al.*, 1999; Yousry *et al.*, 1995), and with regard to its deep relationships, it is particularly related to the floor of the lateral ventricle which is constituted by the superior thalamic surface.

Its corresponding cranial site, which is given by a 2 cm area around the cranial point located 1 cm posterior to the coronal suture and 3 cm lateral to the sagittal suture, can be particularly useful for the correct positioning of craniotomies for frontal and anterior ventricular lesions, which should then be predominantly anterior to the coronal suture as already proposed by other authors (Apuzzo and Amar, 1988; Ehni and Ehni, 1988; Lavyne and Patterson, 1988; Shucart, 1988; Yasargil *et al.*, 1988a; Yasargil *et al.*, 1988b). Anteriorly to the coronal suture, the interhemispheric approaches also have the benefit of dealing with fewer bridging veins (Rhoton, 2003). For interhemispheric anterior transcallosal approaches, the frontal mesial retraction as far as the SFS/PreCS level still avoids the retraction of the paracentral lobule. The callosal section posteriorly to the paracentral lobule level can cause severe disconnection syndromes (Bogen, 1988) and carries the risk of leading into the quadrigeminal cistern, hence posterior to the ventricular body.

Frontal craniotomies for mesial exposure of the anterior aspects of the cingulate gyrus and the corpus callosum, including the most common site of pericallosal aneurysms, may require craniotomies with greater anterior extent.

Central craniotomies for exposure of the pre- and postcentral gyri, the mesial paracentral lobule, and parts of the cingulate gyrus and corpus callosum that are inferior to the paracentral lobule, should be based both in the SFS/PreC key point and in the superior Rolandic point (SRP) that lie underneath the bony area located approximately 5 cm behind the bregma. These craniotomies should then be predominantly posterior to the coronal suture.

In relation to possible surgical neurological impairments pertinent to central craniotomies, besides the evident motor deficits related to damage to the precentral gyrus (Brodal, 1981; Penfield and Rasmussen, 1950b; Penfield and Boldrey apud Brodal, 1981), resections of the postcentral gyrus can cause persistent arm and leg sensory abnormalities such as astereognosis (Hansebout, 1982; Penfield and Rasmussen, 1950b; Rasmussen and Milner, 1975 apud Hansebout, 1982).

3.2.4.1 Anatomical Remarks Pertinent to Common Frontal Transcerebral Procedures

The generally consistent anatomical features of the superior frontal sulcus (SFS) already mentioned make it an important microneurosurgical corridor or landmark particularly for the removal of common tumors of the superior frontal gyrus and supplementary motor area (SMA) (Duffau, 2011a), of the middle frontal gyrus, and for transcerebral approaches to the frontal horn and body of the lateral ventricle.

The frontal interhemispheric approach provides exposure of the medial aspects of the superior frontal and cingulate gyri, and of the callosal cistern which harbors both pericallosal arteries. From this exposure, opening of the corpus callosum provides access to the front and body of the lateral ventricle since the cavities are just next to the midline, and from the lateral ventricle, the third ventricle can then be entered through the foramen of Monro, or through a transchoroidal (Wen *et al.*, 1998), subchoroidal (Lavyne and Patterson, 1988), or interforniceal (Apuzzo and Amar, 1988) route as discussed later.

Exposure of the Superior Frontal Gyrus and Sulcus, and of the Interhemispheric Fissure

For all these approaches, the patient should be set preferably straight, with some degree of neck flexion and head elevation, and a coronal incision or a laterally based U flap should be made. Alternatively, the patient can also be laid laterally positioning the head with the midline oriented horizontally and having the side to be approached on the bottom in order to allow gravity to optimize the interhemispheric exposure (Lawton *et al.*, 1996).

Regarding the craniotomy placement, a few very important anatomical features should be considered:

1) The meeting point of the superior frontal sulcus with the precentral sulcus, hence the anterior aspect of the precentral gyrus, is located approximately 3 cm lateral to the sagittal suture and 2 cm posterior to the coronal suture (Ribas *et al.*, 2006).
2) The central sulcus reaches the midline (superior Rolandic point) about 5 cm posterior to the bregma (Gusmão *et al.*, 2000; Broca, 1876b; Ribas *et al.*, 2006).
3) The lesion should always be understood in relation to the coronal suture, which is known to be related to the interventricular foramina of Monro along the coronal plane of its midline point (Krause, 1912; Pernkoff, 1980; Rhoton, 2003; Rhoton, 1999; Seeger, 1978; Seeger, 1995; Testut and Jacob, 1932; Ebeling *et al.*, 1987; Rowland and Mettler, 1948; Yousry *et al.*, 1995; Apuzzo, 1988; Ehni and Ehni, 1988; Lavyne and Patterson, 1988; Shucart, 1988; Yasargil *et al.*, 1988b), and which transects the corpus callosum just anteriorly to its half length.
4) The cortical veins which drain into the superior sagittal sinus are more numerous and more relevant over the central area (Rhoton, 2003), hence from 2 cm posteriorly to the coronal suture (Ribas *et al.*, 2006).
5) The craniotomy should always expose the superior sagittal sinus to allow comfortable interhemispheric handling; a bony bar of only 1 cm covering the sinus will be covering almost half of the superior frontal gyrus longitudinally.
6) A rather extensive dissection of the interhemispheric fissure along the midline, always preserving the central draining veins, enlarges the surgical exposure and facilitates any surgical maneuver.

It is essential to bear in mind that a transcallosal approach more than 2 cm posteriorly to the coronal suture would require dealing with central veins, retraction of the paracentral lobule, and, since the atriums are away from and lateral to the midline, a more posteriorly callosal opening implies the risk of reaching the pineal cistern and not the ventricular cavity (Ribas *et al.*, 2006). From its posterior end point along the midline, the splenium opens laterally and posteriorly in order to cover and encircle both atriums and occipital horns.

The placement of craniotomies to reach lesions related to the medial aspects of the superior frontal and cingulate gyri, and vascular lesions of the callosomarginal and pericallosal arteries, should also be based on their relationships with the coronal suture, with the genu of the corpus callosum, and with the ventricular cavities.

Since the medial surface of the superior frontal gyrus faces the falx, this cortical surface (superior frontal gyrus) can be easily separated from this dural surface (falx), but both cingulate gyri can be more firmly attached to each other along the inferior margin of the falx, requiring careful separation in order to preserve their pial surfaces. The corpus callosum is easily recognized due to its glistening white color and tiny vessels. While the more superior callosomarginal artery usually runs firmly attached to the pial surface along the cingulate sulcus, both pericallosal arteries run along the corpus callosum cistern (Figures 3.21, 3.22 and 3.23). Koutsarnakis *et al.* studied the sulcal and the subcortical anatomy related to the superior frontal sulcus (SFS), and found that the 5 cms of the SFS immediately anterior to the Precentral Sulcus always overlie the body and the anterior horn of the lateral ventricle, with the distance from the fundus of the sulcus to the ventricular cavity varying from 1.3 to 2.5 cm fibers between its fundus and the ventricle. These authors identified five white matter layers: 1) Arcuate fibers which connect adjacent cortical areas. 2) Fibers of the frontal Asland tract which connect the posterior part of the superior frontal gyrus with the pars opercularis of the inferior frontal gyrus. 3) Fibers of the

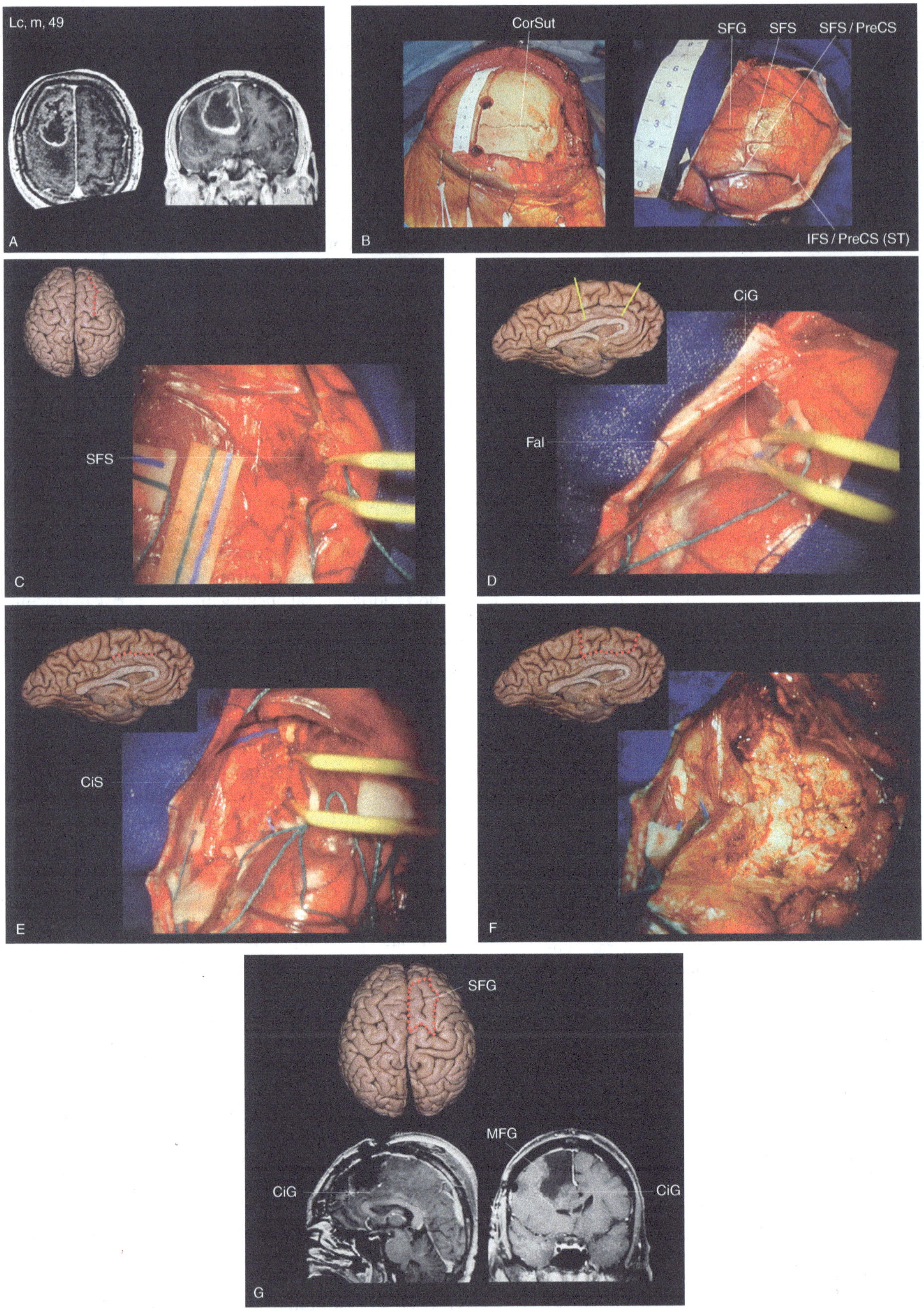

Figure 3.21 Sulcal to sulcal resection of a high grade glioma of the right superior frontal gyrus. (A) MR images of the tumor occupying the superior frontal gyrus; (B) the superior frontal/precentral sulci meeting point which is the posterior limit of the resection, craniotomy extending 2 to 3 cm posteriorly to the coronal suture in order to expose the precentral sulcus; operative view and identification of the main anatomical landmarks; (C) opening of the superior frontal sulcus; (D) identification of the cingulate gyrus within the interhemispheric fissure; (E) opening of the cingulate sulcus; (F) cavity after en bloc removal of the superior frontal gyrus containing the tumor; (G) postoperative MR images.

CiG: cingulate gyrus; CiS: cingulate sulcus; CorSut: coronal suture; Fal: falx; IFS/PreCS(ST): inferior frontal and precentral sulci meeting point underneath the stephanion; ST: stephanion (meeting point of the coronal suture and superior temporal line); MFG: middle frontal gyrus; SFG: superior frontal gyrus; SFS/PreCS: superior frontal and precentral sulci meeting point; SFS: superior frontal sulcus.

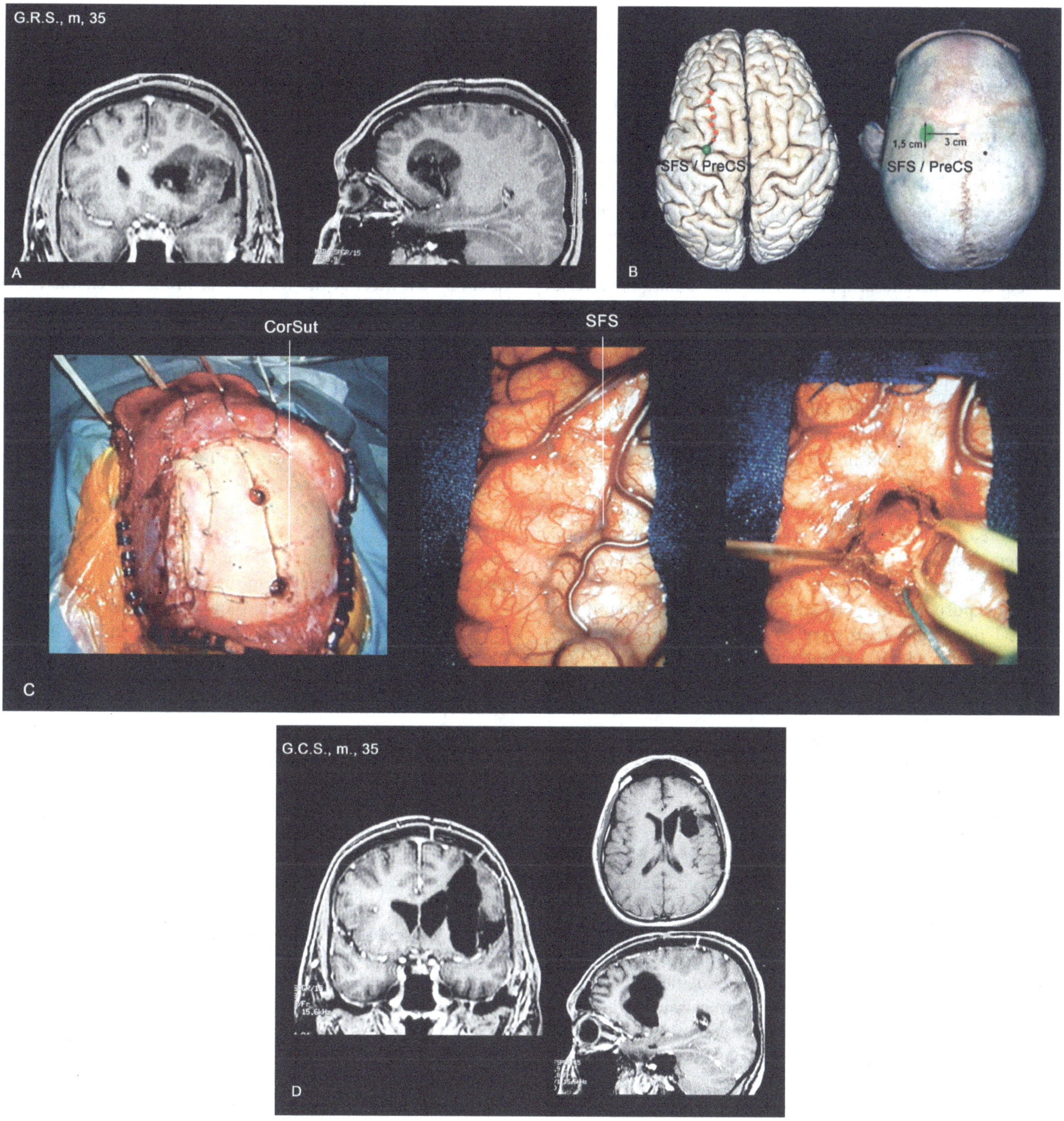

Figure 3.22 Transsulcal (superior frontal sulcus) resection of the residual mass of a left insular low glioma previously operated through the Sylvian fissure. (A) MR images; (B) the superior frontal sulcus and its meeting point with the precentral sulcus; (C) craniotomy extending 2 to 3 cm posteriorly to the coronal suture, identification and opening of the posterior aspect of the superior frontal sulcus for the transsulcal resection; (D) postoperative MR images.
CorSut: coronal suture; SFS: superior frontal sulcus; SFS/PreCS: superior frontal and precentral sulci meeting point.

external capsule. 4) Fibers of the anterior limb of the internal capsule. 5) Callosal fibers which intermingle with the fibers of the internal capsule and which lie over the thin layer of ependyma. These authors found that the horizontal fibers of the superior longitudinal fascicle were always running lateral to the SFS at the level of the middle frontal gyrus, and considered the SFS route towards the ventricle a safe approach (Koutsarnakis *et al.*, 2017).

Transcallosal Approaches to the Lateral Ventricles

Since the foramina of Monro constitute the limit between the frontal and the body of each lateral ventricle which are immediately next to the midline, while the frontal horns are then located just anteriorly to the coronal suture plane, the bodies of the lateral ventricle are situated just posteriorly to the coronal suture plane. Nevertheless, for their correct exposure and protection of the central veins and of the paracentral lobule, the craniotomy should always extend two-thirds anteriorly and one-third posteriorly to the coronal suture (until 2 cm posteriorly to the coronal suture), and the superior sagittal sinus has to be unroofed to allow a proper interhemispheric approach as already previously discussed (Figure 3.24).

For the transcallosal approach, the callosomarginal arteries (which usually run along and close to the cingulate sulcus) should be left intact underneath the arachnoid, and the pericallosal arteries (which run along the callosal cistern) should be dissected and mobilized along their lengths as much as possible. This is to avoid their kinking and their possible tearing during further retractions. Perpendicular small branches should also not be left under tension, and should be divided if necessary.

The glistening and very white corpus callosum can be opened either between both pericallosal arteries, or with both of them displaced medially, which may protect them during posterior lateral brain retractions.

For exposure of the body and frontal horn, the longitudinal callosal opening should have its center at the level of the coronal suture, which corresponds to the interventricular foramen of Monro, and preferably should not exceed more than 2 cm. As already stressed, since the atriums are off midline and already posterior to both thalami, a more posterior callosotomy implies the risk of reaching the pineal cistern and not the ventricular cavity (Ribas *et al.*, 2006).

Just before reaching the ventricle through a callosotomy, the ependyma can be recognized by its darker and purple color.

The identification of the choroid plexus indicates that the body of the lateral ventricle has been entered, once there is no choroid plexus in the frontal horn. The choroid plexus runs along the choroidal fissure separating the fornix medially from the thalamus laterally, and is attached to these two neural structures, respectively, by the taenia fornicis and by the taenia choroidea which are very thin membranes and extensions of the ependyma that cover the choroid plexus.

After the necessary enlargement of the callosotomy, the anatomy of the ventricular body should be identified: the choroid plexus with the fornix medially and the superior surface of the thalamus laterally to it, the white, and at this level short, septum pellucidum in the midline sagittal plane with its base attached to the dorsal aspect of the ipsilateral fornix, the body of the caudate nucleus as the lateral wall of this ventricular portion, and the thalamostriate vein running between the caudate and the superior thalamic surface.

Regarding the important venous anatomy in this region, which helps to orient the neurosurgeon, the thalamostriate vein is the most developed vein of the lateral ventricle, and it runs from posterior to anterior and from lateral to medial along the striothalamic sulcus over the stria terminalis toward the intraventricular foramen of Monro. It is covered by ependyma until it pierces the inferior membrane of the tela choroidea to join the ipsilateral internal cerebral vein already within the velum interpositum cistern, adjacent to the foramen of Monro. The anterior septal vein runs along the septum pellucidum in the midline, from anteriorly to posteriorly, in order to also join the ipsilateral internal cerebral vein usually just next to the thalamostriate vein, with these three veins constituting the so-called venous angle (Taveras and Wood, 1976). When the thalamostriate, anterior septal and internal cerebral vein meet at the foramen of Monro, it characterizes the true venous angle, and when thalamostriate vein enters the choroidal fissure and the velum interpositum posteriorly to the foramen of Monro, the venous configuration is known as the false venous angle (Taveras and Wood, 1976).

The correct identification of the venous pattern indicates if the ipsilateral or contralateral ventricle has been entered, with the striothalamic vein being always lateral when approaching the ipsilateral ventricle.

Anterior and posterior caudate veins, and other subependymal superior thalamic veins which also run through the choroidal fissure to drain into the internal cerebral vein, can also be identified in the body of the lateral ventricle.

Anteriorly to the foramen of Monro lies the frontal horn, with the largest area of the septum containing the septal vein as its medial wall, the bulging head of the caudate as its lateral wall, and the rostrum and genu of the corpus callosum, respectively, as its floor and anterior wall.

If more lateral room is necessary, the exposure can be increased laterally with a partial removal of the medial aspect of the cingulate gyrus and of the underlying corpus callosum, preferably with both pericallosal arteries already previously displaced medially (Figures 3.25 and 3.26).

Transcallosal Approaches to the Third Ventricle

Once having reached the lateral ventricle through a midline transcallosal or through a transcortical route, the third ventricle can then be entered through its roof in many different ways (Apuzzo, 1988), but the approaches that are more frequently used for exposure of the anterior two-thirds of its cavity are the transforaminal, the subchoroidal (Hirsh *et al.*, 1979; Delandsheer *et al.*, 1978; Lavyne and Patterson, 1983), the transchoroidal (Wen *et al.*, 1998), and the interforniceal approach (Apuzzo, 1988). All of these approaches reach the cavity of the third ventricle through the velum interpositum, and should preferably be done through the right side. Nevertheless, given the anatomical complexity of the neural and vascular structures related to these approaches and their variants, some anatomical issues should be emphasized for a better understanding.

Once inside the lateral ventricle, the identification of the choroid plexus and the understanding of the venous pattern should initially lead to the crucial conclusion whether the ipsilateral or the contralateral ventricle has been entered, as discussed in the previous section. Once certainly inside the

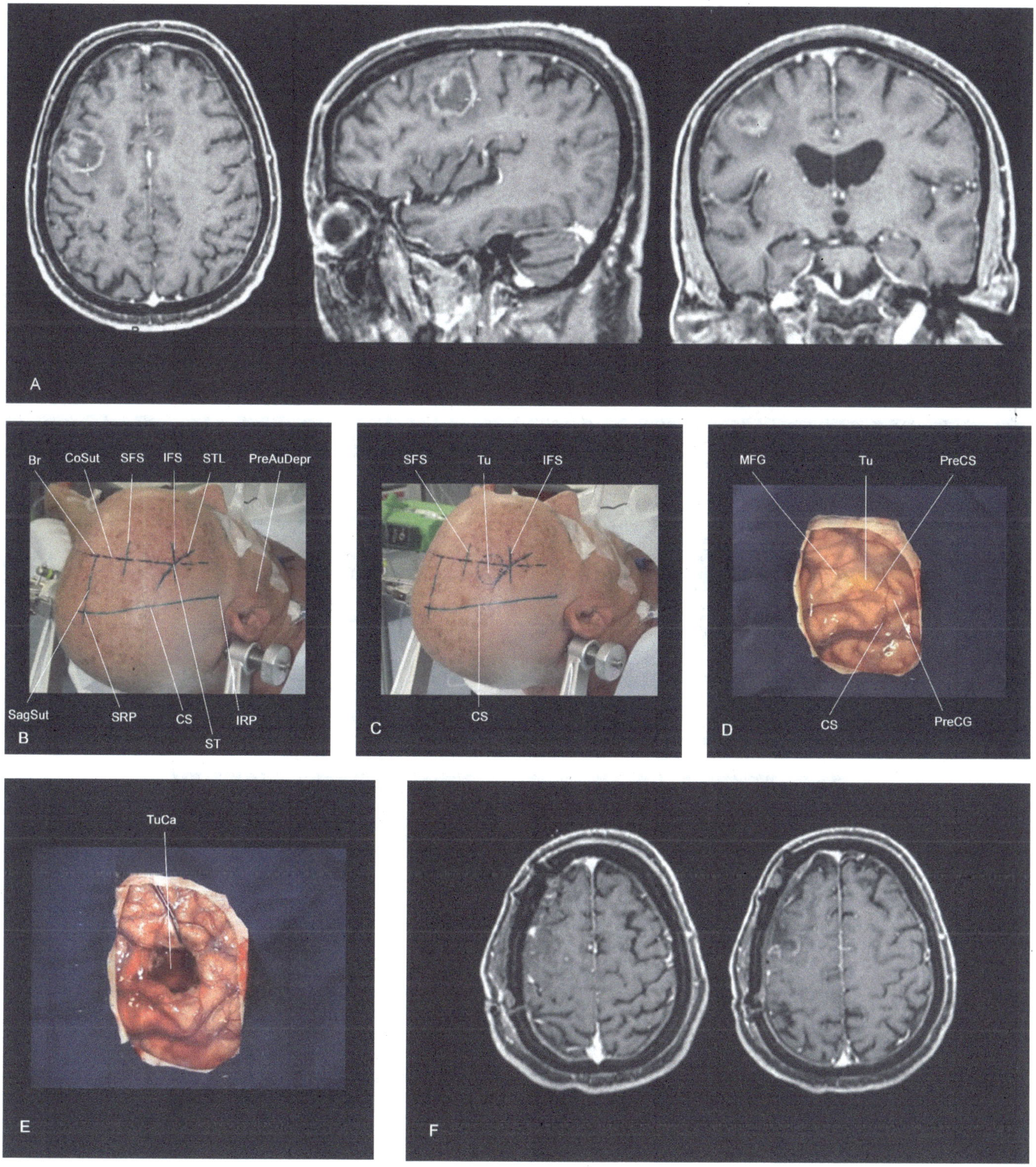

Figure 3.23 Resection of a high grade glioma located in the right middle frontal gyrus just anteriorly to the precentral sulcus. (A) Preoperative MR images; (B) main frontal anatomical landmarks and their related sulci: the central sulcus between the superior Rolandic point (located 5 cm posterior to the bregma) and the inferior Rolandic point (4 cm superior to the preauricular depression), the superior frontal sulcus which runs 2 to 3 cm lateral to the sagittal suture, the most posterior aspect of the inferior frontal sulcus underneath the stephanion (meeting point of the coronal suture with the superior temporal line); (C) location of the tumor in the posterior aspect of the right middle frontal gyrus; (D) exposure of the brain surface and identification of the sulci and gyri; (E) tumor cavity after the resection; (F) postoperative MR images.

Br: bregma; CoSut: coronal suture; CS: central sulcus; IFS: inferior frontal sulcus; IRP: inferior Rolandic point; MFG: middle frontal gyrus; PreAuDepr: preauricular depression; PreCG: precentral gyrus; PreCS: precentral sulcus; SagSut: sagittal suture; SFS: superior frontal sulcus; SRP: superior Rolandic point; ST: stephanion (meeting point of the coronal suture and superior temporal line); STL: superior temporal line; Tu: tumor; TuCa: tumor cavity.

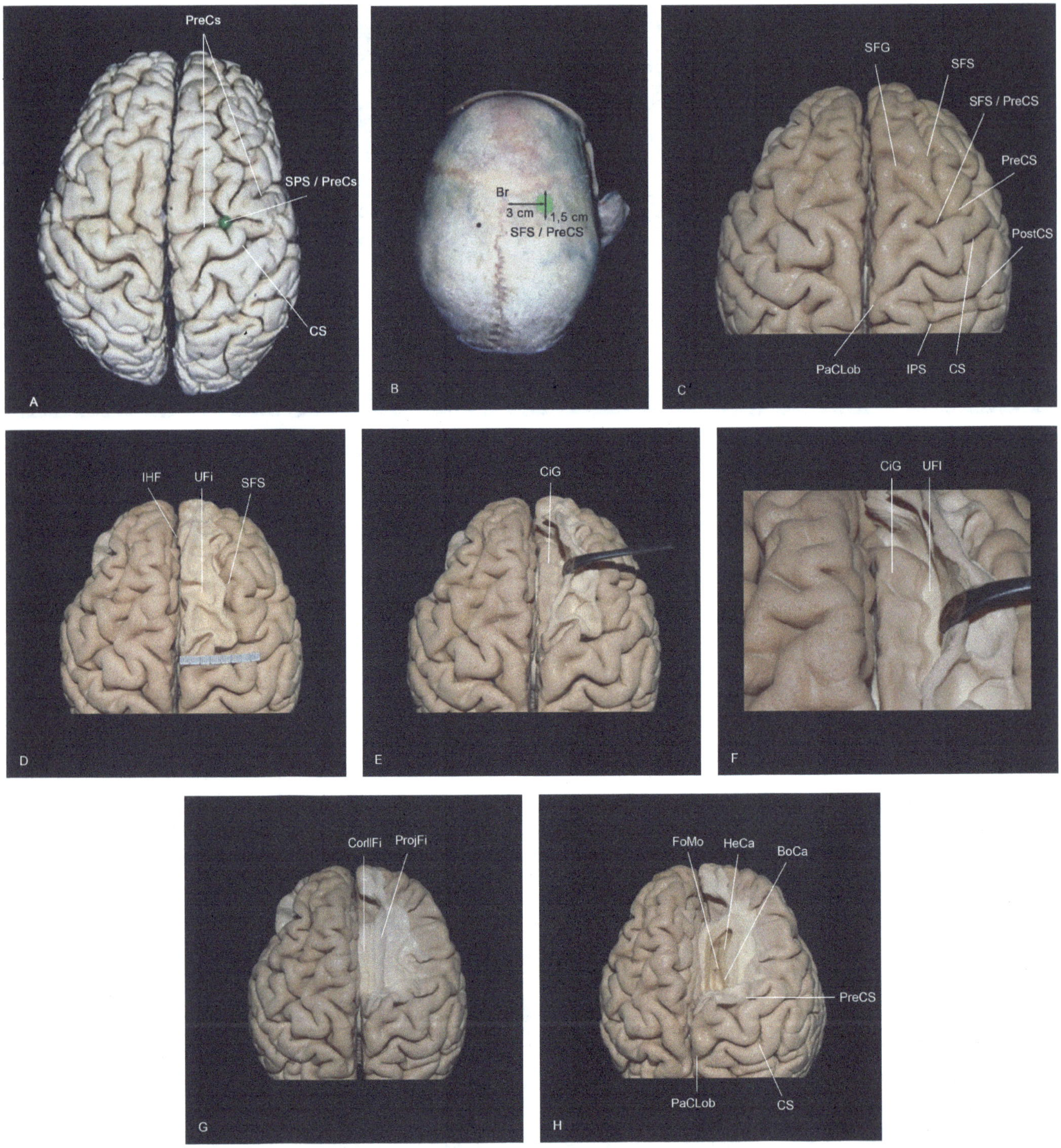

Figure 3.24 The superior frontal gyrus, its underlying white matter fibers, and the lateral ventricle. (A) The superior frontal and precentral sulci meeting point; (B) its corresponding cranial site; (C) the main sulci and gyri landmarks; (D) subcortical U-fibers seen after the removal of the superior frontal gyrus cortex; (E) superior surface of the cingulate gyrus within the cingulate sulcus; (F) U-fibers arising from the cingulate gyrus; (G) callosal and projection fibers seen after the removal of the cingulate gyrus; (H) view of the anterior horn and body of the lateral ventricle underneath the superior frontal gyrus and anteriorly to the paracentral lobule.

BoCa: body of the caudate nucleus; CallFi: callosal fibers; CiG: cingulate gyrus; CiS: cingulate sulcus; CS: central sulcus; FoMo: foramen of Monro; HeCa: head of caudate nucleus; IHF: interhemispheric fissure; IPS: intraparietal sulcus; PaCLob: paracentral lobule; PostCS: postcentral sulcus; PreCS: precentral sulcus; ProjFi: projection fibers; SFG: superior frontal gyrus; SFS/PreCS: superior frontal and precentral sulci meeting point; SFS: superior frontal sulcus; UFi: U fibers.

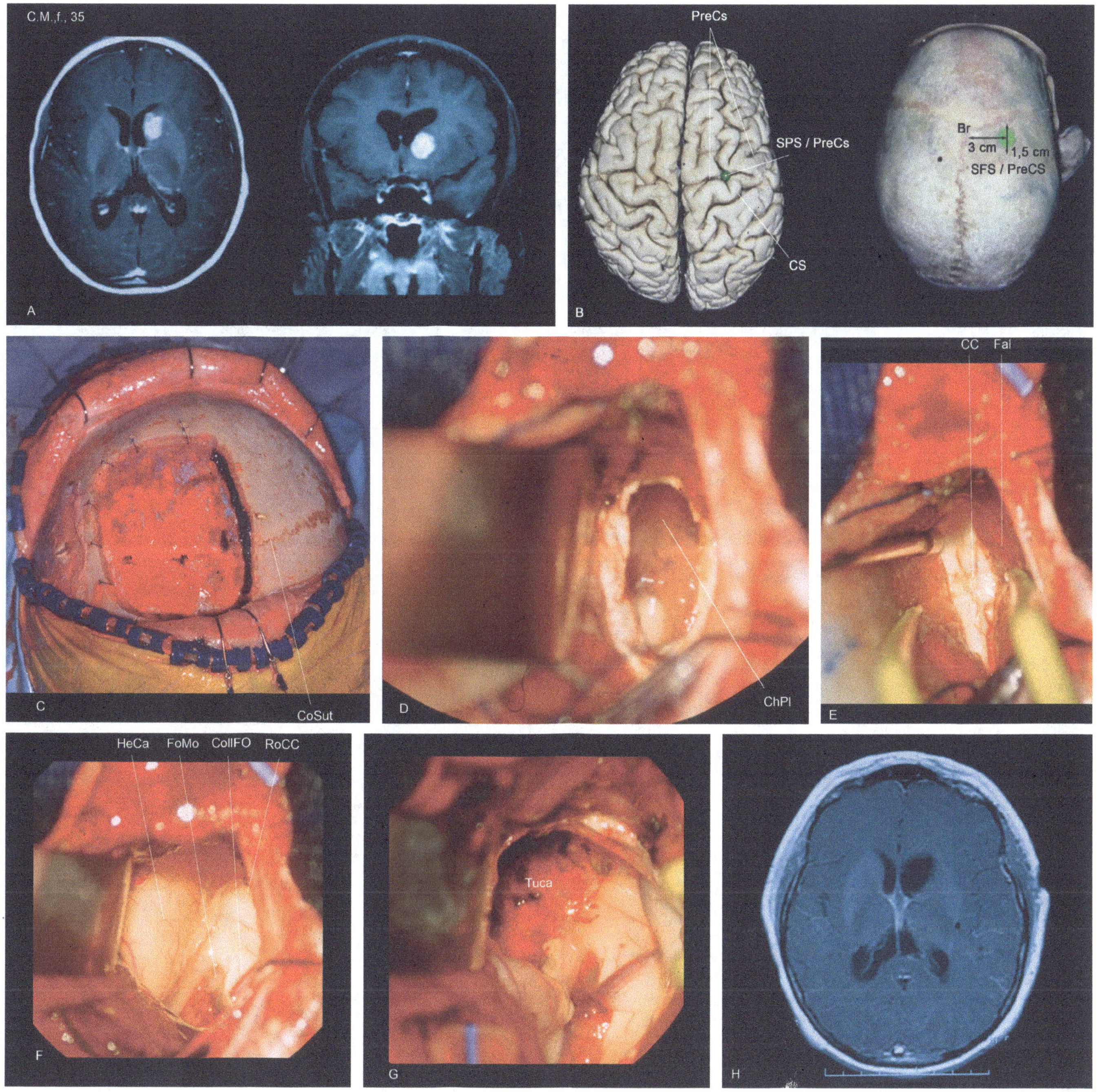

Figure 3.25 Resection of a left head of the caudate nucleus breast cancer metastasis. (A) MR images; (B) the superior frontal and precentral sulci meeting point and its corresponding cranial site: limit of the brain retraction in order not to retract the paracentral lobule; (C) craniotomy extending only until 2 to 3 cm posteriorly to the coronal suture; (D) exposure of the corpus callosum; (E) exposure of the choroid plexus, indicating entrance inside the body of the left lateral ventricle; (F) repositioning of the spatula and exposure of the left anterior horn with the head of the caudate as its lateral wall, the rostrum of the corpus callosum as its floor, and with the column of the fornix constituting the anterior margin of the foramen of Monro; (G) view of the tumor cavity after resection of the lesion; (H) postoperative MR image.

Br: bregma; CC: corpus callosum; ChPl: choroid plexus over the thalamus; CollFo: column of the fornix; CoSut: coronal suture; CS: central sulcus; Fal: falx; FoMo: foramen of Monro; HeCa: head of caudate nucleus; PreCS: precentral sulcus; RoCC: rostrum of the corpus callosum; SFS/PreCS: superior frontal and precentral sulci meeting point; TuCa: tumor cavity.

ipsilateral ventricular body, with the striothalamic vein laterally, attention should be directed to the interventricular foramen of Monro and to the choroid plexus, having particularly in mind that the body of the fornix lies medially to the choroid plexus, the superior surface of the thalamus lies laterally to the choroid plexus, and the choroidal fissure runs underneath the choroid plexus (Figure 3.27).

The roof of the third ventricle, which extends from both interventricular foramina anteriorly to the pineal recess posteriorly, is comprised of five layers: an upper

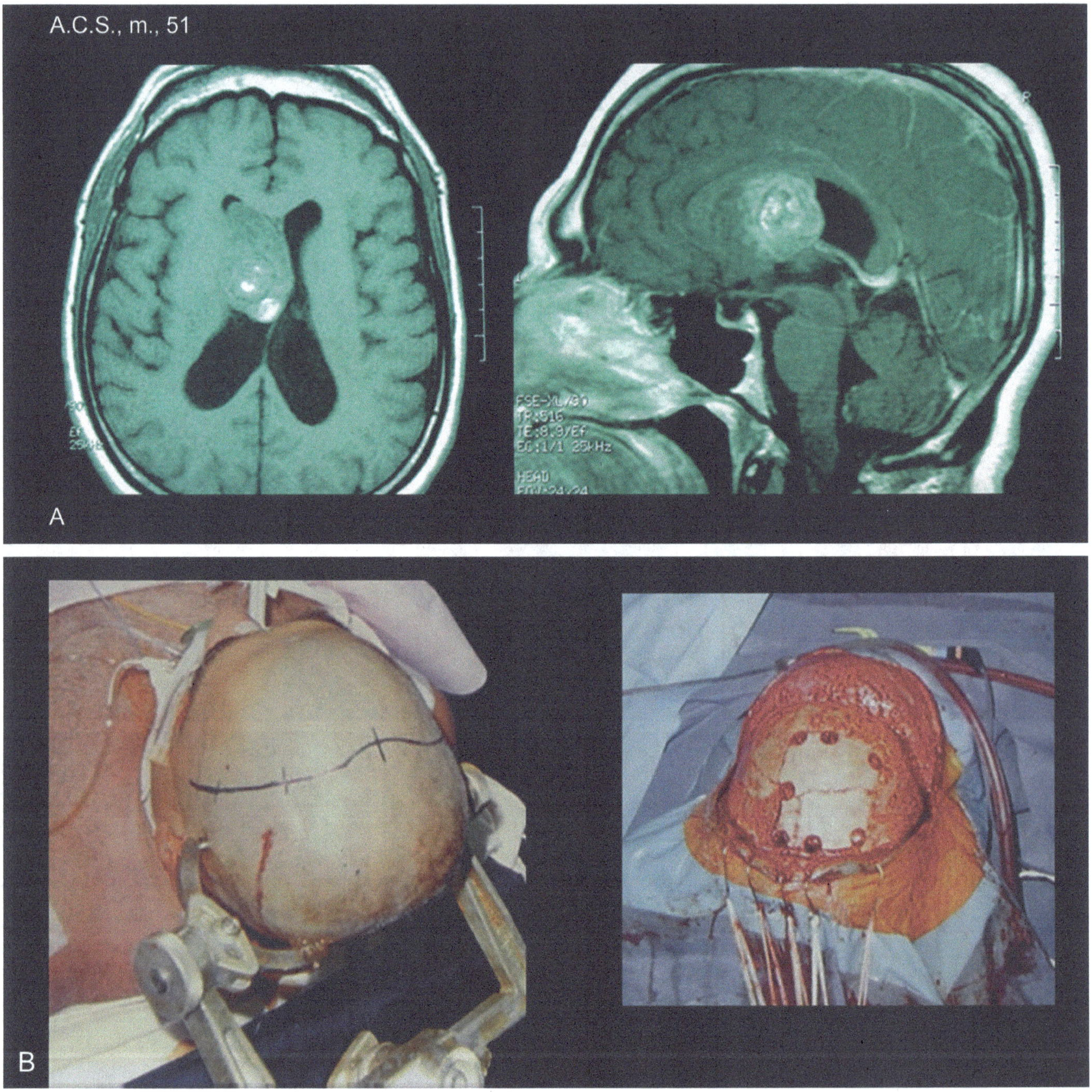

Figure 3.26 Resection of a subependymoma of the body of the right lateral ventricle. (A) MR images; (B) incision and craniotomy extending 2 to 3 cm posteriorly to the coronal suture in order to avoid retraction of the paracentral lobule and frequent cortical central veins; (C) view of the right superior frontal gyrus and of a prominent cortical vein apparently running along the precentral sulcus which is usual; (D) exposure of the corpus callosum with brain retraction being done just anteriorly to the paracentral lobule; (E) opening of the corpus callosum and view of the tumor; (F) view of the floor of the right ventricle after tumor removal, as expected with a mesial frontal retraction done predominantly posteriorly to the coronal suture which is related to the foramen of Monro along its coronal planes.

Br: bregma; BoFo: body of fornix; CC: corpus callosum; ChPl: choroid plexus over the thalamus; CortV: cortical vein; Fal: falx; FoMo: foramen of Monro; SeptV: septal vein; SFG: superior frontal gyrus; Tha: thalamus; Tu: tumor.

and neural layer formed by both fornices, the two (superior and inferior) layers of tela choroidea which harbor the cistern of the velum interpositum in between, and the vascular layer (internal cerebral veins, medial posterior choroidal arteries), with the choroid plexus of the third ventricle attached to the inferior tela choroidea along two pedicles which are continuous through both choroidal fissures (Yamamoto *et al.*, 1981).

It is important to emphasize that all these structures can be displaced due to the presence of a third ventricle mass, including the internal cerebral veins that can be pushed together toward one of the sides favoring the contralateral approach.

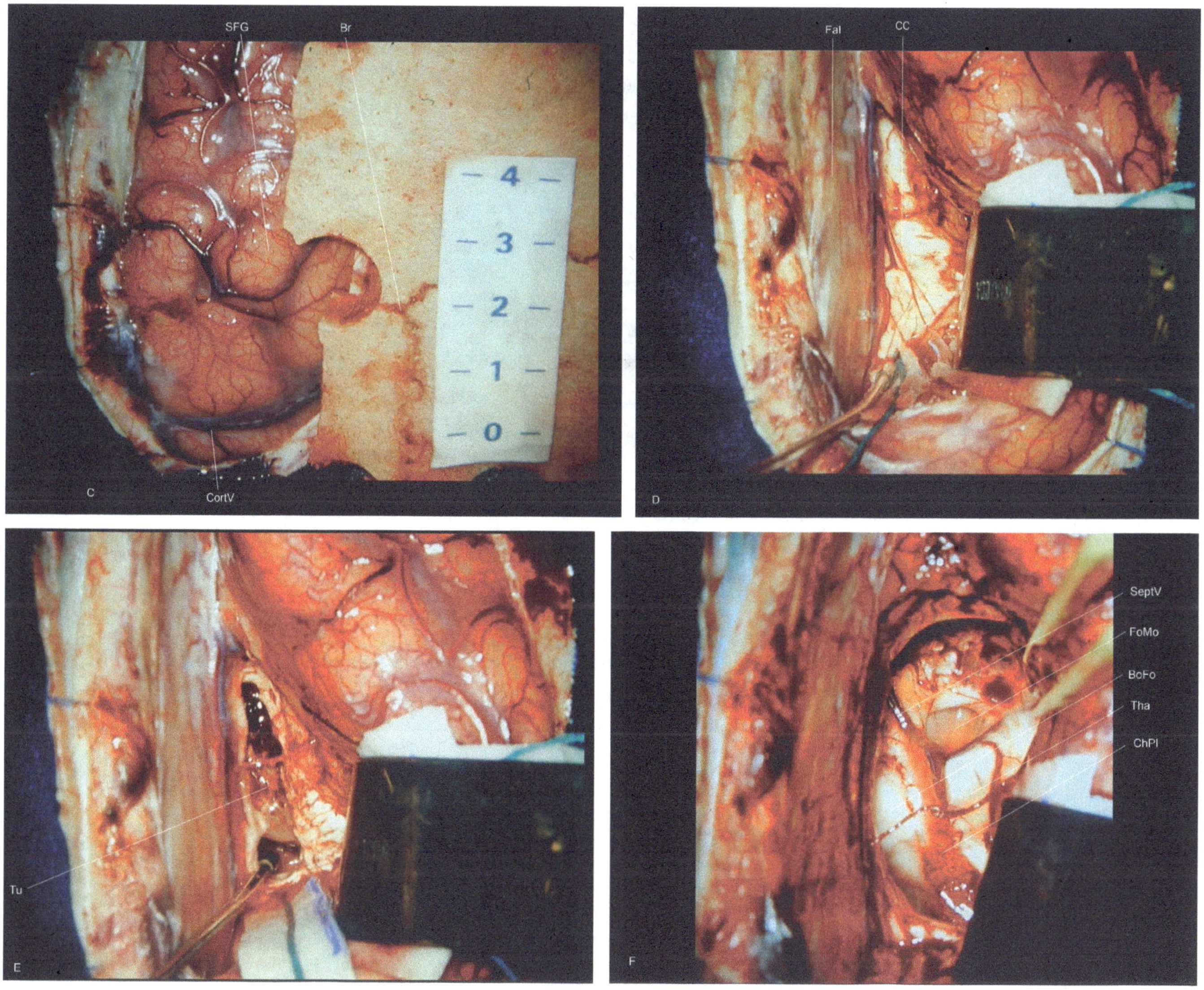

Figure 3.26 (cont.)

The pure transforaminal approach is very limited since both foramina of Monro are located superiorly and very anteriorly within the third ventricle cavity. It can be adequate when the foramen is dilated, and more particularly for the removal of non-giant colloid cysts which usually arise within the velum interpositum, and for dumbbell anterior third ventricular lesions.

Both the subchoroidal and the transchoroidal approaches correspond to a posterior enlargement of the foramen of Monro, since the choroidal fissure is opened and the choroid plexus can be partially coagulated and removed if necessary, and both are done through the velum interpositum (Figure 3.28A and 3.28B).

In the subchoroidal approach, the choroidal fissure is opened and the velum interpositum cistern is entered through the opening of the taenia choroidea, hence along the lateral aspect of the choroid plexus of the lateral ventricle which is then pushed medially, and coagulated and partially removed if necessary. A flat microdissector can then be passed underneath the tela choroidea in order to expose the cleavage plane between the superomedial aspect of the thalamus and the roof of the third ventricle, and the entrance to the velum interpositum should be made by elevating the tela together with the internal cerebral vein (Lavyne and Patterson, 1983). Although not considered to be a major risk by Hirsh *et al.* (1979), Delandsheer *et al.* (1978), and Lavyne and Patterson (1983) who described this technique, the main disadvantage of the subchoroidal route is that it might require the division and sacrifice of the thalamostriate vein, which potentially can cause venous hypertension in the ipsilateral basal ganglia and internal capsule as pointed out by McKissock (1951). The anterior septal vein can be coagulated and removed, if necessary, without consequences. Viale and Turtas described a subchoroidal variant that avoids the division of the thalamostriate vein (Viale and Turtas, 1980).

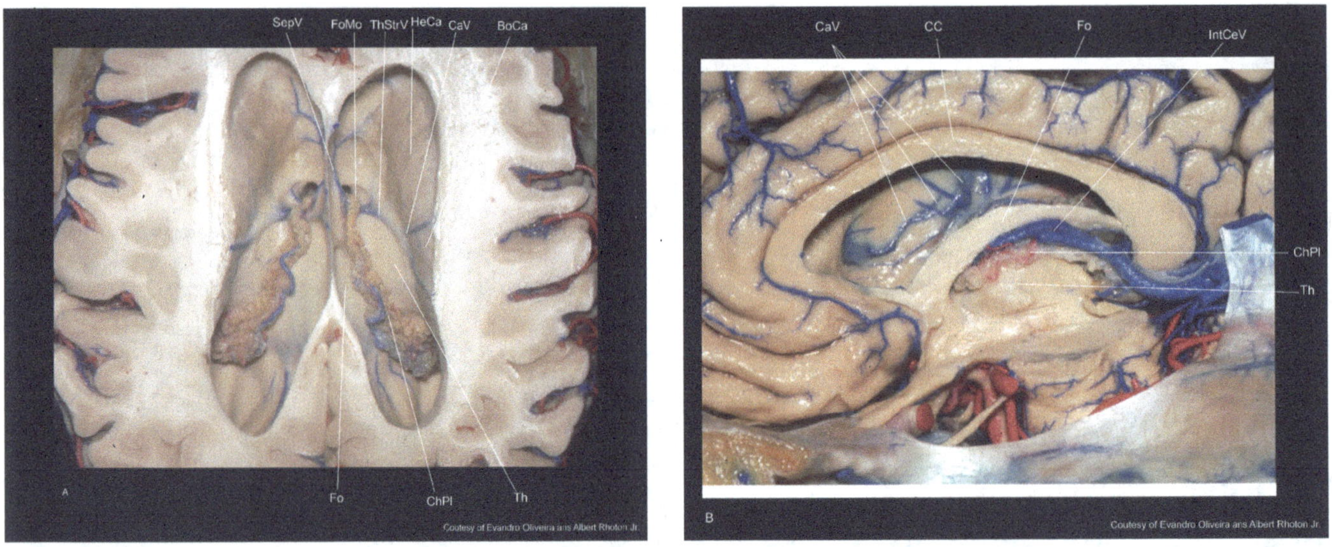

Figure 3.27 (A) Veins on the floor of the lateral ventricle: identification of the choroid plexus running along the choroid fissure toward the foramen of Monro, with the thalamus laterally and the fornix medially, confirms the exposure of the body of the lateral ventricle since there is no choroid plexus in the anterior horn; the thalamostriate vein always run parallel and lateral to the choroid plexus, between the thalamus and the body of the caudate nucleus toward the foramen of Monro or to the choroid fissure posteriorly to the foramen (less common), and the septal vein runs along the midline from the anterior horn toward the foramen of Monro; the right or left positioning of the thalamostriate vein in relation to the choroid plexus then, respectively, indicates exposure of the right or left body of the lateral ventricle; (B) the roof of the third ventricle: the fornix constitutes both the medial aspect of the floor of the body of the lateral ventricle and the upper aspect of the roof of the third ventricle; both internal cerebral veins, together with distal branches of both medial posterior choroidal artéries, run inside the so-called velum interpositum, between the superior and inferior layers of the choroid plexus of the third ventricle which runs attached to the inferior tela already within the third ventricular cavity.

BoCa: body of the caudate nucleus; CaV: caudate vein; CC: corpus callosum; ChPl: choroid plexus over the thalamus; Fo: fornix; FoMo: foramen of Monro; HeCa: head of caudate nucleus; IntCeV: internal cerebral vein; SepV: septal vein; Th: thalamus; ThStrV: thalamostriate vein. (Courtesy of Evandro de Oliveira and Rhoton Collection)

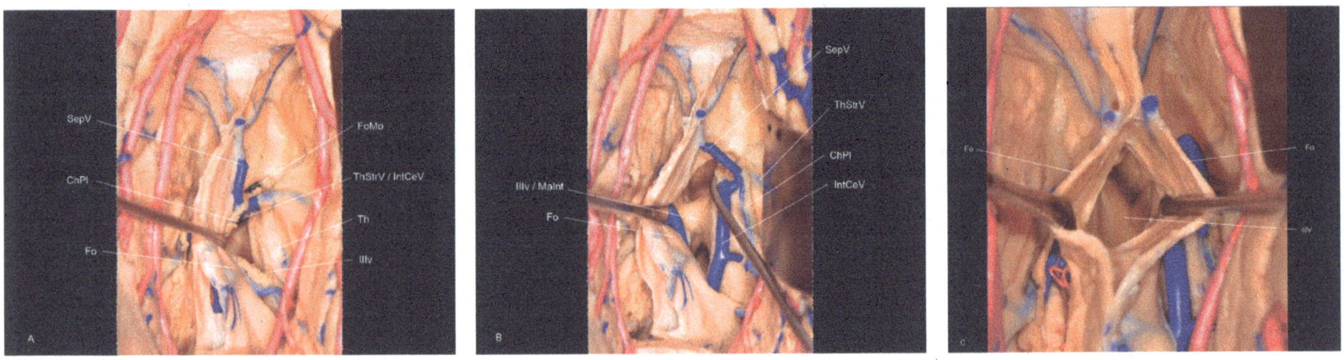

Figure 3.28 Approaches to the third ventricle through the lateral ventricle. (A) Subchoroidal: lateral to the choroid plexus, entering the velum interpositum lateral to the internal cerebral vein and hence having to divide the thalamostriate vein anteriorly in order to connect the opening of the choroidal fissure with the foramen of Monro; more problematic if the thalamostriate vein enters the choroidal fissure posteriorly to the foramen of Monro; (B) transchoroidal or suprachoroidal: medial to the choroid plexus and lateral to the fornix, entering the velum interpositum medial to the ipsilateral internal cerebral vein, creating then a surgical corridor continuous with the ipsilateral foramen of Monro; (C) interforniceal: entering the velum between the bodies of the two fornices and both internal cerebral veins.

ChPl: choroid plexus over the thalamus; Fo: fornix; FoMo: foramen of Monro; IIIv/MaInt: mass intermedia inside third ventricle; IIIv: third ventricle; IntCeV: internal cerebral vein; SepV: septal vein; Th: thalamus; ThStrV/IntCeV: connection of thalamostriate and internal cerebral veins; ThStrV: thalamostriate vein. (Courtesy of Eduardo Santamaria Carvalhal Ribas and Rhoton Collection.)

The transchoroidal approach is performed through the opening of the choroidal fissure through its taenia fornicis, hence along the medial side of the choroid plexus, in order to enter the velum interpositum, and then the third ventricle, between both internal cerebral veins. This route corresponds then to a posterior enlargement of the foramen of Monro without the division of the thalamostriate vein, since the venous angle given by this vein and the ipsilateral internal cerebral vein is displaced laterally (Wen *et al.*, 1998). The anterior septal vein can be sacrificed if necessary.

The interforniceal approach is also a transvelum interpositum approach, performed in between both fornices (Figure 3.28C).

Once inside the body of the lateral ventricle, the raphe can be identified as the basal attachment of the septum pellucidum along the dorsal aspect of the ipsilateral fornix. The development of the interforniceal plane should be started at the level of the medial aspect of the ipsilateral foramen of Monro (Apuzzo and Amar, 1988), since its medial and anterior margins correspond to the forniceal body–column (pillar) transition. This opening from anterior to posterior should not exceed 2 cm in order preserve the hippocampal commissure (Apuzzo and Amar, 1988). The main concern with the interforniceal approach is the possible damage to both fornices with all its consequences.

Since each of the two layers of the septum pellucidum attaches superiorly to the inferior aspect of the corpus callosum and inferiorly to the dorsal aspect of the ipsilateral forniceal body, an occasional cavum of the septum pellucidum can constitute a natural interforniceal surgical corridor with both fornices already apart.

3.2.5 Parietal Key Points

The parietal key points are 1) the intraparietal and postcentral sulci meeting point (IPS/PostCS), 2) the euryon (Eu), and 3) the parieto-occipital incisure (POInc).

3.2.5.1 The Intraparietal and Postcentral Sulci Meeting Point

The relationships of the intraparietal sulcus of Turner (Lockard, 1977) with the postcentral sulcus vary in the literature, since the former is usually constituted by a slightly oblique or longitudinal parietal segment that curves anteriorly and is usually continuous with the more inferior part of the postcentral sulcus (Ebeling and Steinmetz, 1995b; Steinmetz *et al.*, 1990).

While Broca in the nineteenth century described the intraparietal sulcus separately from the inferior aspect of the postcentral sulcus (Gusmão *et al.*, 2000), more recently, Duvernoy (1991) considered the lower aspect of the postcentral sulcus as the anterior ascending segment of the intraparietal sulcus with the postcentral sulcus itself being constituted only by its more superior segment. Ono *et al.* (1990), studying the brain sulci through a more microsurgically oriented point of view, considered them separately like Broca.

The intraparietal sulcus separates the superior from the inferior parietal lobule. While the superior parietal lobule merges and is continuous with the precuneus in the mesial surface, the inferior parietal lobule is comprised by the supramarginal and by the angular gyri, separated by the intermediary sulcus of Jensen (von Economo and Koskinas apud Tamraz and Comair, 2000) which can be an inferior branch of the intraparietal sulcus, a superior distal branch of the superior temporal sulcus, or both.

Anteriorly, the intraparietal sulcus is thus particularly related to and usually continuous with the postcentral sulcus, and posteriorly it is usually continuous with the intra-occipital sulcus (Duvernoy, 1991; Naidich *et al.*, 1995) which is also called the transverse occipital sulcus (Ono *et al.*, 1990; Yasargil, 1994) and superior occipital sulcus (Testut and Jacob, 1932), and which separates the more evident superior from the middle occipital gyrus (Naidich *et al.*, 1995; Testut and Jacob, 1932).

According to the studies about its morphology, the intraparietal sulcus is predominantly parallel to the interhemispheric fissure in about 90 percent of humans, being then transverse in only about 10 percent, and is continuous with the postcentral sulcus in about 80 percent of humans (Ebeling and Steinmetz, 1995b; Ono *et al.*, 1990; Steinmetz *et al.*, 1990; Ribas *et al.*, 2006; Ribas, 2005b).

The intraparietal/postcentral sulci meeting point (IPS/PostCS) then corresponds to the connection or transition point between these two sulci, or to the postcentral sulcus point more particularly related to the most anterior aspect of the intraparietal sulcus level (projection site of the intraparietal sulcus into the postcentral sulcus). When these two sulci are not continuous, the IPS/PostCS constitutes an important neurosurgical key point 1) since it is an evident point that delineates posteriorly the postcentral gyrus, 2) because it can be utilized as a safe starting point for the microsurgical opening of these sulci, and 3) due to its deep relationship with the ventricular atrium or trigone, as also shown by Harkey *et al.* (Harkey *et al.*, 1989; Ribas *et al.*, 2006; Ribas, 2005b) (Figure 3.29).

Despite the sulcal and gyral variability of the parietal opercular region found by Ebeling and Steinmetz (Ebeling and Steinmetz, 1995b; Steinmetz *et al.*, 1990), these authors also concluded that the junction between the PostCS and the IPS is

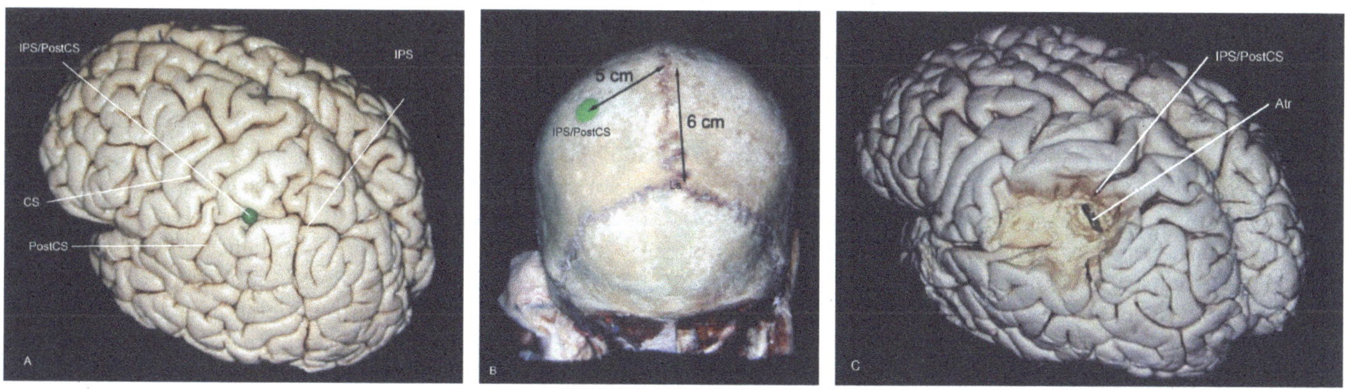

Figure 3.29 (A) Intraparietal and postcentral sulci meeting point, or anterior projection of the intraparietal sulcus on the postcentral sulcus point when there is an interruption between both sulci; (B) its corresponding cranial site; and (C) relationship of the intraparietal and postcentral sulci point with the atrium of the lateral ventricle.

Atr: atrium of lateral ventricle; CS: central sulcus; IPS/PostCS: intraparietal and postcentral sulci meeting point; IPS: intraparietal sulcus; La: lambda; PostCs: postcentral sulcus.

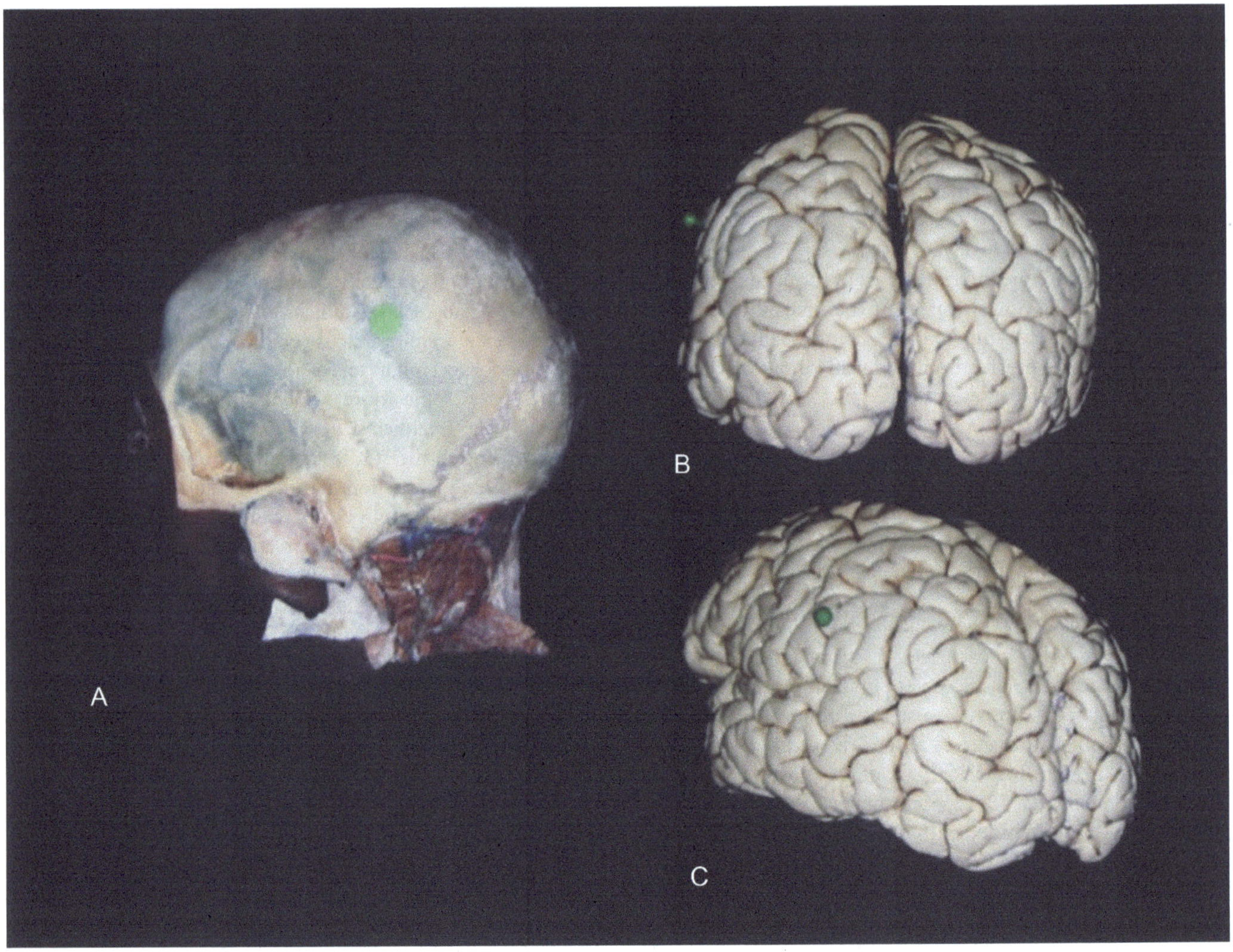

Figure 3.30 The Euryon and the supramarginal gyrus. (A) The Euryon corresponds to the most prominent point of the parietal tuberosity or bossa, and (B) posterior view; (C) oblique view lies over the superior aspect of the supramarginal gyrus.
AG: angular gyrus; Eu: Euryon; IPS: intraparietal sulcus; SMG: supramarginal gyrus.

indeed a prominent sulcal landmark for radiological and surgical purposes (Ebeling and Steinmetz, 1995b).

The IPS/PostCS key point is a mid-parietal point, and its distance from the midline varies roughly from 3.5 to 5.0 cm (Harkey *et al.*, 1989; Ribas *et al.*, 2006; Ribas, 2005b). Due to its variability, it lies underneath the 2 cm diameter cranial area located 6 cm anteriorly to the lambda and 5 cm laterally to the sagittal suture (Ribas *et al.*, 2006; Ribas, 2005b).

Regarding its deep relationship with the ventricular cavity, the IPS/PostCS meeting point, which actually corresponds to the point of the postcentral sulcus most particularly related to the level of the anterior extremity of the intraparietal sulcus, is related to the ventricular atrium along a 30° posteriorly oblique radial approach (Ribas *et al.*, 2006; Ribas, 2005b).

3.2.5.2 The Euryon and the Supramarginal Gyrus

The euryon (Eu) is the craniometric point that corresponds to the center of the parietal tuberosity (Gusmão *et al.*, 2000; Broca, 1876b; Pernkoff, 1980), and is very easily palpated as the most prominent cranial parietal area (Figure 3.30).

The Eu is usually located immediately superiorly to the superior temporal line (STL), and also corresponds to the area of intersection of the STL with a vertical line that passes through the posterior aspect of the mastoid tip and through the meeting point of the squamous and parieto-mastoid sutures (PaMaSut/SqSut) (Ribas *et al.*, 2006; Ribas, 2005b).

In relation to the cortical surface, the Eu always lies over the superior aspect of the supramarginal gyrus, more frequently over its posterior half, hence always posteriorly to the postcentral sulcus (PostCS) (average distance: 1.5–3.0 cm), laterally to the intraparietal sulcus (IPS) (average distance: 1–3 cm), and anteriorly to the intermediary sulcus of Jensen (von Economo and Koskinas apud Tamraz and Comair, 2000) (ISJ) (average distance: 1–2 cm), which separates the supramarginal gyrus (SMG) from the angular gyrus (AG).

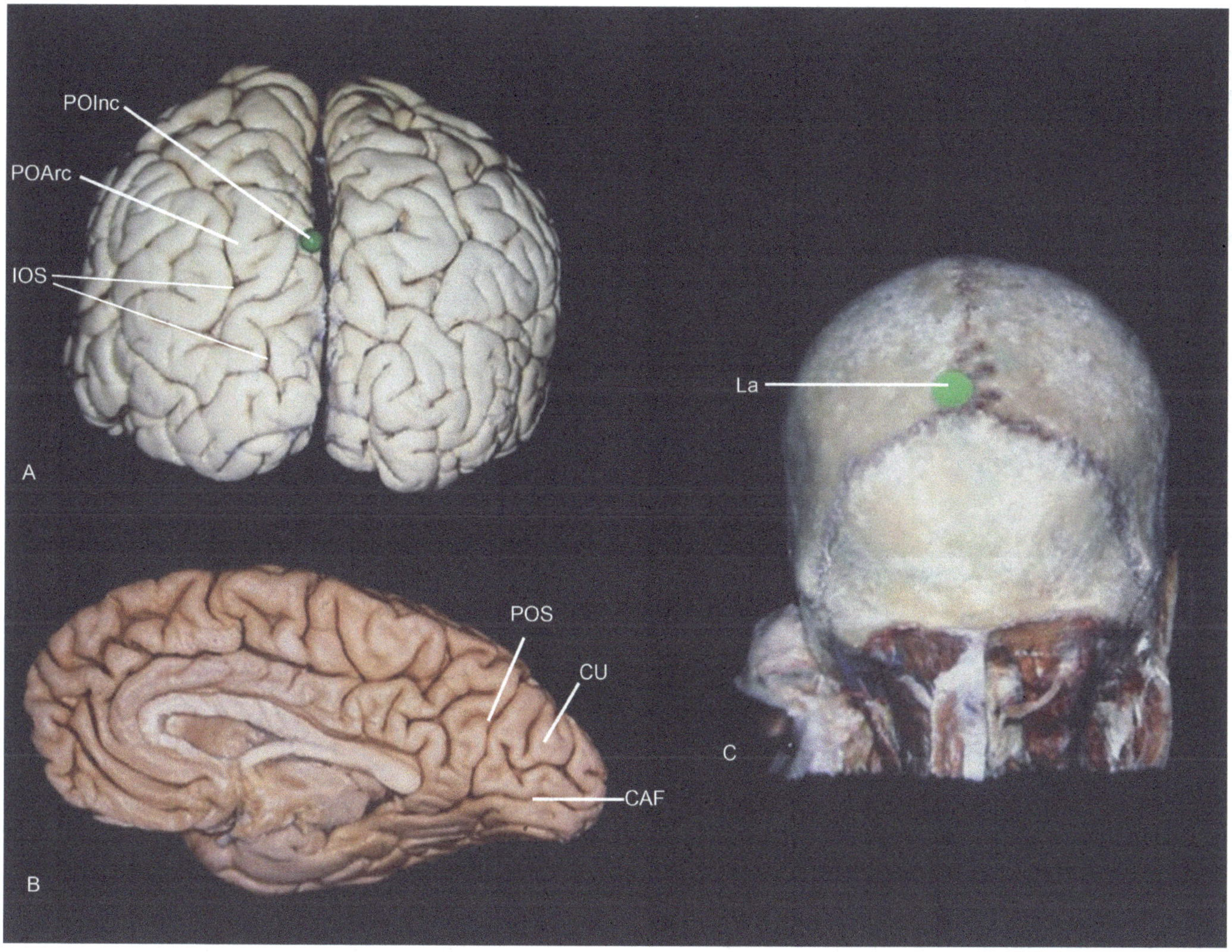

Figure 3.31 The parieto-occipital incisure and the lambda. (A, B) The parieto-occipital incisure corresponds to the depth of the parieto-occipital sulcus on the medial aspect of the superolateral surface of the brain, and (C) lies exactly underneath the cranial site given by the angle between the sagittal and lambdoid sutures on each side of the skull.

CaF: calcarine fissure; CU: cuneus; IOS: intra-occipital sulcus (continuation of the intraparietal sulcus, also named superior occipital sulcus); La: lambda; POArc: parieto-occipital arc, also known as the first parieto-occipital connection of Gratiolet (Broca, 1876b); POInc: parieto-occipital incisure, in the past also known as the external perpendicular fissure (Broca, 1876b); POS: parieto-occipital sulcus.

The posterior Sylvian point (PSP) is then always anterior and inferior to the Eu (average distance 2–3 cm) (Ribas *et al.*, 2006; Ribas, 2005b).

In the dominant hemisphere, the cortical area underneath the Eu is particularly related to the parietal speech zone, that although relatively spread (Ojemann *et al.*, 1989), has its epicenter roughly located 1–4 cm above the Sylvian fissure and from 2 to 4 cm behind the postcentral sulcus (Hansebout, 1982; Rasmussen and Milner, 1975 apud Hansebout, 1982).

3.2.5.3 The Parieto-Occipital Incisure and the Lambda

The parieto-occipital sulcus is a very deep sulcus which runs along the medial surface of the brain hemisphere separating the precuneus from the cuneus, and its depth appears transversally and very evidently on the medial aspect of the hemispheric superolateral surface as the parieto-occipital incisure (POInc) (Petrides, 2012; Ribas *et al.*, 2006).

The parieto-occipital incisure (POInc) lies on the medial aspect of the superolateral surface of the brain, transversally to the interhemispheric longitudinal fissure. It is always inside an also very evident U-shaped convolution currently called the parieto-occipital arcus (Petrides, 2012) (POArc) and classically known as the first or superior parieto-occipital connection of Gratiolet (Testut and Jacob, 1932) (Figure 3.31).

Since, in the past, the parieto-occipital sulcus was also denominated the internal occipital fissure due to its perpendicularity in relation to the calcarine fissure, the POInc was formerly known as the external occipital fissure (Broca, 1876b).

The POInc corresponds to the most superior point of the parieto-occipital sulcus and constitutes a useful surgical landmark since it defines the position of the parieto-occipital sulcus, and hence the posterior aspect of the precuneus along the interhemispheric fissure (IHF) (average longitudinal extent of the precuneus along the IHF: 3.5–4.05 cm) (Ribas *et al.*, 2006;

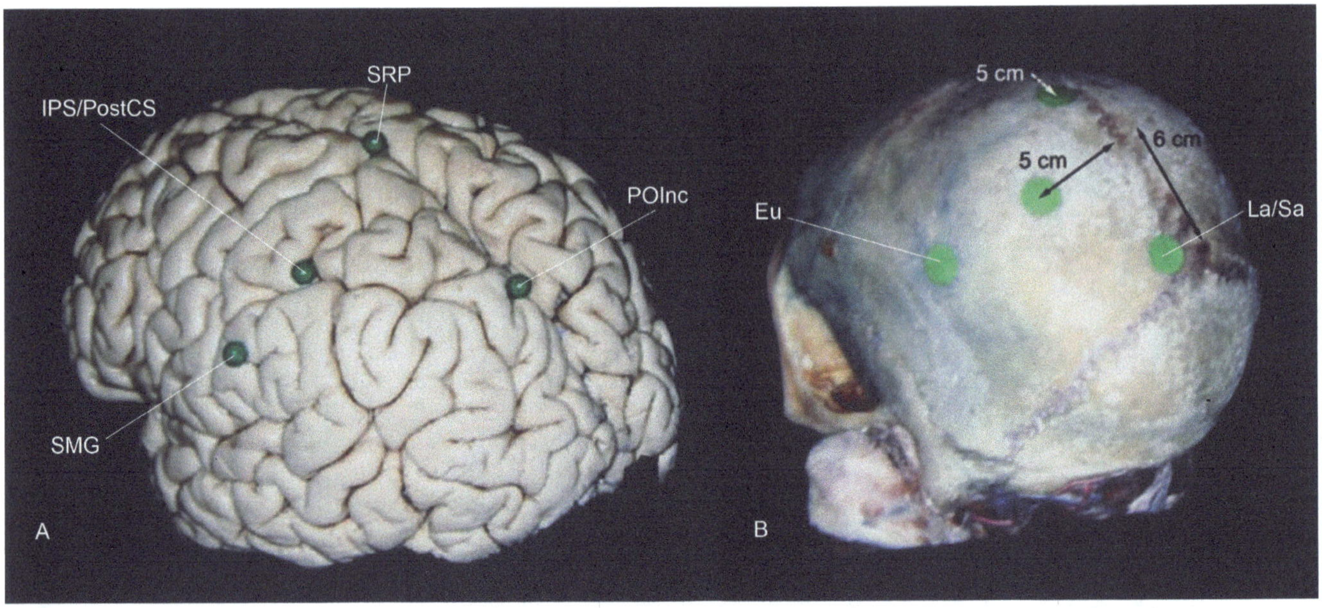

Figure 3.32 The parietal key points altogether. (A, B) The superior aspect of the supramarginal gyrus lies underneath the euryon, which corresponds to the most prominent point of the parietal tuberosity or bossa; the intraparietal and postcentral meeting point lies underneath the cranial area located 6 cm anterior to the lambda and 5 cm lateral to the sagittal suture; the superior Rolandic point lies underneath the cranial area located 5 cm posterior to the bregma along the sagittal suture; and the parieto-occipital incisure, which corresponds to the most superior point of the parieto-occipital sulcus (depth of the parieto-occipital sulcus seen on the superolateral surface of the brain), which lies underneath the angle between the lambdoid and sagittal sutures.

Eu: euryon; IPS/PostCS: intraparietal and postcentral sulci meeting point; La/Sa: angle between the lambdoid and sagittal sutures; POInc: parieto-occipital incisure, in the past also known as the external perpendicular fissure (Broca, 1876b); SMG: supramarginal gyrus; SRP: superior Rolandic point.

Ribas, 2005b). As with other well-developed sulci, it is not uncommon to have a vein running along the POInc.

Regarding its cranial relationships, each POInc lies underneath each paramedian area that corresponds to the angle between the sagittal and each lambdoid suture (La/Sa) (Broca, 1876b; Ribas *et al.*, 2006; Ribas, 2005b) (Figure 3.31C).

3.2.5.4 Parietal Craniotomies

Parietal craniotomies should then have as their main landmarks: 1) the superior Rolandic point (SRO) already described; 2) the intraparietal and the postcentral sulci transition or meeting point (IPS/PostCS), which is located underneath the cranial site 6 cm anterior to lambda and 5 cm lateral to the sagittal suture; 3) the euryon (Eu), which corresponds to the center of the parietal tuberosity, and which always lies over the supramarginal gyrus; and 4) the parieto-occipital incisure (POInc) which corresponds to the emergence of the parieto-occipital sulcus on the interhemispheric fissure (IHF) and which lies underneath and immediately lateral to the lambda (Figure 3.32).

The position of the lambda in adults can be estimated through its distances from the other midline craniometric points (about 24–26 cm posterior to the nasion, 12–14 cm posterior to the bregma and 2–4 cm anterior to the opisthocranion). The close relationships that were found between the euryon (Eu) and the vertical line originating at the posterior aspect of the mastoid tip, and of the euryon with the superior temporal line, previously described, can help its palpatory recognition and its intraoperative localization.

The exposure of the superior parietal lobule (SPL) also requires the knowledge that the superior Rolandic point (SRP) lies underneath the cranial point located 5 cm posteriorly to the bregma (Br), since the SRP and the POInc define the extension of the postcentral gyrus and of the precuneus together along the midline.

The exposure of the inferior parietal lobule (IPL) can be particularly aided by the exposure also of the visually evident distal part of the Sylvian fissure (SyF), since its identification corroborates the identification of the basal aspect of the supramarginal gyrus (SMG), and of its connection with the superior temporal gyrus (STG) that encircles the distal segment of the SyF (Ono *et al.*, 1990; Rhoton, 2003). The posterior Sylvian point (PSyP) lies 2–3 cm anteriorly and inferiorly to the Eu (Ribas, 2005b; Ribas *et al.*, 2006).

On the cortical surface, the most prominent point of the supramarginal gyrus (SMG) that lies underneath the Eu, is located 1.5–2.5 cm posteriorly to the postcentral sulcus (PostCS), and 1.5–2.5 cm lateral to the intraparietal sulcus (IPS) (Ribas, 2005b; Ribas *et al.*, 2006).

Although being more frequently interrupted (Ono *et al.*, 1990), the intraparietal sulcus (IPS) was found to have an evident continuous segment (average length: 3.19±1.17 cm), usually longitudinal in relation to the interhemispheric fissure (Ribas *et al.*, 2006; Ribas, 2005b). Both the intraparietal sulcus, and its frequently continuous postcentral sulcus, are often covered by a cortical vein (Rhoton, 2003).

The intraparietal sulcus (IPS) depth was studied by Ebeling and Steinmetz (1995b) (mean: 20 mm, range: 13–26 mm), and by Harkey *et al.* (1989) (mean: 24 mm,

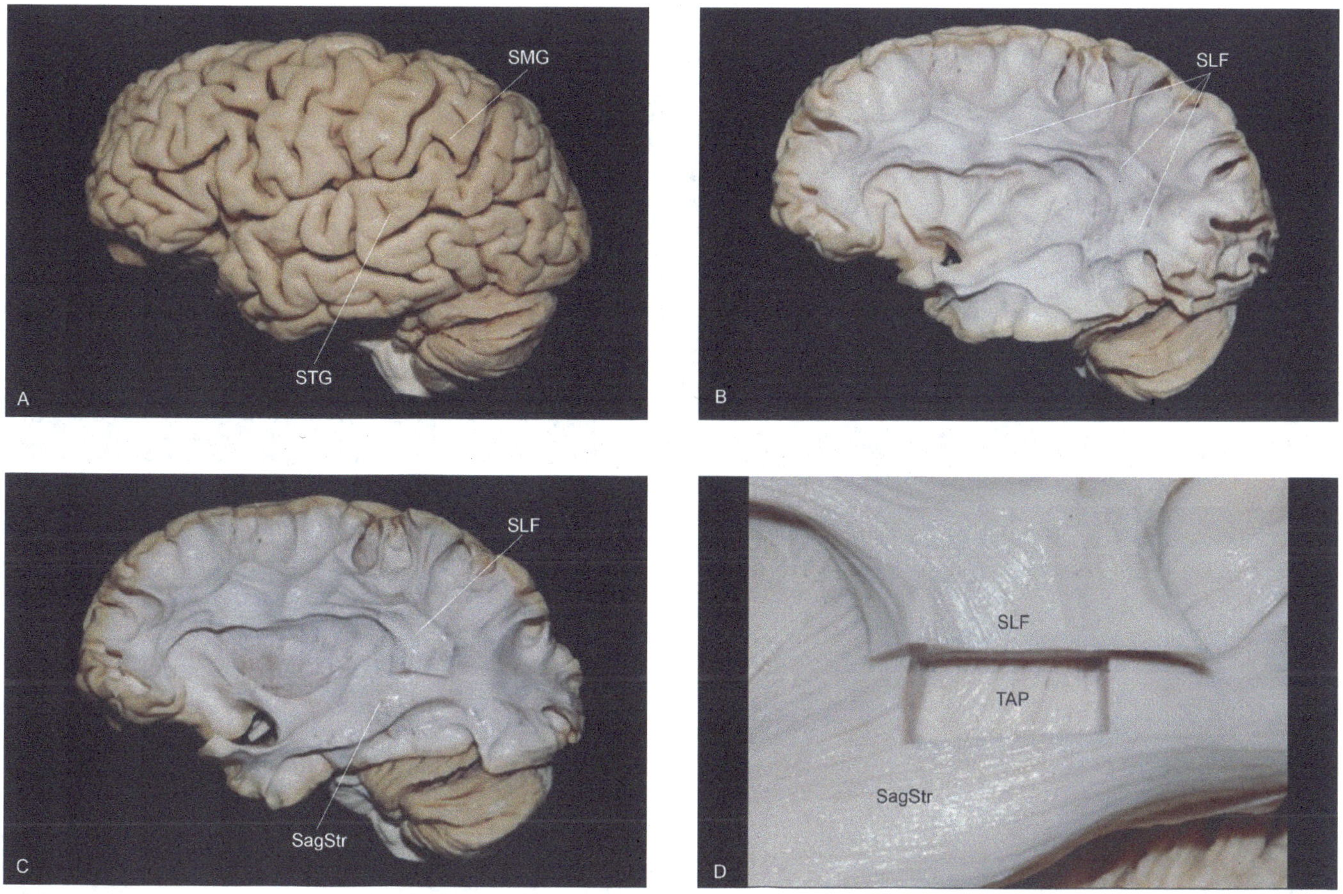

Figure 3.33 Main fiber systems underneath the supramarginal gyrus which cover the atrium. (A) Cortical area of the supramarginal gyrus; (B) exposure of the white matter of the supramarginal gyrus; (C) superficial fibers of the sagittal stratum running underneath the superior longitudinal fascicle; (D) fibers of the tapetum running underneath the sagittal stratum and immediately above the ependyma of the ventricular cavity.

SagStr: sagittal stratum; SLF: superior longitudinal fascicle; SMG: supramarginal gyrus; STG: superior temporal gyrus; TAP: tapetum.

range: 20–27 mm), and shown to be suitable as a microneurosurgical corridor.

For IPS transsulcal approaches to the ventricular cavity, it is important to stress that its closest topographical relationship with the atrium is given particularly by its most anterior part. Since its intersection point or its projection onto the postcentral sulcus is coronally posterior to the atrium and related to the splenium (Spl) (at the level of the Spl: 75 percent, posterior to the Spl: 25 percent; average distance from the Spl: posterior 0.23±0.50 cm), the transsulcal or parasulcal approach to the atrium from the IPS/PostCS is possible only along a 30–45° posteriorly oblique radial approach. The intraparietal sulcus opening posteriorly to the IPS/PostCS key point enlarges its exposure, but definitely runs progressively away from the atrium.

In relation to possible surgical complications resulting from the parietal transsulcal and transgyral approaches, in the dominant hemisphere, language impairments can be related to damage to the supramarginal and angular gyri, and to the subcortical superior longitudinal and arcuate fascicles which lie lateral to the intraparietal sulcus (Hansebout, 1982; Ojemann *et al.*, 1989; Rasmussen and Milner, 1975 apud Hansebout, 1982; Duffau, 2011b) (Figure 3.33). In the non-dominant hemisphere, the parietal damage can cause derangement of complex functions involving somatic as well as psychological elements, which have as a common feature a defective recognition of sensory impressions (neglect, agnosias), and which are especially marked in tasks that require appreciation of spatial relationships (Brodal, 1981) (Figure 3.34).

3.2.5.5 Anatomical Remarks Pertinent to Common Parietal Transcerebral Procedures

The identification of the parietal landmarks for the main sulci and gyri (Figure 3.32) enables the localization and removal of parietal cortical and subcortical lesions, and transparietal approaches toward the atrium of the lateral ventricle.

Since the atriums or trigones of the lateral ventricles are off-midline cavities located behind both thalami, their access requires off-midline approaches. A key anatomical feature to have in mind with regard to the atriums is that, while the most posterior aspect of the splenium within the midline ends covering the pineal or quadrigeminal cistern, its lateral extensions open bilaterally and posteriorly covering both thalamic

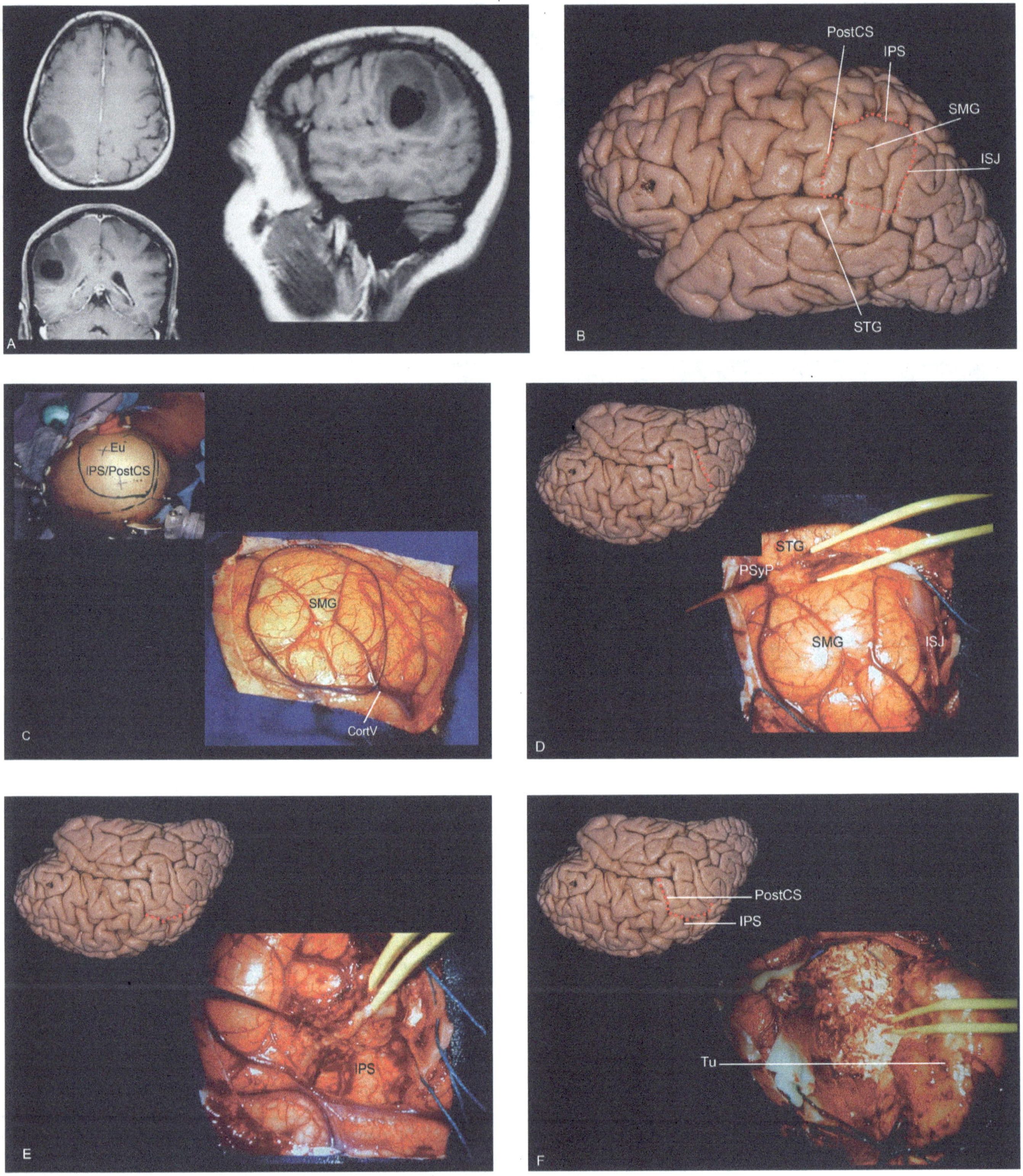

Figure 3.34 Anatomical resection of a right supramarginal gyrus containing a low grade glioma. (A) Preoperative MR images; (B) anatomical delineation of the supramarginal gyrus which is continuous with the superior temporal gyrus along its base; (C) planning the craniotomy with the euryon that lies above the supramarginal gyrus and with identification of the intraparietal sulcus site, and exposure of the supramarginal gyrus with a cortical vein running along the intraparietal sulcus; (D) opening of the intermediary sulcus of Jensen which separates the supramarginal from the angular gyrus; (E) opening of the intraparietal sulcus; (F) opening of the postcentral sulcus which is continuous with the intraparietal sulcus, and en bloc removal of the tumor within the supramarginal gyrus; (G) tumor cavity; and (H) postoperative MR images.

CortV: cortical vein; Eu: euryon; IPS/PostCS: intraparietal and postcentral sulci meeting point; IPS: intraparietal sulcus; ISJ: intermediary sulcus of Jensen; PostCS: postcentral sulcus; PSyP: posterior Sylvian point; SMG: supramarginal gyrus; STG: superior temporal gyrus; Tu: tumor; TuCa: tumor cavity.

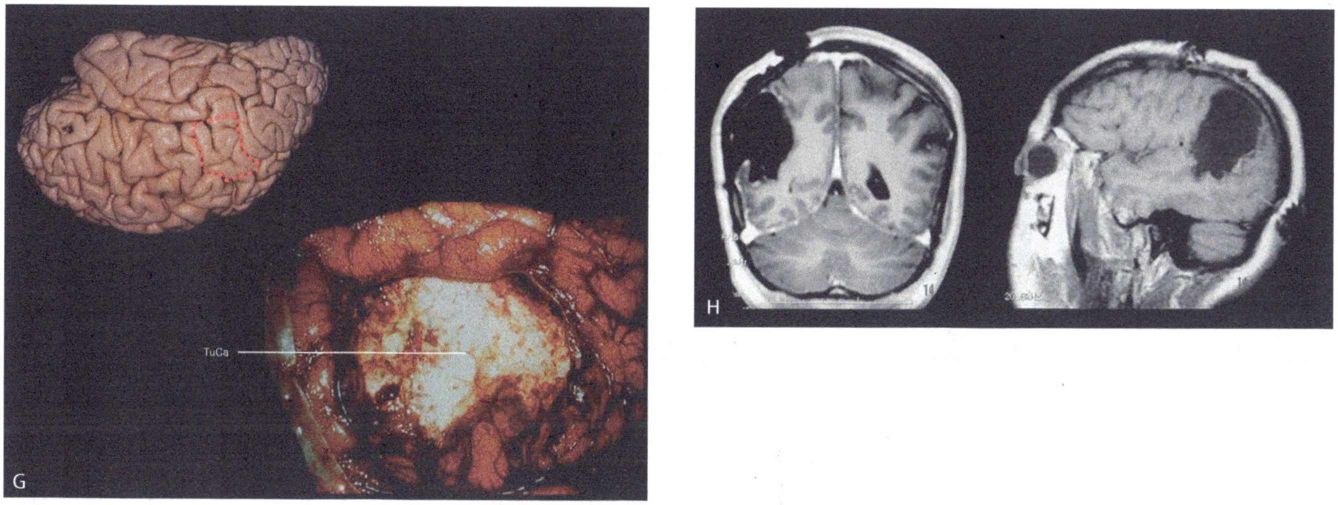

Figure 3.34 (Cont.)

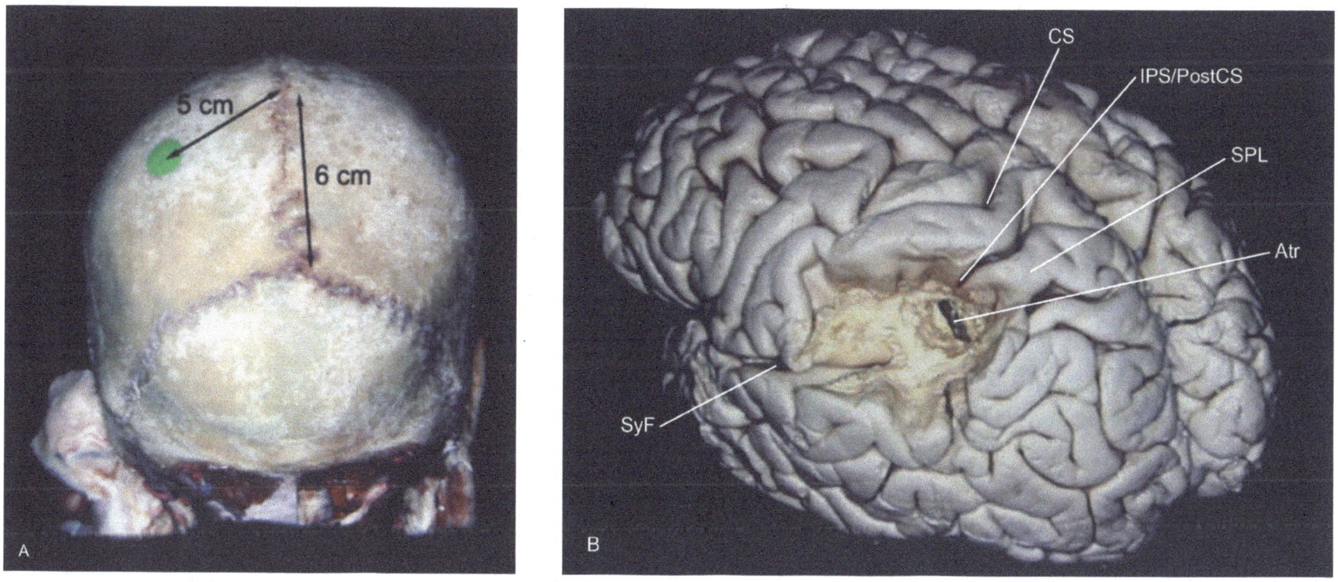

Figure 3.35 Transparietal approach to the atrium seen after anatomical removal of the supramarginal gyrus. (A) The intraparietal and postcentral meeting point lies underneath the 2 cm diameter cranial area located 6 cm anteriorly to the lambda and 5 cm lateral to the sagittal suture, and (B) it corresponds to the closest superficial point to the atrium; the more posterior along the intraparietal sulcus, the more posterior to the atrium.
Atr: atrium of lateral ventricle; CS: central sulcus; IPS/PostCS: intraparietal and postcentral sulci meeting point; SPL: superior parietal lobule; SyF: Sylvian fissure.

pulvinars and encircling both atrial cavities and their variable posterior extensions that constitute the occipital horns, already inside the brain parenchyma and hence posterior to the most posterior aspect of the splenium seen along the midline.

Given this anatomical location, only the most superior and anterior tumors of the atrium can be reached through the anterior transcallosal approaches already described to access the frontal horn and the body of each lateral ventricle, with the other atrial tumors requiring different transcerebral approaches according to their main locations, extensions, and vascularizations. The main approaches to the ventricular atrium are the transparietal, the transtemporal, and the parieto-occipito-interhemispheric.

Transparietal Approach to the Atrium

Although sometimes interrupted, the intraparietal sulcus is a very evident sulcus that transverses the superolateral surface of the parietal lobe, and which is usually continuous with the inferior and downward segment of the postcentral sulcus. Their actual or projected meeting or transition point constitutes the nearest point between the parietal surface and the atrium (Ebeling and Reulen, 1995a; Harkey *et al.*, 1989; Ribas *et al.*, 2006). Nevertheless, the transparietal microneurosurgical approach to the atrium has to be mandatorily initiated through the transitional site between these two sulci, since the more posterior along the intraparietal sulcus, the more posterior in relation to the atrium, particularly if this cavity is not enlarged (Figure 3.35).

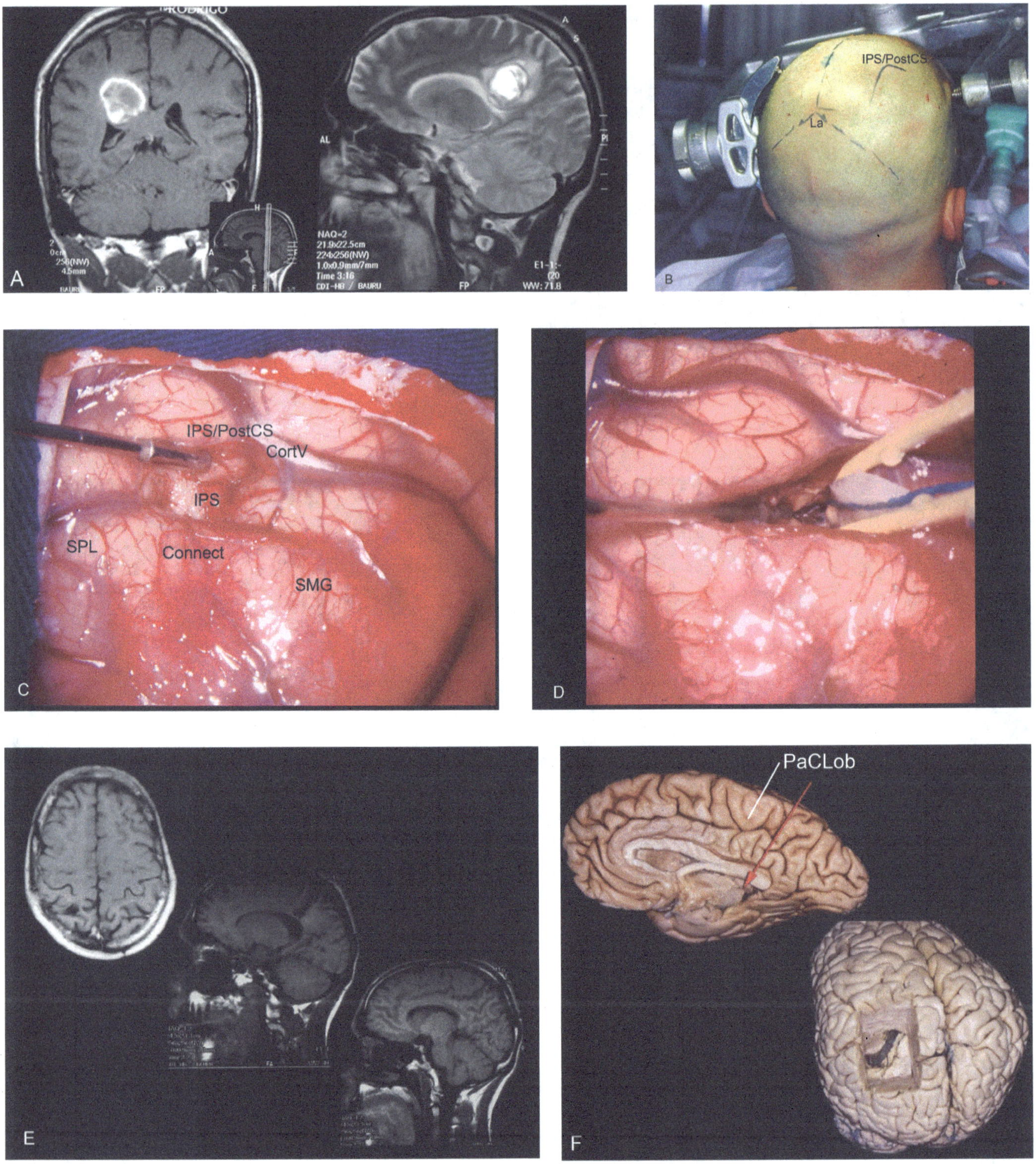

Figure 3.36 Transparietal transsulcal resection of a cavernoma located at the top of the right atrium. (A) Preoperative MR images; (B) planning the craniotomy in order to expose the most anterior aspect of the right intraparietal sulcus, where it is usually continuous with the postcentral sulcus; (C) opening of the most anterior aspect of the intraparietal sulcus, between a cortical vein which is running along the postcentral, central, and a posterior connection between the superior parietal lobule and the supramarginal gyrus; (D) exposure of the cavernoma at the depth of the most anterior aspect of the intraparietal sulcus; (E) postoperative MR images, showing the small opening of the intraparietal sulcus as seen in surgery, and the track toward the atrium; (F) anatomical specimens showing the desired approach direction just posteriorly to the paracentral lobule on the sagittal view, and of the atrium through an exposure centered along the intraparietal sulcus.

Connect: connection between the superior parietal lobule and the supramarginal gyrus; CortV: cortical vein; IPS: intraparietal sulcus; IPS/PostCS: intraparietal and postcentral sulci meeting point; La: lambda; PaCLob: paracentral lobule; SMG: supramarginal gyrus; SPL: superior parietal lobule.

For this approach, the patient should ideally be in the semi-sitting position, and the craniotomy should be done having as its center the cranial projection of the actual transition point of both sulci, or of the projected point of the most anterior segment of the intraparietal into the postcentral sulcus, which is located approximately 6 cm superior to the lambda along the sagittal suture and 5 cm laterally to it (Ribas *et al.*, 2006).

Preoperatively, both the shape and interruptions of both sulci, as well as their joining site, can be estimated through careful study of 3D rendered MR images of the patient. The projection of their joining site on the skull surface can be better estimated through a fusion of the patient's CT and MR images, if available.

Intraoperatively, after identifying the visible segments of the intraparietal and postcentral sulci considering their usual or known courses as carefully seen in MR images, their actual or projected meeting or transition point can usually be identified as a variable enlargement of the sub-arachnoid space, and this should also be confirmed with the aid of neuronavigation if available. It is very frequent to find veins running along or immediately next to both sulci (Figure 3.36).

The transparietal approach to the atrium can be performed transsulcally, subpially or transgyrally, but always considering that: 1) the transition site between the postcentral and the intraparietal sulci constitutes the nearest and easiest surface site to reach the atrium more securely, 2) the surgical route has to follow the sulcal orientation which always leads toward the nearest ventricular cavity (Ebeling and Reulen, 1995a; Harkey *et al.*, 1989; Ribas *et al.*, 2006), and 3) surgery has to be performed along a 30-degree posteriorly oblique radial approach (Ribas *et al.*, 2006). Both neuronavigation and intraoperative ultrasound can be very helpful to confirm the route toward the atrium.

Once having reached the ventricular cavity, the surgical corridor can be enlarged, if necessary, by removing more brain tissue posteriorly along the intraparietal sulcus orientation and preferably medially from the superior parietal lobule, in order to avoid further damage to the superior longitudinal and arcuate fascicles which run mainly laterally to the intraparietal sulcus, mostly already within the inferior parietal lobule.

Having studied the anatomy related with the intraparietal sulcus (IPS) approach to the atrium, Koutsarnakis *et al.* found that the anterior half of this sulcus always lies above the atrium, and there are four consecutive layers of fiber tracts between the IPS fundus and the atrium: 1) The U-shaped fibers that connect adjacent gyri. 2) The arcuate segment of the superior longitudinal fascicle (SLF) which is located only deep to the IPS most anterior portion. 3) Fibers of the external capsule and parietopontine fibers of the corona radiata on their way to the internal capsule. 4) Fibers of the tapetum running over the ventricular ependyma. For these authors there are no optic radiation fibers over the roof of the atrium, and the depth of the parieto-occipital sulcus seen on the superolateral surface (parieto-occipital incisure) demarcates the transition of the atrium to the occipital horn, where the optic radiation fibers sweep around the lateral wall of the atrium to reach the roof of the occipital horn. Considering their findings, Koutsarnakis *et al.* suggest the approach to be taken through the very middle of the sulcus in order to avoid both arcuate and visual fibers. (Koutsarnakis *et al.*, 2017).

Regarding the side, non-dominant parietal damage is more particularly related to left hemineglect and anosognosia, spatial disorientation, construction and dressing apraxias. Dominant parietal damage can be responsible for dysphasias, dyslexia, dyscalculia, apraxia, tactile agnosia, and a possible Gerstmann syndrome (Figure 3.37).

3.2.6 Posterior Temporal Key Point

3.2.6.1 The Posterior Extremity of the Superior Temporal Sulcus

The superior temporal sulcus is a long, deep, and frequently continuous (Ono *et al.*, 1990) sulcus, and usually ends as a trifurcation with its middle and most horizontal branch penetrating inside the angular gyrus. Just before its bifurcation or trifurcation, its most distal segment and extremity (postSTS) is always located 2–3 cm posteriorly and inferiorly to the posterior Sylvian point (PSyP; end point of the lateral or Sylvian fissure), hence posteriorly to the insula, to the posterior limb of the internal capsule, and to the thalamus.

The postSTS lies underneath the cranial area located 3 cm above the evident squamosal and parietomastoid suture meeting point (Ribas *et al.*, 2006) (Figure 3.38).

At its depth, the postSTS is related to the atrium of the lateral ventricle (Harkey *et al.*, 1989; Ribas *et al.*, 2006).

Regarding the anatomical relationships of the atrium of the lateral ventricle, it is important to bear in mind that, while the supramarginal gyrus covers the most superior aspect of the atrium, the posterior part of the superior temporal gyrus covers its most inferior aspect (Figure 3.39).

3.2.6.2 Posterior Temporal Craniotomies

Posterior temporal craniotomies for posterior temporal and inferior parietal cortical exposures, and for approaches to the atrium and to the posterior aspect of the inferior horn, can then be centered at the posterior portion of the superior temporal sulcus (postSTS). The postSTS is situated underneath the cranial site located 3 cm vertically above the very evident transition point between the horizontal parietomastoid suture and the oblique posterior aspect of the squamous suture (Harkey *et al.*, 1989; Ribas *et al.*, 2006).

The concomitant exposure of the distal aspect of the Sylvian fissure, located 2–3 cm anteriorly and superiorly to this cranial point, is very helpful to corroborate the identification of the sulci and gyri in this region.

The basal aspect of posterior temporal craniotomies should be immediately superior to the evident parietomastoid and squamous suture transition point mentioned above, since this point is related to the superior surfaces of the petrous bone and of the tentorium transition (Ribas, 1991; Ribas *et al.*, 2005a).

In order to reach the ventricular cavity, the distal STS transsulcal or subpial parasulcal approach should be

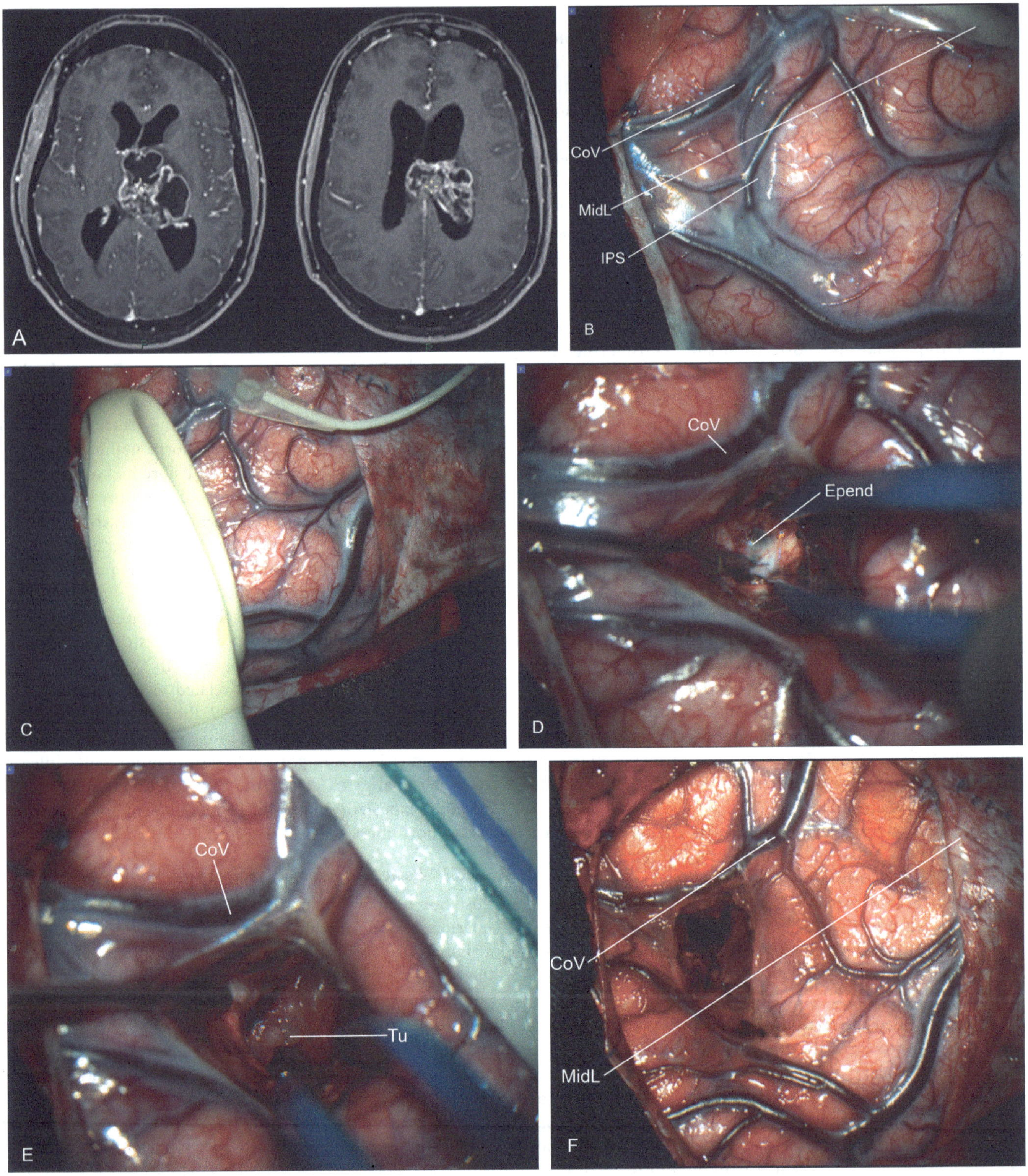

Figure 3.37 Transparietal transsulcal resection of a left thalamic and atrial astrocytoma. (A) Preoperative MR images; (B) view of the anterior aspect of the intraparietal sulcus and a large anterior cortical vein apparently running along the postcentral sulcus; (C) Use of brain mapping and ultrasound; (D) opening of the intraparietal sulcus and reaching the ependyma with its dark appearance; (E) view of the tumor within the atrium; (F) transsulcal view after resection; (G) postoperative MR images showing the site of entrance, the track of the approach, and the atrium free of tumor.

CoV: cortical vein apparently running along the postcentral sulcus; Epend: ependyma; IPS: intraparietal sulcus; MidL: midline dura mater; Tu: tumor.

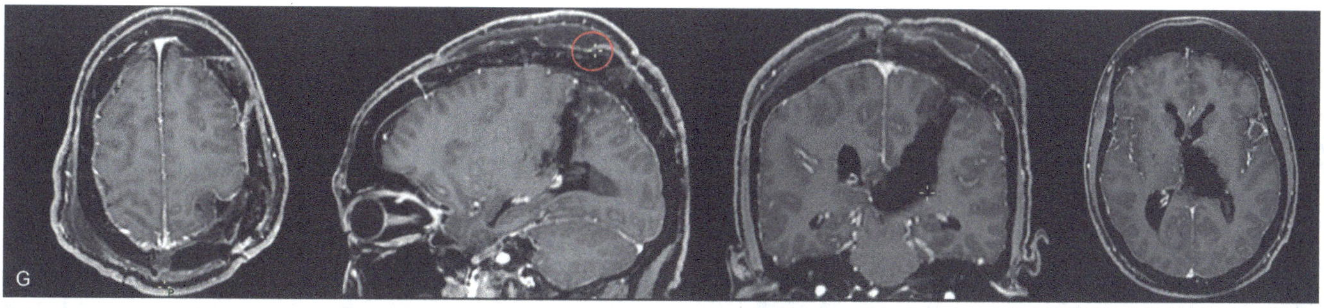

Figure 3.37 (Cont.)

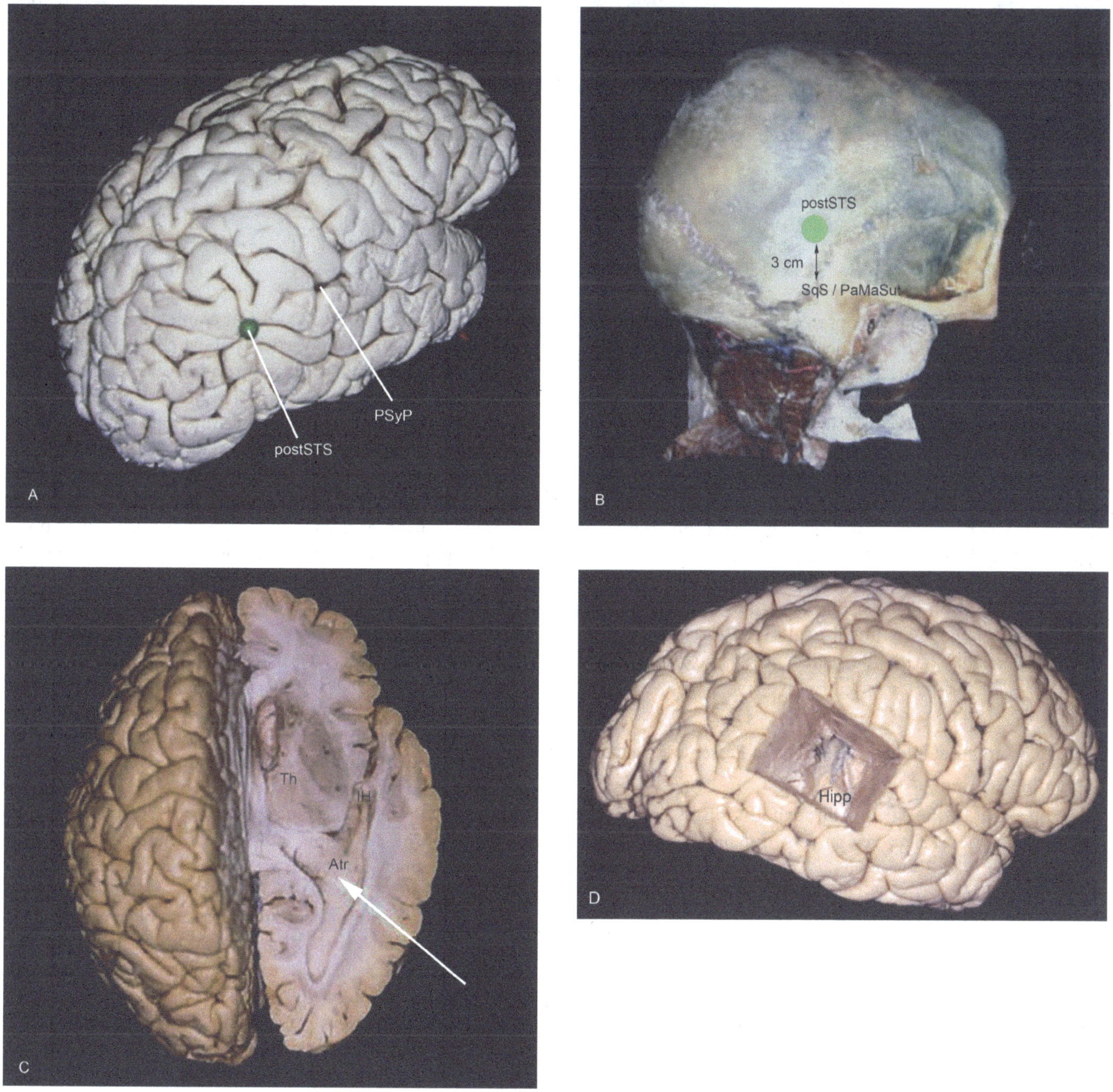

Figure 3.38 The posterior segment of the superior temporal sulcus. (A) Before its usual distal trifurcation, the most posterior segment of the superior temporal sulcus is located posterior and inferior to the distal aspect of the Sylvian fissure, and (B) it lies underneath the cranial area located 3 cm above the evident meeting point of the squamosal and parietomastoid suture; (C) a radially and anteriorly oriented approach through the opening of the posterior segment of the superior temporal sulcus leads to the atrium; (D) exposure of the atrium through a window centered in the most posterior segment of the superior temporal sulcus and view of the most posterior part of the hippocampus.

Atr: atrium of lateral ventricle; Hipp: hippocampus; IH: inferior horn; postSTS: distal extremity of the posterior segment of the superior temporal sulcus; PSyP: posterior Sylvian point; SqS/PaMaSut: meeting point of squamosal and parietomastoid sutures; Th: thalamus.

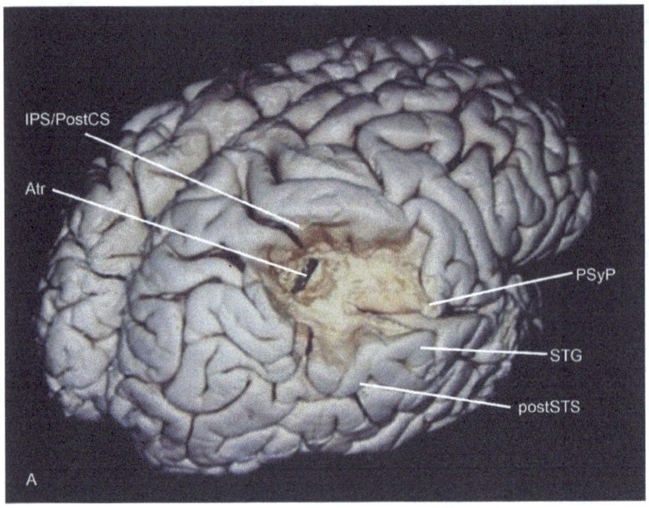

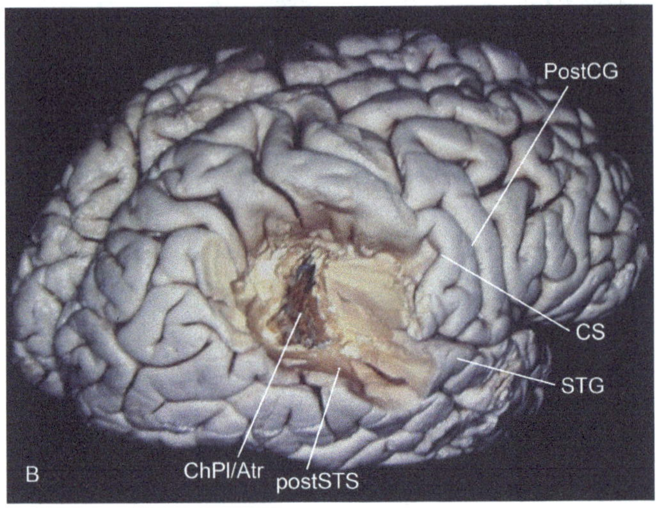

Figure 3.39 Exposure of the atrium. (A) Exposure of the superior aspect of the atrium after the anatomical removal of the supramarginal gyrus; (B) further exposure of the inferior aspect of the atrium with removal of the posterior part of the superior temporal gyrus guided by the identification of the posterior segment of the superior temporal sulcus.

Atr: atrium of lateral ventricle with choroid plexus over the thalamus; ChPl/Atr: choroid plexus within the atrium; CS: central sulcus; IPS: intraparietal sulcus; IPS/PostCS: intraparietal and postcentral sulci meeting point; PostCG: postcentral gyrus; PostCS: postcentral sulcus; postSTS: distal extremity of the posterior segment of the superior temporal sulcus ; PSyP: posterior Sylvian point; STG: superior temporal gyrus.

performed radially along an approximately 30° to 40° posteriorly inclined coronal plane (Ribas *et al.*, 2006) (Figure 3.40).

Other than for atrial lesions, this posterior temporal approach is also adequate for non-dominant ventricular atrial lesions that extend inferiorly toward the inferior horn and eventually also to the ambient and quadrigeminal cisterns through the choroidal fissure. Although always damaging optic radiation fibers (Ebeling and Reulen, 1988), this approach, when limited, can ultimately cause no significant clinical visual deficits (Hugher *et al.*, 1999).

Transcerebral posterior temporal approaches should be avoided in the dominant hemisphere due to their possible consequent language impairments (Ojemann *et al.*, 1989), unless done with the patient awake (Duffau, 2011b) (Figure 3.41).

3.2.6.3 Anatomical Remarks Pertinent to Posterior Temporal Approaches

The approach to the atrium through the distal part of the superior temporal sulcus region (Ebeling and Reulen, 1995a; Harkey *et al.*, 1989; Ribas, 2006) is more appropriate for more inferior atrial tumors, particularly when these lesions extend toward the temporal horn and/or receive significant blood supply from the anterior choroidal artery. Nevertheless, this approach can damage more significantly the optic radiations that run along the lateral wall of the atrium, and the Wernicke area with its underlying language-related fibers which lie predominantly within the posterior aspect of the superior temporal gyrus and within the supramarginal gyrus when in the dominant hemisphere. Awake craniotomies, when feasible, can minimize such damage.

As already mentioned, the most distal point of the superior temporal sulcus before its usual trifurcation lies about 2 to 3 cm posteriorly and inferiorly to the posterior Sylvian point (end of the Sylvian fissure) (Ribas, 2006). For craniotomy purposes, this area is located about 3 cm vertically above the meeting point of the horizontal parietomastoid suture and the ascending posterior aspect of the squamous suture. This is a site that can usually be palpated as a slight depression over the superior aspect of the mastoid process (Ribas, 2006; Ribas and Rodrigues, 2007).

Once a horizontal sulcal segment just inferiorly and posteriorly to the end of the Sylvian fissure has been identified, an adjoining transparenchymal approach can be performed transsulcally, subpially or transgyrally, 30 to 40 degrees anteriorly and radially oriented (Ribas, 2006; Ribas, 2005b). The ventricular route can be more securely aided by neuronavigation and with the use of intraoperative ultrasound. Further brain tissue can be removed as necessary for a proper exposure.

Since Heschl's gyrus bounds the triangular temporal plane anteriorly and obliquely, with its inner apex immediately next to the atrium, opening of the most posterior aspect of the Sylvian fissure can also lead to the atrium. Nevertheless, this opening is technically difficult due to the flatness of the fissure at this level. This approach necessitates further removal of the superior temporal intraopercular surface (auditory primary cortical area), and/or the base of the supramarginal gyrus.

More basal temporal approaches can be made, namely through a window created by removal of the posterior part of the inferior temporal gyrus and of its medially adjacent fusiform gyrus which corresponds to the floor of the posterior aspect of the temporal horn and of the atrium. These approaches can spare both the optic radiations and the language areas within the dominant hemisphere, but are much more suitable for inferior lesions already also occupying the temporal horn. For these approaches, it is important to bear in mind that the inferior temporal gyrus, although broad, is short in height, and its exposure requires a very low temporal craniotomy. Since the fusiform gyrus lies predominantly over

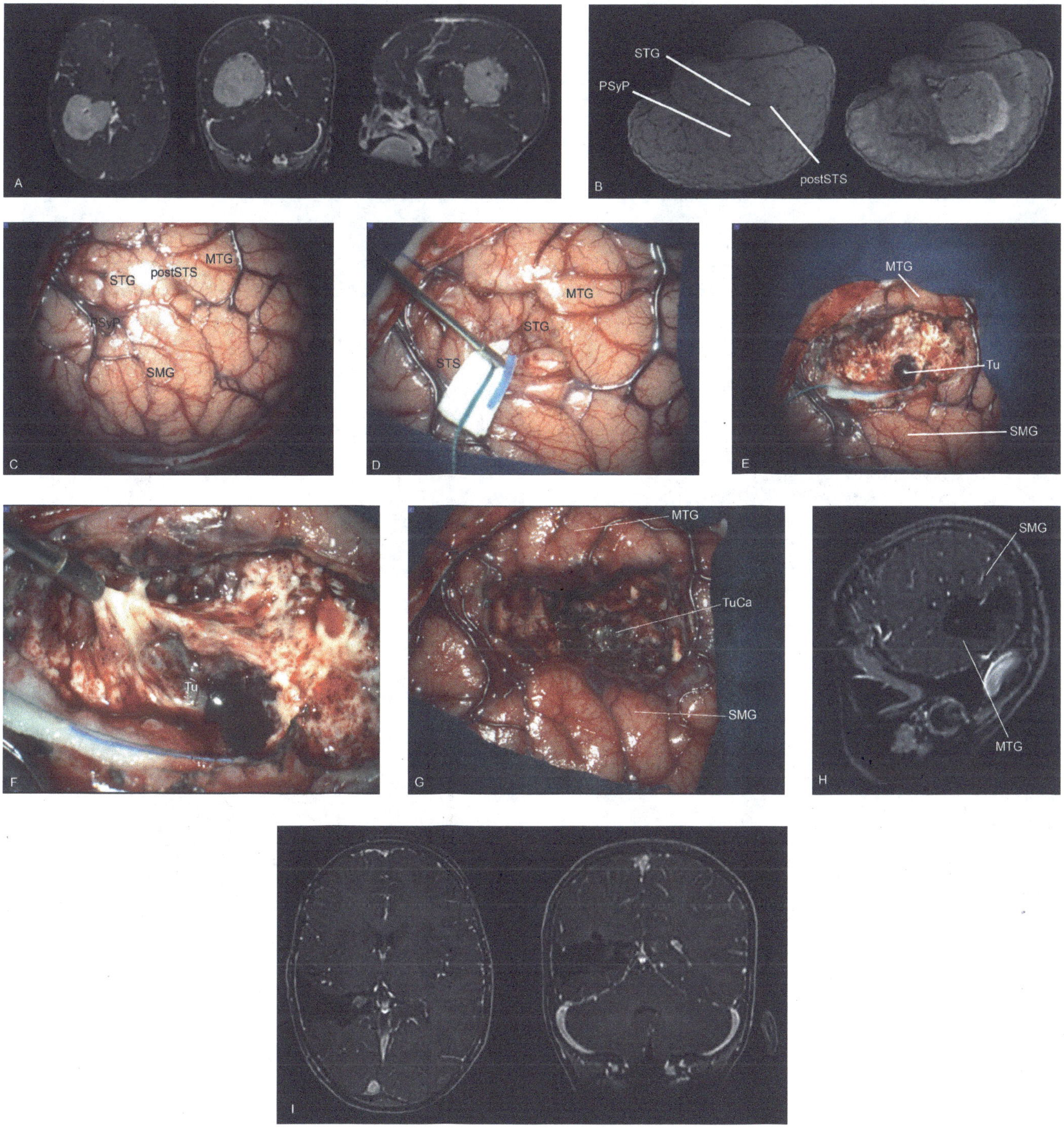

Figure 3.40 Resection of a right intra-atrium choroid plexus papilloma through the opening of the posterior segment of the right superior temporal sulcus and resection of its adjacent part in the superior temporal gyrus. (A) Preoperative MR images; (B) 3D rendered MR images of the projection of the tumor on the brain surface, in the operative position; (C) surgical exposure of the right posterior temporal surface; (D) opening of the distal or posterior aspect of the superior temporal sulcus; (E) white matter and tumor seen through a window given by a partial resection of the posterior part of the right superior temporal gyrus; (F) further exposure of the tumor; (G) postoperative cavity; (H) postoperative sagittal MR image showing the removal of the posterior part of the right superior temporal gyrus; (I) postoperative axial and coronal MR images showing the surgical corridor for the right atrium tumor removal.

MTG: middle temporal gyrus; postSTS: distal extremity of the posterior segment of the superior temporal sulcus; PSyP: posterior Sylvian point; SMG: supramarginal gyrus; STG: superior temporal gyrus; STL: superior temporal line; STS: superior temporal sulcus; Tu: tumor; TuCa: tumor cavity.

the superior surface of the petrous bone, the craniotomy base should include the extent between the preauricular depression (the upper surface of the most posterior aspect of the zygomatic root, just anteriorly to the tragus), and the meeting point of the horizontal parietomastoid and the posterior and ascending portion of the squamous suture, located at the upper aspect of the mastoid process (Ribas and Rodrigues, 2007).

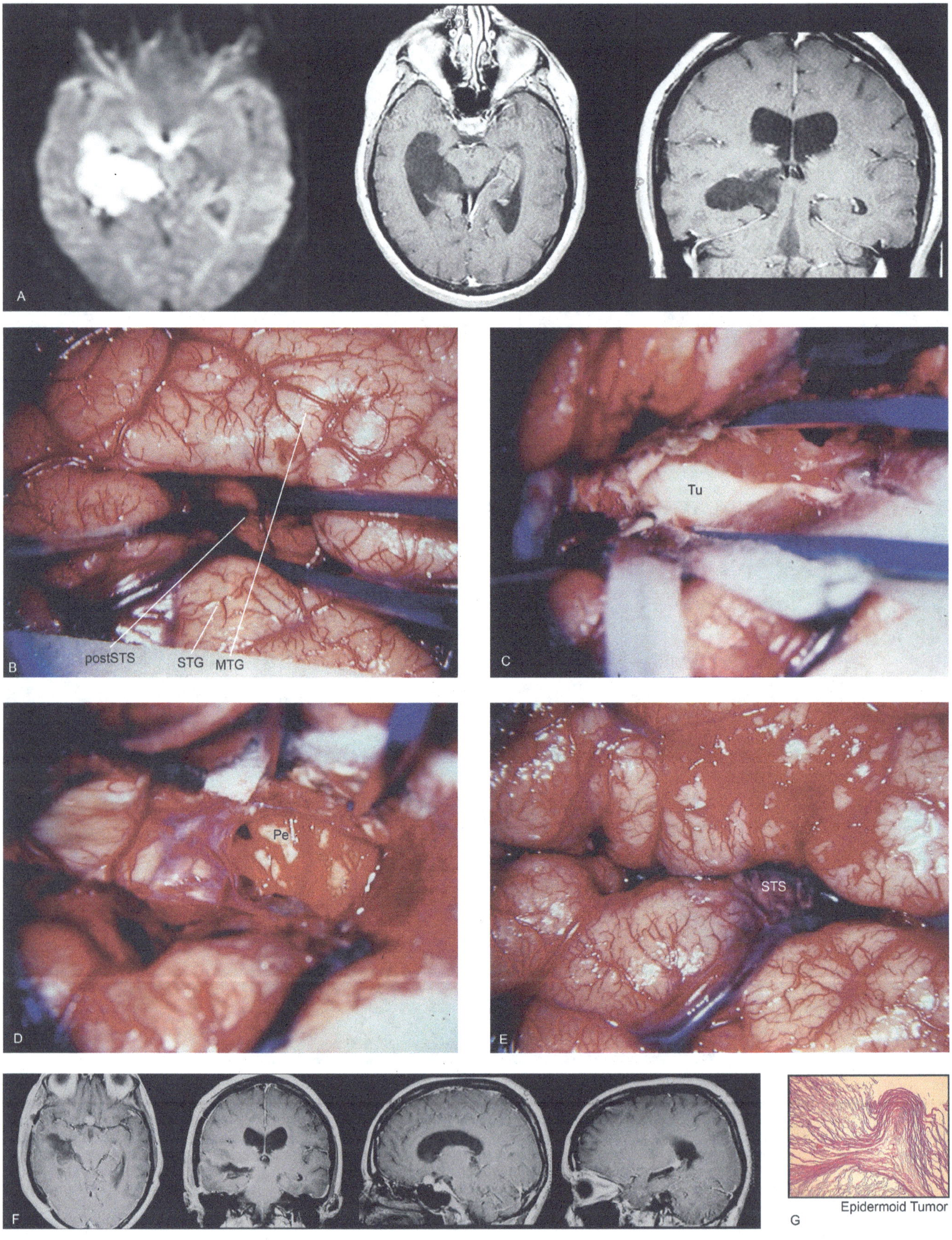

Figure 3.41 Resection of a right ventricular and cisternal epidermoid tumor through the posterior segment of the right superior temporal sulcus. (A) Diffusion-weighted and T1 MR images of the tumor occupying the right inferior horn and reaching the ambient and pineal cisterns through the opening of the choroidal fissure, and the atrium along the ventricular cavity; (B) opening of the distal segment of the superior temporal sulcus; (C) exposure of the epidermoid tumor inside the ventricular cavity; (D) view of the cerebral peduncle after resection and removal of the tumor from the already described communicating compartments; (E) view of the transsulcal approach after the resection; (F) postoperative MR images showing the already described communicating compartments free from tumor; note that the thalamus is not compressed as previously; (G) typical histological aspect of the epidermoid tumor.

MTG: middle temporal gyrus; Pe: cerebral peduncle midbrain; postSTS: distal extremity of the posterior segment of the superior temporal sulcus; STG: superior temporal gyrus; STS: superior temporal sulcus; Tu: tumor.

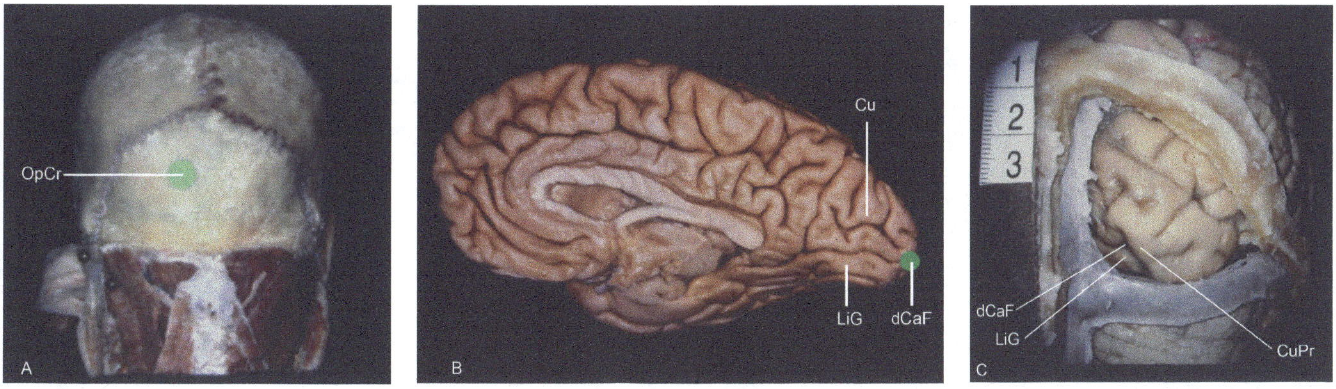

Figure 3.42 The opisthocranion and the distal extremity of the calcarine fissure. (A) The opisthocranion corresponds to the most prominent point of the occipital bossa, and (B, C), it lies exactly over the distal extremity of the calcarine fissure and hence of the posterior cuneal prominence.
Cu: cuneus; CuPr: posterior cuneal prominence; dCaF: distal extremity of the calcarine fissure; LiG: lingual gyrus; OpCr: opisthocranion.

3.2.7 Occipital Key Point

Together with the parieto-occipital incisure (POInc) already described, the opisthocranion (OpCR) constitutes the other important landmark for occipital exposures.

3.2.7.1 The Opisthocranion

The opisthocranion (OpCr) is the craniometric point that corresponds to the most prominent occipital cranial point along the midline(Gusmão *et al.*, 2000; Broca, 1876b; Pernkoff, 1980), and is an important landmark because its area always overlies the superior aspect of the calcarine fissure, hence the base of the cuneus, within the occipital pole.

The distance of approximately 2 cm from the OpCr to the occipital base indicates the height of the lingual gyrus.

3.2.7.2 Occipital Craniotomies

Occipital craniotomies that intend to expose the surface and/or the medial aspect of the occipital lobe, and occipital craniotomies for transtentorial approaches to the retrocallosal area and pineal region which require the uplifting of the occipital pole from the oblique falcotentorial transition, should place the opisthocranion (OpCr) as their center. This is because this cranial point is located over the base of the cuneus (Cu) and hence over the distal part of the calcarine fissure (dCaF), which should constitute the center of their cortical exposures (Figure 3.42).

Along the midline, these craniotomies should then expose: 1) superiorly, the superior extremity of the parieto-occipital sulcus, which also corresponds to the parieto-occipital incisure (POInc) located underneath the sagittal and lambdoid suture angle (La/Sa), and 2) inferiorly, the occipital base, which is externally related to the external occipital prominence, or inion (Broca, 1876b; Pernkoff, 1980), over the torcula (Ribas *et al.*, 2005a). This will leave the OpCr, with its underlying cuneal prominence (Cu) and distal extremity of the calcarine fissure (dCaF), at the center of the cranial and cortical exposures, as already also illustrated by Seeger (1978) and by McComb and Apuzzo (1988).

Given the occasional difficulty in palpating the inion (In) and estimating the position of the lambda (La), and given the usual prominence of the opisthocranion (OpCr), it is important to bear in mind that the La is usually located 2 to 4 cm above the OpCr (Ribas, 2006; Ribas, 2005b), and the In 6 to 8 cm inferiorly to the La (Ribas, 1991).

Along the midline, while the cuneus then projects between the La/Sa and the OpCr, the lingual gyrus projects between the OpCr and the In (Ribas *et al.*, 2006) (Figure 3.43).

Interhemispheric approaches through occipital craniotomies done below the La usually have the advantage of dealing with fewer bridging veins than those through parietal craniotomies (Rhoton, 2003). It is interesting to point out that, along the occipital mesial surface, the opisthocranion, the distal half of the calcarine fissure, the isthmus of the cingulate gyrus, and the splenium are roughly at the same level.

The lateral extent of the craniotomy depends on the necessary occipital cortical exposure.

The intra-occipital sulcus (Duvernoy, 1991; Naidich *et al.*, 1995), which is also called the transverse occipital sulcus (Ono *et al.*, 1990; Yasargil, 1994) and the superior occipital sulcus (Testut and Jacob, 1932), is usually a predominantly vertical continuation of the intraparietal sulcus inferior to the parieto-occipital incisure (POInc), which separates the usually more evident and vertical superior occipital gyrus (SOG) from the more variable middle occipital gyrus (MOG) (Naidich *et al.*, 1995; Testut and Jacob, 1932; Alves, 2012; Ribas, 2010). The lateral occipital sulcus (Ono *et al.*, 1990; Yasargil, 1994) or inferior occipital sulcus (Testut and Jacob, 1932; Alves, 2012; Ribas, 2010) separates the middle and inferior occipital gyri, and the lunate sulcus, when present, lies anteriorly to the occipital pole (Ono *et al.*, 1990; Yasargil, 1994; Alves, 2012; Ribas, 2010).

For a better understanding of the occipital gyral architecture, it is important to bear in mind that, just as the superior parietal lobule is continuous along the midline with the precuneus, the superior occipital gyrus is continuous with the cuneus, and the inferior occipital gyrus is continuous with the lingual gyrus. The inferior temporal, the inferior occipital, the lingual, and the parahippocampal

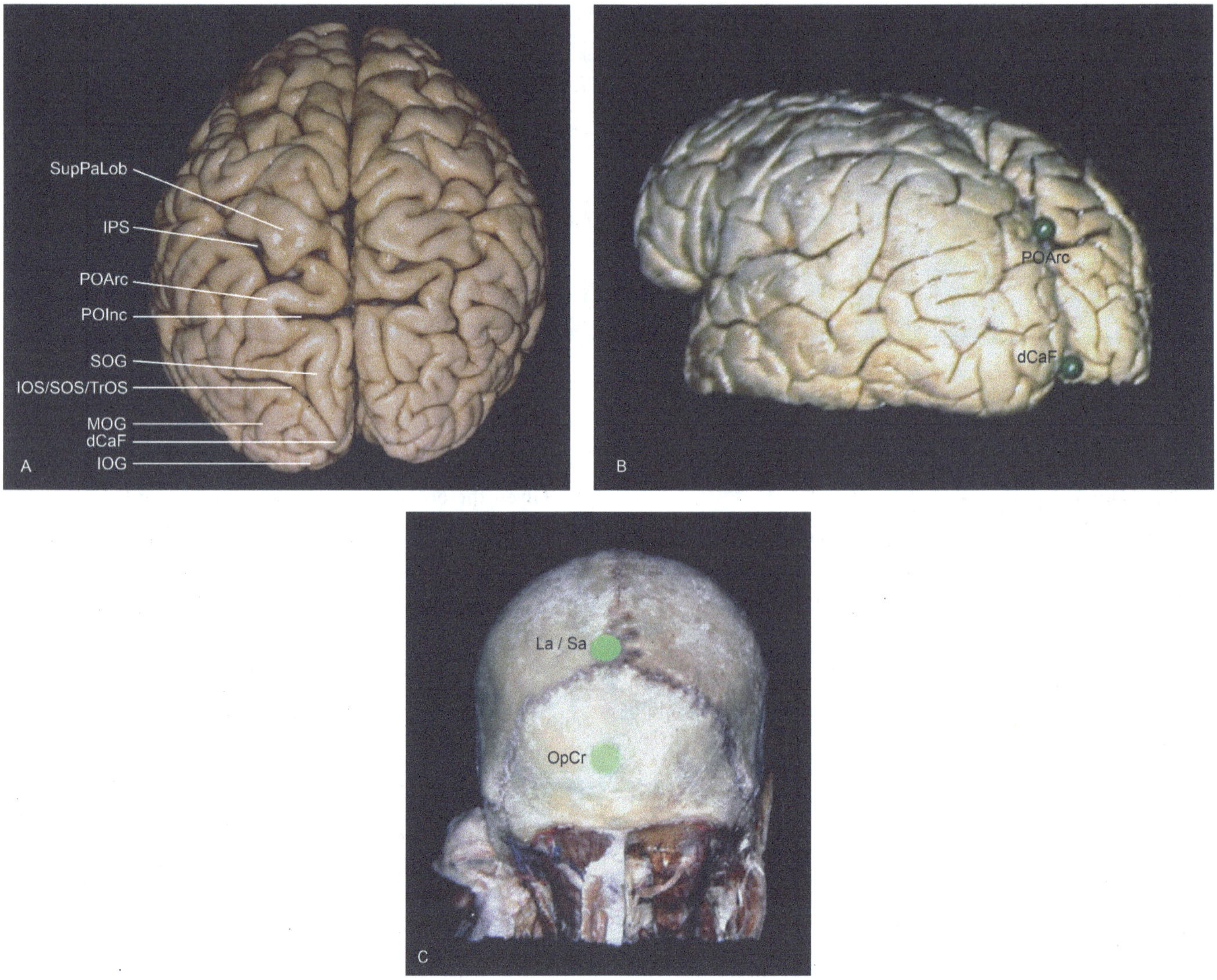

Figure 3.43 The parieto-occipital surface and its related cerebral and cranial key points. (A) Parieto-occipital sulci and gyri: the intra-occipital (or superior occipital, or transverse occipital) sulcus is a continuation of the intraparietal sulcus; the parieto-occipital incisure corresponds to the depth of the parieto-occipital sulcus; the parieto-occipital arc, or parieto-occipital connection of Gratiolet, connects the superior parietal lobule with the superior occipital gyrus; while the superior parietal lobule is continuous with the precuneus along the midline, the always vertical superior occipital gyrus is continuous with the cuneus, and the inferior occipital gyrus is continuous with the lingual gyrus; (B) parieto-occipital sulcal key points; and (C) their related cranial points.

dCaF: distal extremity of the calcarine fissure; IOG: inferior occipital gyrus; IOS: inferior occipital sulcus; IOS/SOS/TrOS: intra-occipital sulcus/superior occipital sulcus/transverse occipital sulcus; IPS: intraparietal sulcus; La/As: angle between the lambdoid and sagittal sutures; MOG: middle occipital gyrus; OpCr: opisthocranion; POArc: parieto-occipital arc, also known as the first parieto-occipital connection of Gratiolet (Broca, 1876b); POInc: parieto-occipital incisure, in the past also known as the external perpendicular fissure (Broca, 1876b); SOG: superior occipital gyrus; SupPaLob: superior parietal lobule; SOS: superior occipital sulcus.

gyri, are all longitudinal and continuous gyri which altogether comprise a basal ring in each cerebral hemisphere.

Occasional significant cortical visual impairments pertinent to occipital approaches are usually secondary to damage to the distal half of the calcarine fissure (Brodal, 1981).

3.2.7.3 Anatomical Remarks Pertinent to Common Occipital Transcerebral Procedures

Occipital Lobectomy

An anatomical occipital lobectomy consists of the removal of the occipital pole, and requires the resection of the superior occipital gyrus and its adjoining cuneus, of the posterior aspects of the middle and inferior occipital gyri, and of the adjoining lingual gyrus, with the patient in the sitting or ventral position.

Since the superior limit of the resection is given by the parieto-occipital incisure, which corresponds to the depth of the parieto-occipital sulcus on the dorsal or superolateral brain surface, the superior limit of the craniotomy should be above the angle that there is in between the sagittal and lambdoid sutures which overlies the parieto-occipital incisure.

The inferior limit of the craniotomy should be at the level of the inion, which corresponds to the level of the transverse sinus and of the tentorium.

The medial extent of the craniotomy should expose the sagittal sinus in order to allow the interhemispheric exposure, and its lateral extent is dependent on the required lateral parenchymal removal.

While the medial and basal occipital surfaces are easily detached and lifted, respectively, from the falx and the tentorium, the superior aspect of the resection should be guided by the parieto-occipital sulcus. A transsulcal section can start at the parieto-occipital incisure on the medial aspect of the superolateral surface, and proceed through its depth along the whole parieto-occipital sulcus, and then extend laterally through the division of the parieto-occipital incisure as far as necessary. A subpial resection should follow the same landmarks.

The lateral section should be made through a transparenchymal vertical incision dividing the middle and inferior occipital gyri as far as the tentorium.

The depth of the subcortical resection is variable, but the point of origin of the parieto-occipital sulcus along the calcarine fissure, which corresponds roughly to its midpoint, can serve as a landmark.

Since the occipital pole harbors both the cuneal and lingual margins of the distal half of the calcarine fissure and their related optic radiations, its removal causes or augments visual hemianoptic defects (Figure 3.44).

Occipital Interhemispheric Approach to the Atrium

The parieto-occipital intrahemispheric approach to the atrium as proposed by Yasargil (1996) is unique in the sense that it is the only approach which does not damage the optic radiations. Nevertheless, it is not quite a direct route, and the surgical corridor is rather limited by the possible degree of occipital retraction.

Since the approach is performed interhemispherically along the cuneus, the patient ideally should be in the semi-sitting position, and the craniotomy along the midline should extend from the lambda, which corresponds to the most distal point of the parieto-occipital sulcus, to the opisthocranion, which is the most prominent cranial point of the occipital bossa and which corresponds to the most distal point of the calcarine fissure. In adults, while the opisthocranion is usually located 3 to 4 cm above the inion, the lambda is usually located between 2 and 4 cm above the opisthocranion and 12 to 14 cm posteriorly to the bregma (Ribas *et al.*, 2006).

The occipital interhemispheric approach is facilitated by the fact that the cortical parieto-occipital veins usually have an ascending course parallel to the superior sagittal sinus for a few centimeters before joining the sinus (Yasargil, 1996; Oka *et al.*, 1985). The access should be made between the falx-tentorium transition and the cuneal surface toward the splenium. It should be borne in mind that the anterior apex of the cuneus, where the parieto-occipital sulcus joins the calcarine fissure and their respective arteries usually also meet, is located at the axial level of the splenial base. Further lateral occipital retraction can be favored by the sacrifice of small draining veins if necessary, and, mainly, by the opening of the parasplenial cisterns and release of CSF. Once the very whitish splenium and the vein of Rosenthal have been identified, the ipsilateral isthmus of the cingulate gyrus is easily seen wrapping the splenium together with the immediately posteriorly adjoining precuneal base, which altogether constitute the opening site of the transcerebral approach to the atrium.

Since the atrial cavity lies laterally, a window has to be made along a lateral and anterior orientation until the ventricular cavity is reached with identification of the tumor and/or the whitish pulvinar of the thalamus that constitutes the anterior wall of the atrium, with the choroid plexus glomus attached.

The main limitation of this approach is given by the degree of occipital retraction, and, as for any other ventricular approach, it is facilitated if there is ventriculomegaly. Since it requires a significant brain retraction and is done through an indirect route, neuronavigation and intraoperative ultrasound are not as helpful as for other approaches, and its accomplishment depends basically on the recognition of anatomical landmarks and orientation (Figure 3.45).

3.3 The Basal Supratentorial Key Points

The basal supratentorial key points delineate the basal aspect of the cerebral hemisphere, and can be used as strategic sites for the placement of basal burr holes of supratentorial basal craniotomies in neurosurgical practice. They are the frontozygomatic process, the anterior temporal, the preauricular depression, the parietomastoid and squamosal suture meeting point, and the asterion.

3.3.1 The Frontozygomatic Process Key Point

The zygomatic process of the frontal bone is the lateral extent of the frontal supra-orbital margin, and it articulates inferiorly with the zygomatic bone through the frontozygomatic suture. The line that arises along its superior and posterior edge curves upwards and backwards giving rise to the superior and inferior temporal lines (Williams and Warwick, 1980). Detachment of the temporal fascia and temporal muscle below and behind the temporal lines reveals the temporal surface of the frontal bone (Williams and Warwick, 1980) which is slightly concave and extends as far as the sphenofrontal suture (Figure 3.46).

While the classic McArthur keyhole (McArthur, 1912 apud Altay and Couldwell, 2012; McArthur, 1918 apud Altay and Couldwell, 2012; Altay and Couldwell, 2012) made just posteriorly to the zygomatic process (approximately 5 mm behind and 7 mm above the zygomatic sutures (Shimizu *et al.*, 2005; Tubbs *et al.*, 2010) exposes both the orbital and the intracranial cavities, a standard burr hole placed 1.0 cm posteriorly to zygomatic process and superiorly to the level of the sphenofrontal suture already exposes only the intracranial compartment, just above the orbital part of the frontal bone which corresponds to the floor of the anterior cranial fossa and to the roof of the orbital cavity. The intracranial surface of the orbital part of the frontal bone is predominantly convex, but such a burr hole exposes the anterior fossa just next to its most lateral aspect which is markedly concave, and

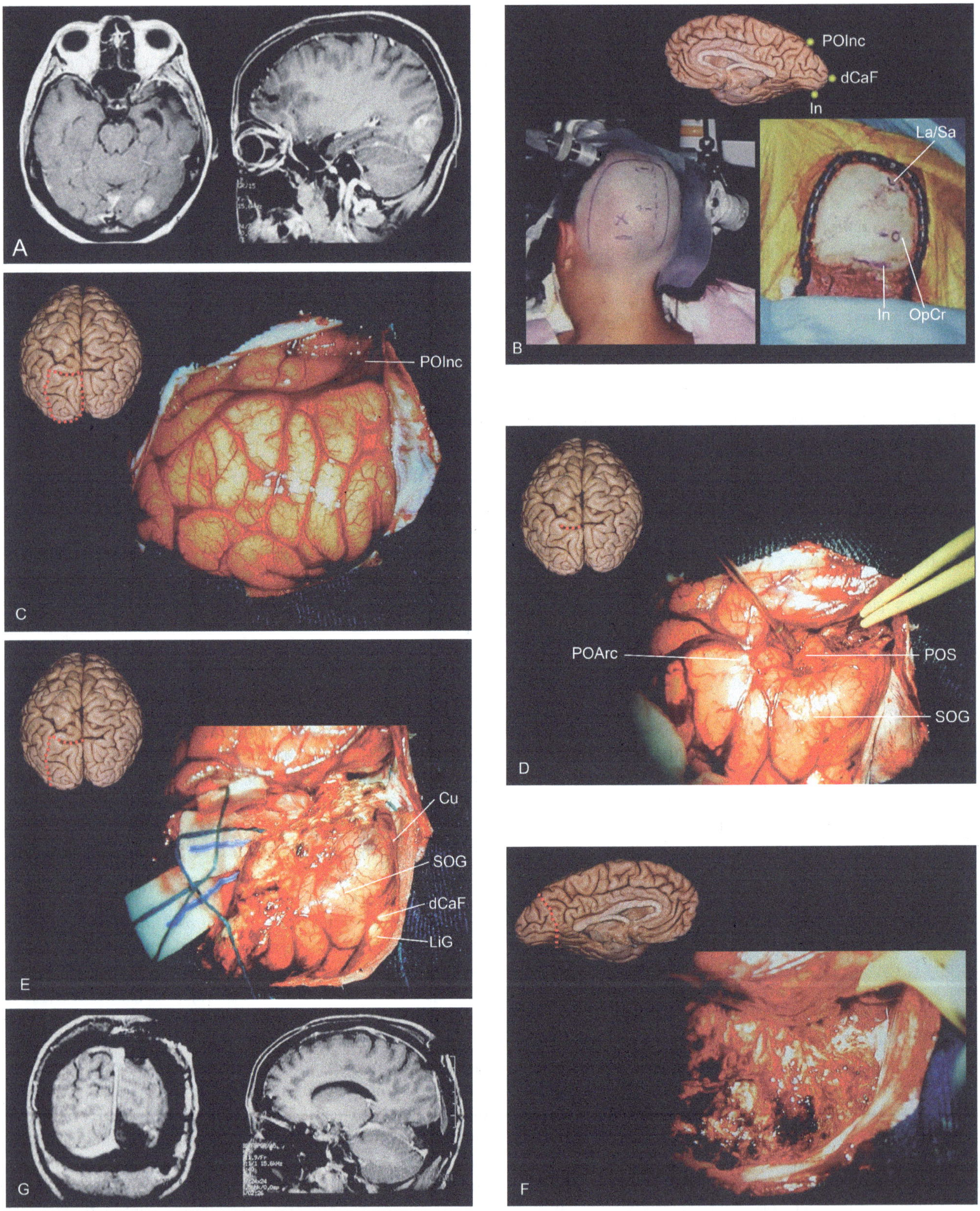

Figure 3.44 Left occipital lobectomy for the resection of a left occipital glioblastoma multiforme (GBM) in a patient with a right hemianopsia and previously operated for the resection of a left anterior temporal GBM. (A) preoperative MR images; (B) parieto-occipital key points and their exposure; (C) anatomical sketch of the surgical planning, and parieto-occipital exposure with vein running along the parieto-occipital incisure; (D) opening of the parieto-occipital sulcus started at the parieto-occipital incisure; (E) section of the parieto-occipital arc, and division of the middle and inferior occipital gyri; (F) view after the resection of the left occipital pole; (G) postoperative MR images.

Cu: cuneus; dCaF: distal extremity of the calcarine fissure; In: inion; La/Sa: angle between the lambdoid and sagittal sutures; LiG: lingual gyrus; OpCr: opisthocranion; POArc: parieto-occipital arc or parieto-occipital connection of Gratiolet; POInc: parieto-occipital incisure, in the past also known as the external perpendicular fissure (Broca, 1876b); POS: parieto-occipital sulcus; SOG: superior occipital gyrus.

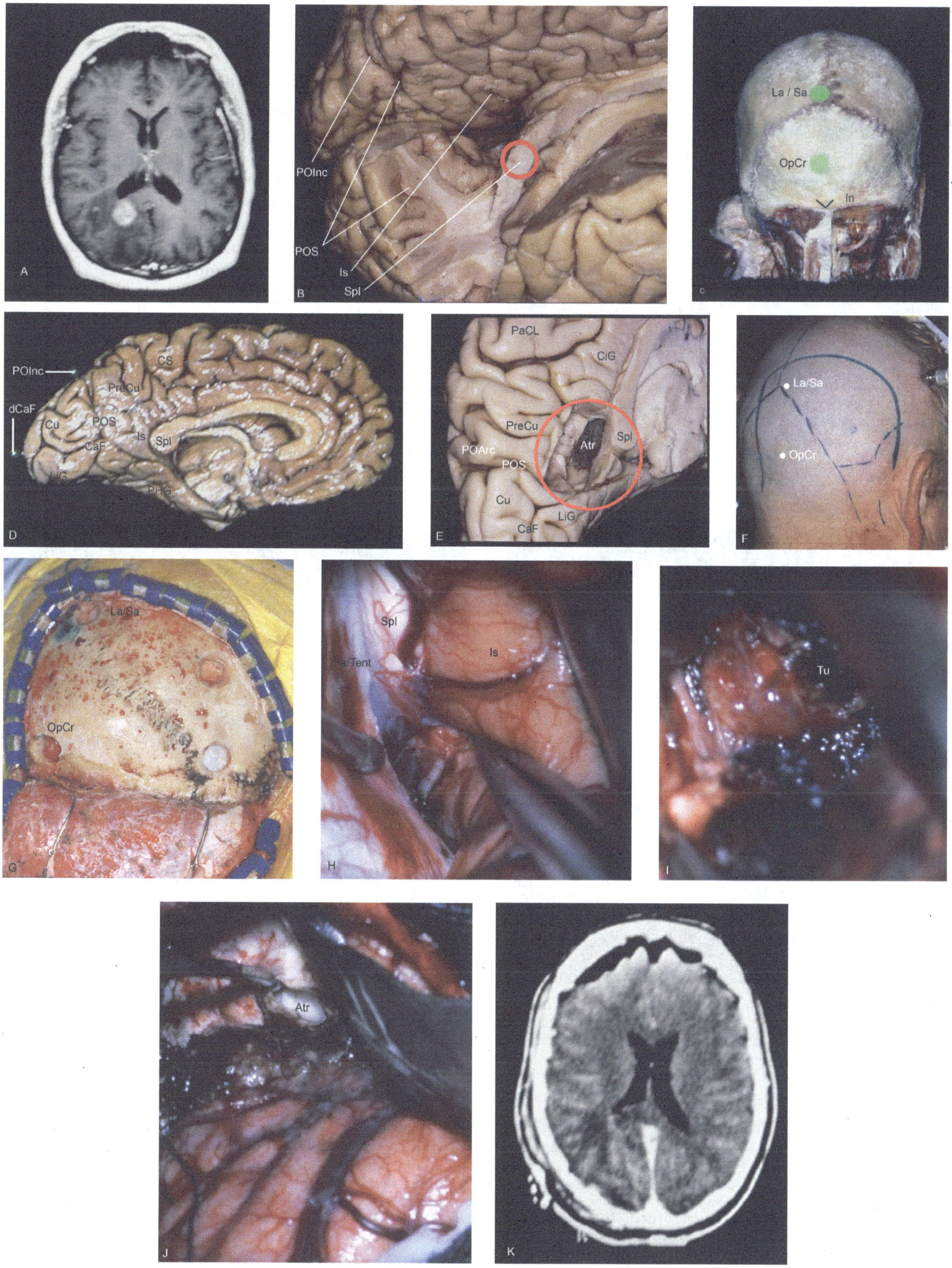

Figure 3.45 Parieto-occipital interhemispheric approach for the resection of a hypernephroma metastatic lesion located posterior to the right atrium. (A) Preoperative MR image; (B) location of the lesion in the right lateral aspect of the splenium which corresponds to the posterior wall of the right atrium; (C) cranial key

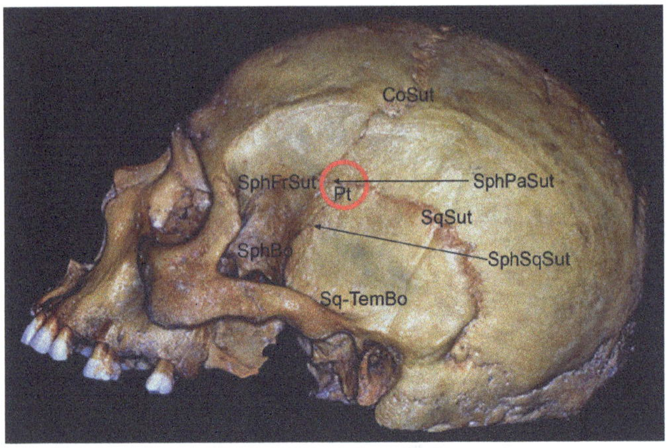

Figure 3.46 The pterion corresponds to the frontotemporal cranial area located around the central bar of its H-shaped set of sutures.

CoSut: coronal suture; Pt: pterion, within the red circle; SphBo: temporal surface of the sphenoid bone; SphFrSut: sphenofrontal suture; SphPaSut: sphenoparietal suture; SphSqSut: sphenosquamosal suture; SqSut: squamosal suture; Sq-TempBo: squamosal part of the temporal bone.

which characterizes a real groove that leads to the suprasellar region (Figure 3.47).

3.3.2 The Anterior Temporal Key Point

The temporal fossa is bounded superiorly by the temporal lines, anteriorly by the frontal process of the zygomatic bone, inferiorly by the zygomatic bone itself, and is inferiorly continuous with the infratemporal fossa through the gap underneath the zygomatic arch, with both fossae harboring the temporal muscle (Williams and Warwick, 1980).

Detachment of the temporal muscle exposes a rather constant H-shaped set of cranial sutures over the surface of the anterior part of the temporal fossa that brings together the frontal, parietal, sphenoidal, and temporal bones, along the coronal, sphenofrontal, sphenoparietal, squamosal, and sphenosquamosal sutures (Williams and Warwick, 1980; Federative Committee on Anatomical Terminology, 1998).

The sphenoparietal suture corresponds to the central and horizontal bar of the H which separates the antero-inferior angle of the parietal bone from the superior margin of the greater wing of the sphenoid bone. A small circular area

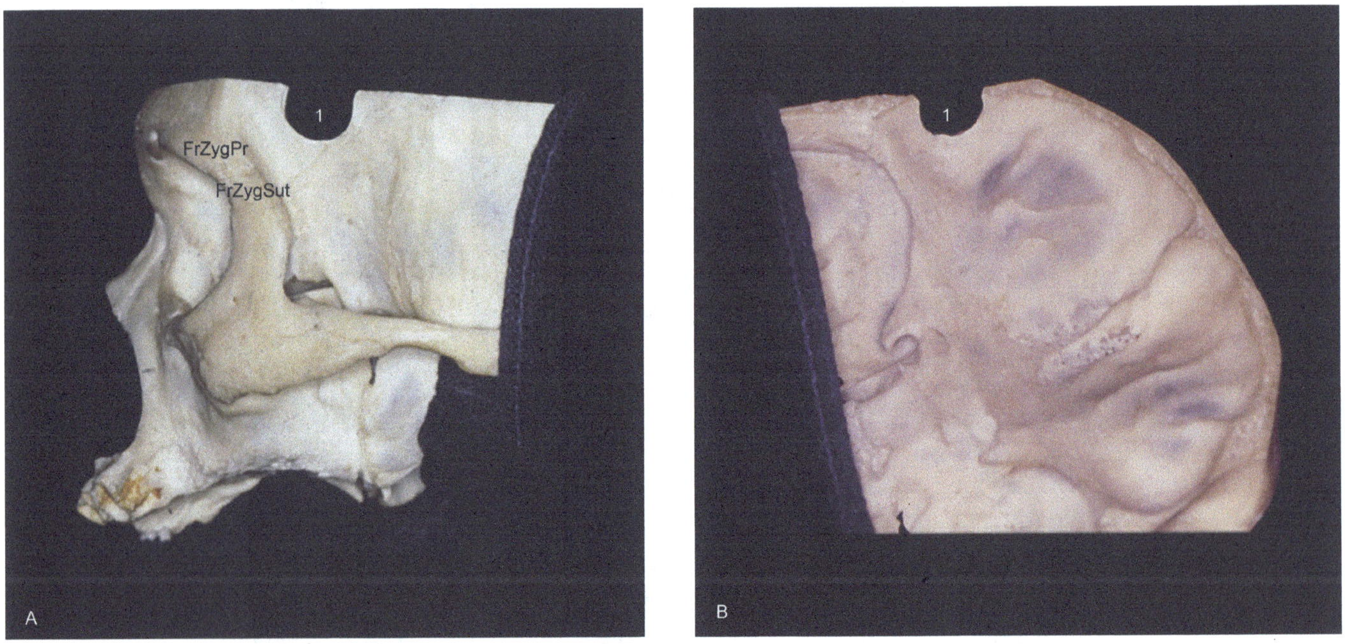

Figure 3.47 Frontozygomatic process key point. (A) A regular burr hole placed 1 cm posteriorly to the zygomatic process of the frontal bone; (B) burr hole reaches the lateral and most concave aspect of the orbital roof/floor of the anterior fossa.

1: frontozygomatic burr hole; FrZygPr: frontozygomatic process of the frontal bone; FrZygSut: frontozygomatic suture.

Caption for Figure 3.45 (cont.)

points for the craniotomy; (D) sulcal key points underneath the cranial key points, and medial parieto-occipital sulci and gyri; (E) site of the window to be made on the isthmus of the cingulate gyrus and lateral aspect of the splenium in order to expose the atrium; (F) incision over the cranial key points; (G) craniotomy burr holes; (H) occipital interhemispheric approach with exposure of isthmus of the cingulate gyrus which encircles the splenium; (I) exposure of the metastatic lesion known to be within the splenium; (J) exposure of the atrium with view of the pulvinar of thalamus after removal of the lesion; (K) postoperative MR images.

Atr: atrium; CaF: calcarine fissure; CiG: cingulate gyrus; CiSMR: cingular sulcus marginal ramus; CS: central sulcus; Cu: cuneus; dCaF: distal extremity of the calcarine fissure; Fa/Tent: falx continuous with tentorium; In: inion; Is: isthmus of cingulate gyrus; La/Sa: angle between the lambdoid and sagittal sutures, over the POInc; LiG: lingual gyrus; OpCr: opisthocranion, over the dCaF; PaCL: paracentral lobule; PHG: parahippocampal gyrus; POArc: parieto-occipital arc; POInc: parieto-occipital incisure, equivalent to the most superior point of the parieto-occipital sulcus; POS: parieto-occipital sulcus; PreCu: precuneus; Spl: splenium of corpus callosum; Tu: tumor.

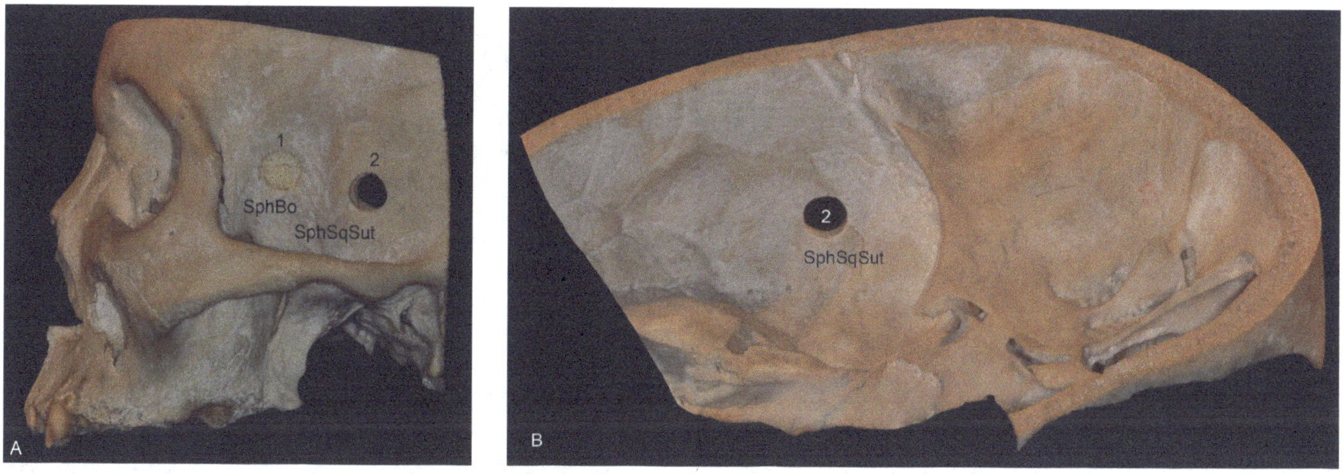

Figure 3.48 Anterior temporal key point. (A) The temporal surface of the sphenoid bone corresponds to the lateral projection of the sphenoid wing, and a regular burr hole placed anteriorly to the sphenosquamosal suture will still run into bone to some extent (1); (B) a regular burr hole placed posteriorly to this suture (2) will reach the temporal fossa more easily and more accurately.
1 & 2: location of burr holes; SphBo: temporal surface of the sphenoid bone; SphSqSut: sphenosquamosal suture.

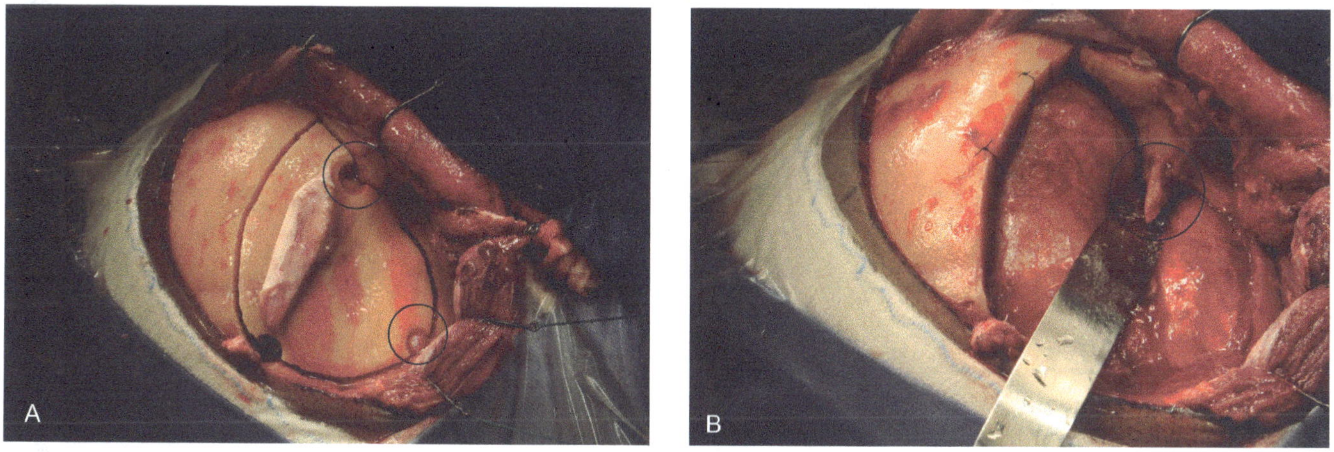

Figure 3.49 The frontotemporal/pterional craniotomy. (A) A frontal lateral burr hole placed posteriorly to the zygomatic process of the frontal bone along the most anterior aspect of the superior temporal line, and an anterior temporal burr hole, are the starting sites for the pterional craniotomy, (B) since the sphenoid wing lies between these two anterior burr holes. Adapted from Chaddad-Neto *et al.* (2012).

around the sphenoparietal suture that includes all of the four adjoining bones is referred to as the pterion (Broca, 1861 apud Finger, 1994; Williams and Warwick, 1980; Altay and Couldwell, 2012). The pterion lies approximately 4.0 cm above the zygomatic arch and 3.5 cm posterior to the frontozygomatic suture (Williams and Warwick, 1980), and is an important landmark since it overlies the lesser wing of the sphenoid which runs anterior and parallel to the stem of the lateral (Sylvian) fissure (Figure 3.47).

The temporal surface of the sphenoid bone lies below the sphenoparietal suture, posteriorly to the sphenofrontal suture and anteriorly to the sphenosquamosal suture. Since it corresponds to the outer aspect of the great wing of the sphenoid bone which is curved and superiorly more compact, a burr hole made over this surface might still run into bone not exposing the intracranial compartment correctly (Figure 3.48A, burr hole 1).

In order to reach the middle fossa fully, a burr hole should be placed on the squamosal surface of the temporal bone, hence posteriorly to the sphenotemporal suture (Chaddad-Neto *et al.*, 2012; Yasargil, 1984a; Yasargil *et al.*, 1975) (Figures 3.48A and B, burr hole 2). If this burr hole is to be connected with the previous frontozygomatic burr hole, it should not be placed too low since the posterior ridge of the sphenoid wing lies between them. An adequate basal frontotemporal craniotomy requires further drilling in order to flatten the orbital roof, the sphenoid wing, and the temporal base (Chaddad-Neto *et al.*, 2012; Yasargil, 1984a; Yasargil *et al.*, 1975). Since this cranial exposure is centered in the pterion, it is classically known as pterional craniotomy (Hamby, 1964 apud Altay and Couldwell, 2012; Altay and Couldwell, 2012; Yasargil *et al.*, 1975; Yasargil, 1984a) (Figure 3.49).

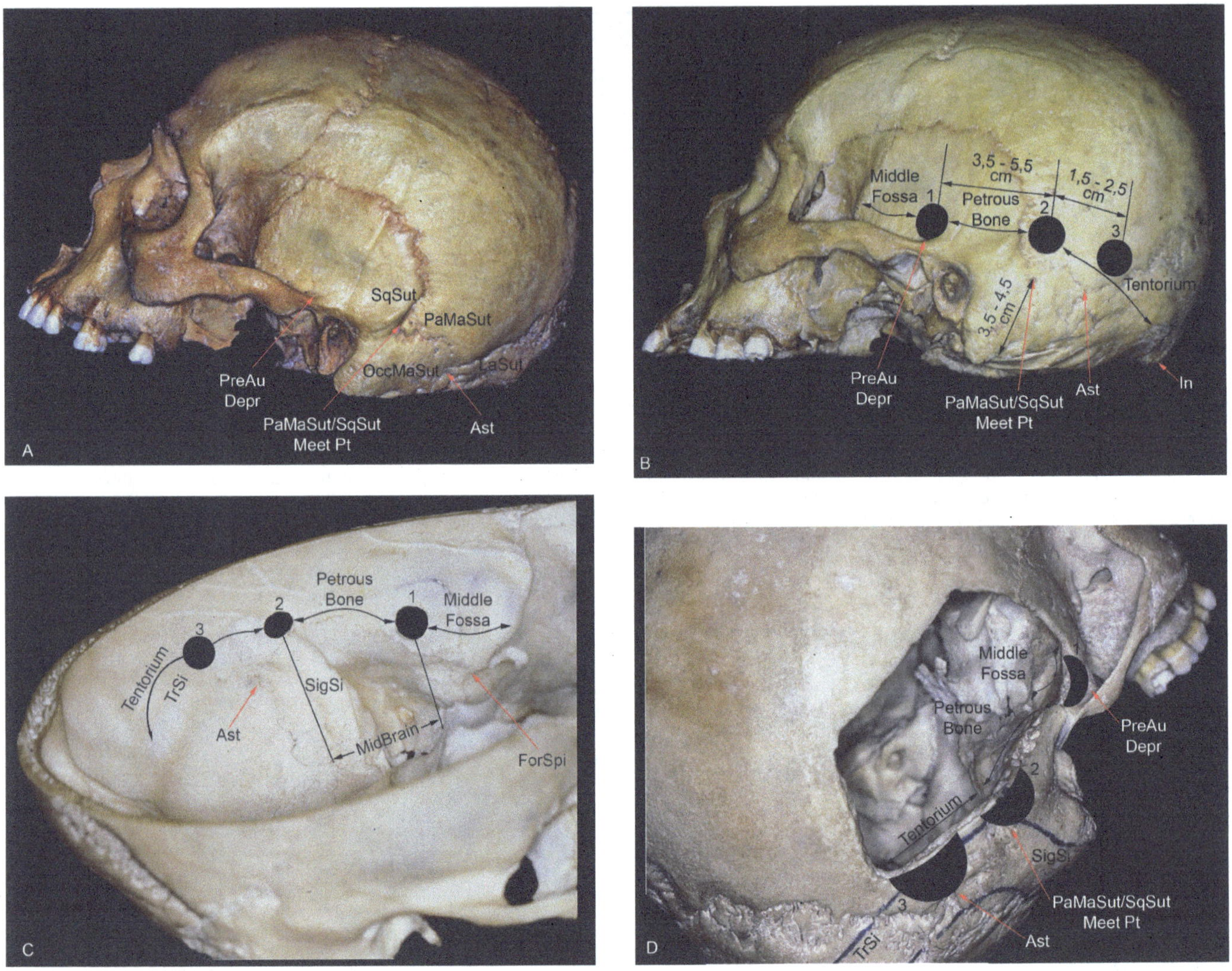

Figure 3.50 Suprapetrosal and asterion key points. (A) The preauricular depression (PreAuDepr) corresponds to the upper portion of the most posterior aspect of the zygomatic process, which is located just anterior to the tragus and external acoustic meatus. The asterion (Ast) corresponds to the junction of the parietomastoid, lambdoid, and occipitomastoid sutures (PaMaSut, LaSut, and OccMaSut, respectively). The point at which the parietomastoid and squamosal sutures meet (PaMaSut/SqSutMeetPt) can usually be felt on palpation like a slight depression; (B) two burr holes – the preauricular burr hole, located immediately above the preauricular depression (1), and the burr hole whose base is located 1 cm above the point at which the parietomastoid and squamosal sutures meet (2), delimit the external projection of the petrous portion of the temporal bone (Petrous Bone); hence, the middle fossa floor (Middle Fossa) lies anterior to the first burr hole, and the superior surface of the tentorium lies posterior to the second burr hole. The burr hole whose base is located 1 cm above the asterion (3) is usually completely, or at least mostly, supratentorial. The line provided by the external occipital protuberance, that corresponds to the inion (In), and the asterion (Ast), roughly indicates the position of the transverse sinus and can be relied on to orient further posterior extensions of supratentorial exposures; (C) and (D) intracranially, the first burr hole (1), located just above the preauricular depression, is situated adjacent to the foramen spinosum (ForSpi). The second burr hole (2), lies 1 cm above the meeting point of the parietomastoid and the squamosal sutures. Intracranially, these two burr holes delimit the most lateral aspect of the superior surface of the petrous portion of the temporal bone (Petrous Bone) and also the lateral aspect of the brainstem (MidBrain). The concave middle fossa floor lies anterior to the first burr hole, and the superior tentorial surface (Tentorium) lies posterior to the second burr hole. a third burr hole (3), whose base lies 1 cm above the asterion, is related to the superior aspect of the transverse sinus (TrSi) and, hence, also to the superior tentorial surface.

1, 2, & 3: burr holes; Ast: asterion; ForSpi: foramen spinosum; In: inion; LaSut: lambdoid suture; MidBrain: superior part of the brainstem; Middle Fossa: concave middle fossa floor; OccMaSut: occipitomastoid suture; PaMaSut: parietomastoid suture; PaMaSut/SqSutMeetPt: parietomastoid and squamosal suture meeting point; Petrous Bone: petrous part of the temporal bone; PreAuDepr: preauricular depression; SigSi: sigmoid sinus; SqSut: squamosal suture; Tentorium: superior tentorial surface; TrSi: transverse sinus. Adapted from Ribas and Rodrigues (2007).

3.3.3 The Preauricular Depression Key Point

The preauricular depression (PreAuDepr) is easily palpable just anteriorly to the tragus and to the external acoustic meatus, over the upper aspect of the most distal portion of the zygomatic process where the superficial temporal artery is usually palpable (Figure 3.50A). Internally, it corresponds to the anterior aspect of the petrous part of the temporal bone, and a burr hole placed just above the PreAuDepr exposes the posterior aspect of the middle fossa floor, at the level of the foramen spinosum (Ribas and Rodrigues, 2007) (Figures 3.50B, C and D).

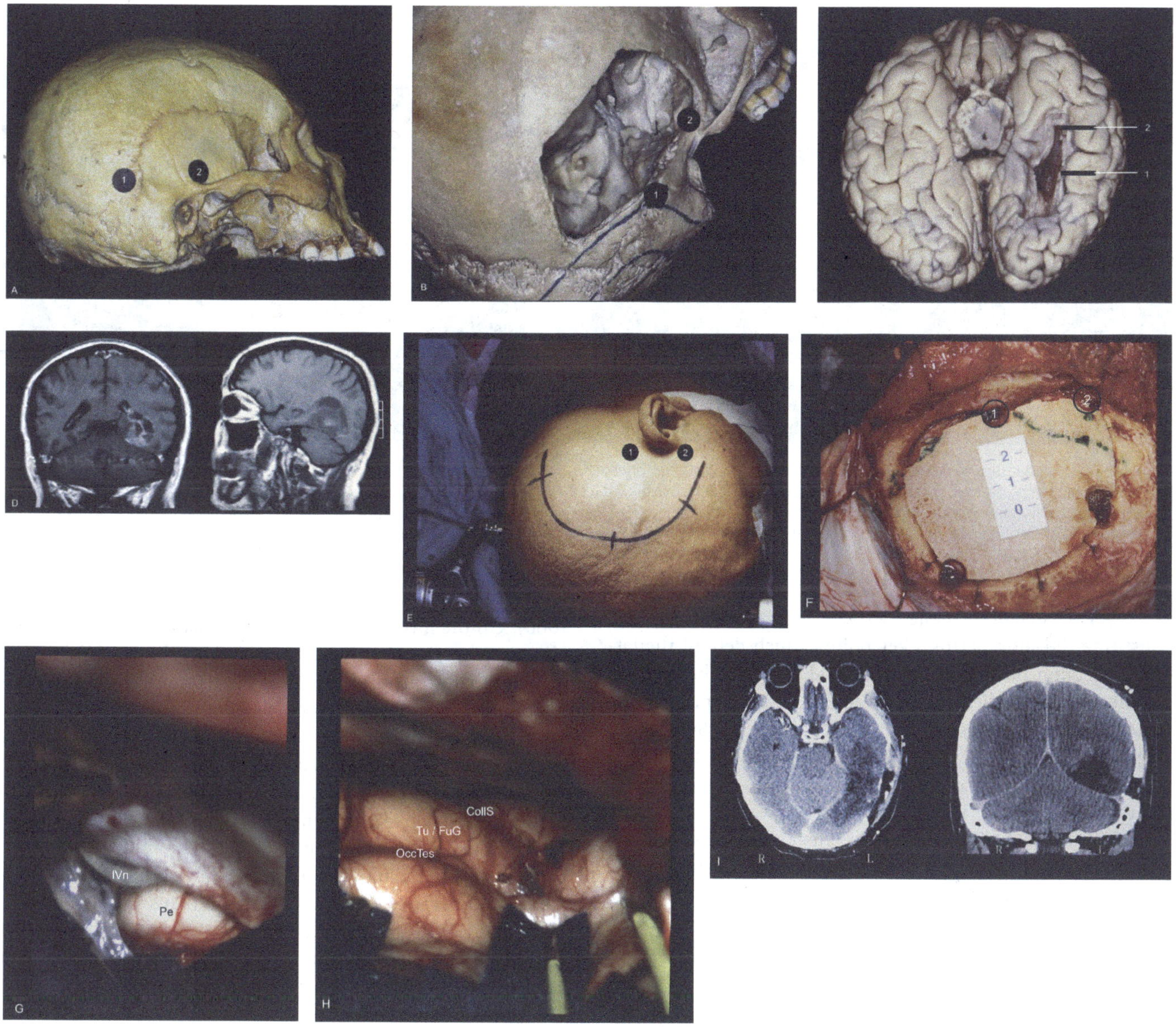

Figure 3.51 (A) The burr holes made (1) just above the parietomastoid and squamous suture meeting point and (2) above the preauricular depression (B) delimit the external projection of the petrous part of the temporal bone, (C) which lies underneath the anterior half of the fusiform gyrus; since the fusiform gyrus constitutes the floor of the atrium, the tumor protrudes inside this cavity; (D) MR coronal and sagittal images showing a left high grade glioma tumor within the posterior part of the fusiform gyrus since it lies already over the tentorium, hence posterior to the petrous bone; (E) scalpel incision and (F) craniotomy site, to expose both the superior surface of the petrous bone (between the burr holes made above the preauricular depression and above the parietomastoid and squamous suture meeting point) and the upper tentorium surface (posterior half of the craniotomy base); (G) subtemporal exposure of the IVth nerve and of the midbrain peduncle after opening of the ambient cistern in order to remove CSF; (H) basal temporal exposure of the fusiform gyrus bulging between the collateral and occipitotemporal sulci; (I) postoperative CT images showing removal of the basal aspect of the left inferior temporal gyrus and removal of the left fusiform gyrus which harbored the tumor.
1: burr hole above the parietomastoid and squamous suture meeting point; 2: burr hole above the preauricular depression; FuG: fusiform gyrus; CollS: collateral sulcus; IVn: fourth cranial nerve; OccTeS: occipitotemporal sulcus; Pe: cerebral peduncle midbrain; Tu/FuG: tumor within the fusiform gyrus.

3.3.4 The Parietomastoid and Squamosal Suture Meeting Point

Since the parietomastoid suture is always horizontal and the posterior part of the squamosal suture is vertical, its meeting point (PaMaSut/SqSutMeetPt) is always very evident and, usually, also palpable because the mastoid or postero-inferior angle of the parietal bone (Williams and Warwick, 1980) is frequently lower than the upper portion of the mastoid process (Ribas and Rodrigues, 2007; Ribas *et al.*, 2005b) (Figure 3.50A). Internally, the PaMaSut/SqSutMeetPt corresponds to the posterior aspect of the petrous part of the temporal bone, and a burr hole placed above it exposes the junction of the petrous upper surface with the tentorium, just superiorly to the transition between the transverse and the sigmoid sinuses (Ribas and Rodrigues, 2007) (Figure 3.50B, C and D).

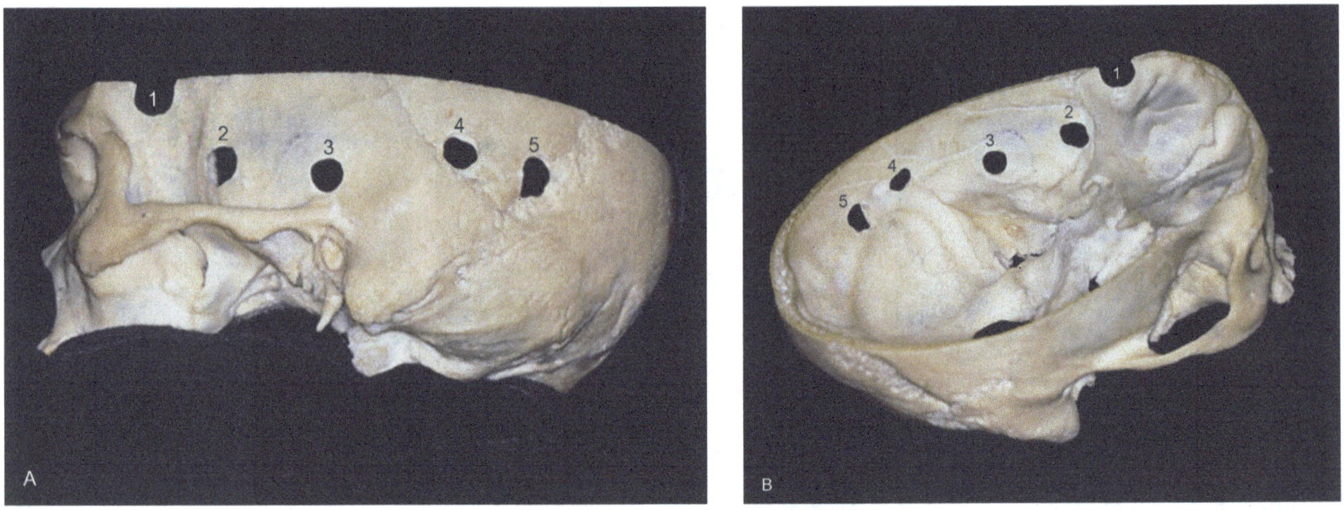

Figure 3.52 Altogether, the cranial basal supratentorial key points can orient the placement of basal burr holes for craniotomies that require exposure of the cerebral frontal, temporal, and occipital basal surfaces. (A) External view; (B) intracranial view.

1: burr hole posterior to the frontozygomatic process; 2: anterior temporal burr hole; 3: burr hole above the preauricular depression; 4: burr hole above the parietomastoid and squamosal suture meeting point; 5: burr hole above the asterion.

The PreAuDepr and the PaMaSut/SqSutMeetPt together constitute the suprapetrosal key points which delimit the lateral projection of the superior petrosal surface. The concave middle fossa floor lies anteriorly to the PreAuDepr, and the tentorium lies just posteriorly to the PaMaSut/SqSutMeetPt. These two key points also correspond roughly to the lateral projection of the midbrain (Ribas and Rodrigues, 2007) (Figure 3.50).

While the anterior part of the fusiform gyrus and the inferior horn lie mostly over the superior petrous surface, the posterior part of the fusiform gyrus and the atrium lie over the tentorium.

3.3.5 The Asterion

The asterion (Ast) is the craniometric point that corresponds to the meeting point of the lambdoid, occipitomastoid, and parietomastoid sutures (Broca, 1875; Williams and Warwick, 1980). On the intracranial surface, the Ast is related to a dural plicature that lies over the preoccipital notch, which is a small incisure that arbitrarily separates the temporal from the occipital lobe (Williams and Warwick, 1980).

While a 1 cm burr hole centered in the Ast exposes the transverse sinus at least partially, a burr hole with its base placed 1 cm above the Ast is completely or mostly superior to the sinus, and hence supratentorial (Ribas *et al.*, 2005b) (Figure 3.50B, C and D). The line provided by the inion (In), which corresponds to the most prominent point of the external occipital protuberance (Broca, 1875; Williams and Warwick, 1980), and by the Ast, roughly indicates the position of the transverse sinus and can be relied on to orient further posterior extensions of supratentorial exposures through basal burr holes with their bases located at least 1 to 2 cm above this line (Ribas and Rodrigues, 2007; Ribas *et al.*, 2005b) (Figures 3.50, 3.51 and 3.52).

References

Altay, T. & Couldwell, W. T. (2012). The frontotemporal ("pterional") approach, and historical perspective. *Neurosurgery*, **71**, 481–91.

Alves, R. V., Ribas, G. C., Párraga, R. G. & Oliveira, E. (2012). The occipital lobe convexity sulci and gyri. *Journal of Neurosurgery*, **166**, 1014–23.

Anderson, D. M. (1999). *Dorland Dicionário Médico Ilustrado*, São Paulo: Manole.

Apuzzo, M. J. (1988). *Surgery of the Third Ventricle*, 2nd edn, Baltimore: Williams and Wilkins, pp. 421–52.

Apuzzo, M. J. & Amar, A. P. (1988). Transcallosal interforniceal approach. In M. J. Apuzzo, ed., *Surgery of the Third Ventricle*, 2nd edn. Baltimore: Williams and Wilkins, pp. 421–52.

Auburtin, S. A. E. (1861). Reprise de la discussion sur la forme et le volume du cerveau. *Bulletin de la Société d'Anthropologie*, **2**, 209–20 apud Catani, M. and Schotten, M. T. (2012). Surface neuroanatomy. In *Atlas of Human Brain Connections*. New York: Oxford University Press, ch. 2, pp. 7–20.

Azevedo, F. A. C., Carvalho, L. R. B., Grinberg, L. T., *et al.* (2009). Equal numbers of neuronal and nonneuronal cells make the human brain an isometrically scaled-up primate brain. *Journal of Comparative Neurology*, **513**(5), 532–41.

Baillarger, J. (1840). Recherches sur la structure de la couche corticale des circonvolutions du cerveau.*Mémoires de l'Académie Royale de Médecine*, **8**, 149–83. [Translated in Clarke, E. and O'Malley, C. D., eds. (1996). *The Human Brain and Spinal Cord: A Historical Study. Illustrated by Writings from Antiquity to the Twentieth Century*, San Francisco: Norman Publishing.]

Bartholin, C. (1641). *Intitutiones anatomicae novis recentiorum opinionibus et observationnibus, quarum innumerae hactenus editae non sunt figurisque auctae ab autorius filio Thoma Bartholino*. Leiden: Lug. Batavorum apud Catani, M. and Schotten, M. T. (2012). Surface neuroanatomy. In *Atlas of Human Brain Connections*. New York: Oxford University Press, pp. 7–20.

Berger, M. S., Cohen, W. A. & Ojemann, G. A. (1990). Correlation of motor cortex brain mapping data with magnetic resonance imaging. *Journal of Neurosurgery*, **72**, 383–7.

Bernal, B. & Altman, N. (2010). The connectivity of the superior longitudinal fasciculus: a tractography DTI study. *Magnetic Resonance Imaging*, **28**, 217–25.

Bernal, B. & Ardila, A. (2009). The role of the arcuate fasciculus in conduction aphasia. *Brain*, **132**, 2309–16.

Bischoff, Th. L. W. (1868). *Die Grosshirnwindungen des Menschen*. Munich apud Broca, P. (1876). Sur la topographie crânie-cérébrale ou sur les rapports anatomiques du crâne et du cerveau. *Revue d'Anthropologie*, **5**, 193–248.

Black, K. L. & Pikul, B. K. (1997). Gliomas: past, present and future. *Clinical Neurosurgery*, **45**, 160–3.

Black, P. M., Moriarty, T., Alexander, E., *et al.* (1997). Development and implementation of intraoperative MRI and its neurosurgical applications. *Neurosurgery*, **41**, 831–42.

Bogen, E. (1988). Physiological consequences of complete or partial commissural section. In M. J. Apuzzo, ed., *Surgery of the Third Ventricle*, 2nd edn. Baltimore: Williams and Wilkins, pp. 167–87.

Boling, W. & Oliver, A. (2004). Localization of hand sensory function to the "plis de passage" moyen of Broca. *Journal of Neurosurgery*, **101**, 278–83.

Boling, W., Olivier, A., Bittar, R. G. & Reutens, D. (1999). Localization of hand motor activation in Broca's "plis de passage" moyen. *Journal of Neurosurgery*, **91**, 903–10.

Boling, W., Parsons, M., Kraszpulski, M., Cantrell, C. & Puce, A. (2008). Whole-hand sensorimotor area: cortical stimulation localization and correlation with functional magnetic resonance imaging. *Journal of Neurosurgery*, **108**, 491–500.

Borden, N. M., Forseen, S. E. & Stefan, C. (2016). *Imaging Anatomy of the Human Brain*. New York: Dermos Medical.

Bouchet, A., Goutelle, A. & Fischer, G. (1966). La fissure transversal du cerveau (fissure transversa cerebri) ou fente cérébrale de Bichat. *Archives d'anatomie, d'histologie et d'embryologie normales et experimentales*, **49**(5), 455.

Bouillaud, J. B. (1825). Recherches cliniques propres à démontrer que la perte de la parole correspond à la lesion des lobules antérieurs du cerveau, et à confirmer l'opinion de M. Gall, sur le sige de l'organe du langage articulé. *Archives générales de médecine*, **8**, 25–45 apud Catani, M. and Schotten, M. T. (2012). Surface neuroanatomy. In *Atlas of Human Brain Connections*. New York: Oxford University Press, ch. 2, pp. 7–20.

Breasted, J. H. (1930). *The Edwin Smith Surgical Papyrus*. Chicago, IL: University of Chicago Press apud Catani, M. and Schotten, M. T. (2012). Surface neuroanatomy. In *Atlas of Human Brain Connections*, New York: Oxford University Press, pp. 7–20.

Brennan, C. A., Li, T. R., Bender, M., Hsiung, F. & Moses, K. (2001). Broad-complex, but not Ecdysone receptor, is required for progression of the morphogenetic furrow in the Drosophila eye. *Development*, **128**(1), 1–11.

Broca, P. (1861). Perte de la parole, ramollissement chronique et destruction partielle du lobe antérieur gauche: sur le siège de la faculté du langage. *Bulletin de la Société d'Anthropologie*, **2**, 235–8, apud Finger, S. (1994). *Origins of Neuroscience*. New York: Oxford University Press.

Broca, P. (1861). Sur les rapports anatomiques des divers points de la surface du crâne et des diverses parties des hémisfères cérébraux. *Bulletin de la Société d'Anthropologie*, **2**, 340 apud Gusmão, S., Silveira, R. L. & Cabral, G. (2000). [Broca and the birth of modern surgery.] [Portuguese] *Arquivos de neuro-psiquiatria*, **58**, 1149–52.

Broca, P. (1875). *Instructions crâniologiques et crâniométriques de la Société d'Anthropologie*. Paris: G. Masson.

Broca, P. (1876a). Diagnostic d'un abcès situé au niveau de la région du langage, trépanation de cet abcès. *Revue d'Anthropologie*, **5**, 244–8 apud Stone, J. L. (1991). Paul Broca and the first craniotomy based on cerebral localization. *Journal of Neurosurgery*, **75**, 154–9.

Broca, P. (1876b). Sur la topographie crânio-cérébrale ou sur les rapports anatomiques du crâne et du cerveau. *Revue d'Anthropologie*, **5**, 193–248.

Broca, P. (1877). Sur la circonvolution limbique et al scissure limbique. *Bulletin de la Société d'Anthropologie*, **12**, 646–57 apud Finger, S. (1994). *Origins of Neuroscience*. New York: Oxford University Press.

Broca, P. (1888). *Mémoires sur le cerveau de l'homme et dês primates.* Paris: Reinwald, pp. 739–804 apud Boling, W. and Oliver, A. (2004). Localization of hand sensory function to the "plis de passage" moyen of Broca. *Journal of Neurosurgery*, **101**, 278–83.

Brodal, A. (1981). *Neurological Anatomy in Relation to Clinical Medicine*, 3rd edn, New York: Oxford University Press.

Brodal, P. (2010). *The Central Nervous System, Structure and Function*, 4th edn, New York: Oxford University Press.

Brodmann, K. (1909) (reprinted 1925). *Verleichende Lokalisations Lehre der Grosshirnrinde in Ihren Prinzipien dar Gestellt auf Grund des Zellenbanes.* Leipzig: J. A. Barth, v. **12**, pp. 324 apud Penfield, W. (1952). *Cerebral Cortex of Man.* New York: Macmillan.

Burdach, K. (1819–1822–1826). *Von Baue und Leben des Gehirns.* Leipzig: Dyk'schen Buchhandlung apud Catani, M. and Schotten, M. T. (2012). Surface neuroanatomy. In *Atlas of Human Brain Connections.* New York: Oxford University Press, pp. 7–20.

Burdach, K. F. (1844). *Umrisse einer Physiologie des Nervensystems.* Leipzig: Leopold Boss apud Türe, U., Yasargil, M. G., Friedman, A. H. & Al-Mefty, O. (2000). Fiber dissection technique: lateral aspect of the brain. *Neurosurgery*, **47**, 417–27.

Butler, A. B. & Hodos, W. (2005). *Comparative Vertebrate Neuroanatomy: Evolution and Adaptation*, 2nd edn, Hoboken: John Wiley & Sons.

Cannestra, A. F., Blodd, A. J., Black, K. M. & Toga, A. W. (1996). The evolution of optical signal in human and rodent cortex. *Neuroimage*, **3**, 202–8.

Carpenter, M. B. (1991). *Core Text of Neuroanatomy*, 4th edn, Baltimore: Williams & Wilkins.

Carpenter, M. B. & Sutin, J. (1983). *Human Neuroanatomy.* Baltimore: Williams & Wilkins.

Catani, M. & Schotten, M. T. (2012). Surface neuroanatomy. In *Atlas of Human Brain Connections*, New York: Oxford University Press, pp. 7–20.

Catani, M. & Thiebaut de Schotten, M. (2008). A diffusion tensor imaging tractography atlas for virtual in vivo dissections. *Cortex*, **44**, 1105–32.

Catani, M., Howard, R. J., Pajevic, S. & Jones, D. K. (2002). Virtual in vivo interactive dissection of white matter fasciculi in the human brain. *Neuroimage*, **17**, 77–94

Catani, M., Jones, D. K., Donato, R. & Ffytche, D. H. (2003). Occipitotemporal connections in the human brain. *Brain*, **129**, 2093–107.

Catani, M., Jones, D. K. & Ffytche, D. H. (2005). Perisylvian language networks of the human brain. *Annals of Neurology*, **57**, 8–16.

Chaddad-Neto, F., Campos Filho, J. M., Doria Netto, H. L., *et al.* (2012). The pterional craniotomy: tips and tricks. *Arquivos de neuro-psiquiatria*, **70**, 727–32.

Chang, E. F., Gabriel, R. A., Potts, M. B., Berger, M. S. & Lawton, M. T. (2011). Supratentorial cavernous malformations in eloquent and deep locations: surgical approaches and outcomes. *Journal of Neurosurgery*, **114**, 814–27.

Chi, J. G., Dooling, E. C. & Gilles, F. H. (1977). Gyral development of the human brain. *Annals of Neurology*, **1**, 86–93.

Chin, L. S., Levy, M. L. & Apuzzo, M. L. J. (1999). Principles of stereotatic neurosurgery. In J. R. Youmans, ed., *Neurological Surgery*, 4th edn, Philadelphia: WB Saunders, pp. 767–85.

Choi, C. Y., Han, S. R., Yee, G. T. & Lee, C. H. (2010). A understanding of the temporal stem. *Journal of Korean Neurosurgical Society*, **47**, 365–9.

Choi, C. Y., Han, S. R., Yee, G. T. & Lee, C. H. (2011). Central core of the cerebrum. *Journal of Neurosurgery*, **114**, 463–69.

Cianchi, M. & Breschi, G. (1997). *Leonardo anatomia.* Firenze: Giuti Gruppo Editoriale.

Cirillo, R. A., Horel, J. A. & George, P. J. (1989). Lesions of the anterior temporal stem and the performance of delayed match-to-sample and visual discriminations in monkeys. *Behavioural Brain Research*, **34**, 55–69.

Clarke E. & Dewhurst K. (1975). *Histoire illustrée de la fonction cérébrale.* Paris: Les Editions Roger Dacosta.

Clarke, E. & O'Malley, C. D., eds. (1996). *The Human Brain and Spinal Cord: A Historical Study. Illustrated by Writings from Antiquity to the Twentieth Century.* San Francisco: Norman Publishing.

Clayton, M. (1992). *Leonardo da Vinci, the Anatomy of Man.* Boston: Bulfinch Press/ Little. Brown.

Collice, M., Collice, R. & Riva, A. (2008). Who discovered the Sylvian fissure? *Neurosurgery*, **63**, 623–8.

Cunningham, D. (1892). *Contribution to the Surface Anatomy of the Cerebral Hemispheres.* Dublin: Hodges Figgis apud Yousry, T. A., Schmid, U. D., Alkadhi, H., *et al.* (1997). Localization of the motor hand area to a knob on the precentral gyrus: a new landmark. *Brain*, **120**, 141–57.

Curran, E. J. (1909). A new association fiber tract in the cerebrum. With remarks on the fiber dissection method of studying the brain. *Journal of Comparative Neurology*, **19**, 645–57 apud Catani,M. and Schotten, M. T. (2012). Surface neuroanatomy. In *Atlas of Human Brain Connections*, New York: Oxford University Press, pp. 7–20.

de Oliveira, J. G., Párraga, R. G., Chaddad-Neto, F., Ribas, G. C. & de Oliveira, E. P. (2012). Supracerebellar transtentorial approach – resection of the tentorium instead of an opening-to provide broad exposure of the mediobasal temporal lobe: anatomical aspects and surgical applications: clinical article. *Journal of Neurosurgery*, **116** (4), 764–72.

de Olmos, J. S. (1972). The amygdaloid projection field in the rat as studied with the cupric silver method. In B. E. Eleftheriou ed., *The Neurobiology of the Amygdala.* New York: Plenum. pp. 145–204 apud Heimer, L. (2003). A new anatomical framework for neuropsychiatric disorders and drug abuse. *American Journal of Psychiatry*, **160**, 1726–39.

de Olmos, J. S. & Heimer, L. (1999). The concept of ventral striatopallidal system and extended amygdala. *Annals of the New York Academy of Sciences*, **877**, 1–32.

De Ribet, R. M. (1957). *Systématisation des centres nerveux et de leurs connexions.* Paris: G. Doin et cie apud Peltier, J., Verclytte, S., Delmaire, C., *et al.* (2011). Microsurgical anatomy of the anterior commissure: correlations with diffusion tensor imaging fiber tracking and clinical relevance. *Neurosurgery*, **69**, ONS241–ONS247.

Debernardi, A., Sala, E., D'Aliberti, G., *et al.* (2010). Alcmaeon of Croton. *Neurosurgery*, **66**, 247–52.

Debierre, C. (1907). *Le cerveau et la moelle épinière.* Paris: Félix Alcan, Librarie Germer Baillière apud Peltier, J., Verclytte, S., Delmaire, C., *et al.* (2011). Microsurgical anatomy of the anterior commissure: correlations with diffusion tensor imaging fiber tracking and clinical relevance. *Neurosurgery*, **69**, ONS241–ONS247.

Déjérine, J. (1892). Contribution a l'étude anatomo-pathologique et clinique des differentes variétés de cécité-verbale. *Mém Soc Biol*, **4**, 61–90 apud Catani, M. and Schotten, M. T. (2012). Surface neuroanatomy. In *Atlas of Human Brain Connections.* New York: Oxford University Press, pp. 7–20.

Déjérine, J. (1895). *Anatomie des centres nerveux.* Paris: Rüeff.

Delandsheer, J. M., Guyot, J. F., Jomin, M., Sherpereel, B. & Laine, I. (1978). Acces au triosième ventricle par voie inter-thalamo-trigonale. *Neurochirurgie*, **24**, 419–21.

Dobson, J. (1925). Herophilus of Alexandria. *Proceedings of the Royal Society of Medicine*, **18**, 19–32 apud Catani, M. & Schotten, M. T.

(2012). Surface neuroanatomy. In *Atlas of Human Brain Connections*, New York: Oxford University Press, pp. 7–20.

Dolenc, V. V. (1985). A combined epi- and subdural direct approach to carotido-ophthalmic artery aneurysms. *Journal of Neurosurgery*, **62**, 667–72.

Dolenc, V. V. (1989). *Anatomy and Surgery of the Cavernous Sinus*. Vienna: Springer-Verlag.

Dorward, N. L., Alberti, O., Palmer, J. D., Kitchen, N. D. & Thomas, D. G. T. (1999). Accuracy of true frameless stereotaxy: in vivo measurement and laboratory phantom studies. *Journal of Neurosurgery*, **90**, 160–8.

Duffau, H. (2011a). *Brain Mapping: from Neural Basis of Cognition to Surgical Applications*. Vienna: Springer-Verlag.

Duffau, H. (2011b). Awake mapping and tumors surgery. In H. Duffau, ed., *Brain Mapping: From Neural Basis of Cognition to Surgical Applications*. Vienna: Springer-Verlag, pp. 305–18.

Duvernoy, H. M. (1991). *The Human Brain*. Vienna: Springer.

Duvernoy, H. M. (1998). *The Human Hippocampus*, 2nd edn, Berlin: Springer.

Ebeling, U. & Reulen, H. J. (1988). Neurosurgical topography of the optic radiation in the temporal lobe. *Acta Neurochirurgica*, **92**, 29–36.

Ebeling, U. & Reulen, H. J. (1992b). Subcortical topography and proportions of the pyramidal tract. *Acta Neurochirurgica*, **118**, 164–71.

Ebeling, U. & Reulen, H. J. (1995a). Space-occupying lesions of the sensory-motor region (review) (106 ref.). *Advances and Technical Standards in Neurosurgery*, **22**, 137–81.

Ebeling, U. & Steinmetz, H. (1995b). Anatomy of the parietal lobe: mapping the individual pattern. *Acta Neurochirurgica*, **136**, 8–11.

Ebeling, U., Eisner, W., Gutbrod, K., *et al.* (1992a). Intraoperative speech mapping during resection of tumors in the posterior dominant temporal lobe. *Journal of Neurology*, **369**, 104.

Ebeling, U., Rikli, D., Huber. P. & Reulen, H. J. (1987). The coronal suture, a useful landmark in neurosurgery? Cranio-cerebral topography between bony landmarks on the skull and the brain. *Acta Neurochirurgica*, **89**, 130–4.

Ebeling, U., Steinmetz, H., Huang, Y. & Kahn, T. (1989). Topography and identification of the inferior precentral sulcus in MR imaging. *AJNR American Journal of Neuroradiology*, **10**, 937–42.

Ecker, A. (1869). *Die Hirnwindungen des Menschen*. Braunschweig: Vieweg.

Ehni, G. & Ehni, B. L. (1988). Considerations in transforaminal entry. In M. J. Apuzzo, ed., *Surgery of the Third Ventricle*, 2nd edn. Baltimore: Williams & Wilkins, pp. 391–420.

Excerpta Medica Foundation (1975). *Nomina Anatomica*, 4th edn, Amsterdam.

Excerpta Medica Foundation (1980). *Nomina Anatomica*, 6th edn, Amsterdam.

Falconer, M. A., Hill, D., Meyer, A., Mitchell, W. & Pond, D. A. (1955). Treatment of temporal lobe epilepsy by temporal lobectomy: survey of findings and results. *Lancet*, **1**, 827–35 apud Hansebout, R. R. (1977). Surgery of epilepsy, current technique of cortical resection. In H. H. Schmidek and W. H. Sweet, eds., *Current Techniques in Operative Neurosurgery*. New York: Grune and Stratton, ch. 9, pp. 101–17.

Federative Committee on Anatomical Terminology (1998). *International Anatomical Terminology*. Stuttgart: Thieme.

Feindel, W. & Rasmussen T. (1991) Temporal lobectomy with amygdalectomy and minimal hippocampal resection: review of 100 cases. *Canadian Journal of Neurological Science*, **18**, 603–5.

Fernández-Miranda, J. C., Rhoton, A. L. Jr., Kakizawa, Y., Choi, C. & Alvarez-Linera, J. (2008). The claustrum and its projection system in the human brain: a microsurgical and tractographic anatomical study. *Journal of Neurosurgery*, **108**, 764–74.

Ferreira, A. G. (1966). [Latin-Portuguese Dictionary] [Portuguese]. Porto: Porto Editora.

Ferrier, D. (1873). Experimental researches in cerebral physiology and pathology. *West Riding Lunatic Asylum Medical Report*, **3**, 30–96 apud Finger, S. (1994). *Origins of Neuroscience*. New York: Oxford University Press.

Ferrier, D. (1876). *The Functions of the Brain*. London: Smith, Elder & Co. (also reprinted in facsimile in London: Dawsons of Pall Mall, 1966) apud S. H. Greenblatt, ed. (1997). *A History of Neurosurgery*. Park Ridge: The American Association of Neurological Surgeons.

Finger, S. (1994).*Origins of Neuroscience*. New York: Oxford University Press.

Fitzgerald, D. B., Cosgrove, G. R., Ronner, S., *et al.* (1997). Location of language in the cortex: a comparison between functional MR imaging and electrocortical stimulation. *AJNR American Journal of Neuroradiology*, **18**, 152–39.

Forkel, S. J., Schotten, M. T., Kawadler, J. M., *et al.* (2014). The anatomy of fronto-occipital connections from early blunt dissections to contemporary tractography. *Cortex*, **56**, 73–84.

Foxman, B. T., Oppenheim, J., Petito, C. K. & Gazzaniga, M. S. (1986). Proportional anterior commissure area in humans and monkeys. *Neurology*, **36**, 1513–7 apud Peltier, J., Verclytte, S., Delmaire, C., et al. (2011). Microsurgical anatomy of the anterior commissure: correlations with diffusion tensor imaging fiber tracking and clinical relevance. *Neurosurgery*, **69**, ONS241–ONS247.

Fritsch, G. & Hitzig, E. (1960). Über die elektrische Erregbarkeit desGosshirns. *Archiv für Anatomie und Physiologie*, 300–332. In G. von Bonin, ed., *Some Papers on the Cerebral Cortex*. Translated as "On the electrical excitability of the cerebrum." Springfield, IL: Charles C. Thomas. pp. 73–96 apud Finger, S. (1994). *Origins of Neuroscience*. New York: Oxford University Press.

Fujii, K., Lenkey, C. & Rhoton, A. L. Jr. (1980). Microsurgical anatomy of the choroidal arteries: lateral and third ventricles. *Journal of Neurosurgery*, **52**, 165–88.

Fujitsu, K. & Kuwabara, T. (1985). Zygomatic approach for lesions in the interpenducular cistern. *Journal of Neurosurgery*, **62**, 340–3.

Gall, F. J. & Spurzheim, J. C. (1810–1819). *Anatomie et physiologie du système nerveux en général, et du cerveau en particulier*. Paris: Schoell apud Catani, M. & Schotten, M. T. (2012). Surface neuroanatomy. In *Atlas of Human Brain Connections*. New York: Oxford University Press, pp. 7–20.

Gibo, H., Carver, C. C., Rhoton, A. L. Jr., Lenkey, C. & Mitchell, R. J. (1981a). Microsurgical anatomy of the middle cerebral artery. *Journal of Neurosurgery*, **54**(2), 151–69.

Gibo, H., Lenkey, C. & Rhoton, A. L. Jr. (1981b). Microsurgical anatomy of the supraclinoid portion of the internal carotid artery. *Journal of Neurosurgery*, **55**(4), 560–74.

Glasser, M. F. & Rilling, J. K. (2008). DTI tractography of the human brain's language pathways. *Cerebral Cortex*, **18**, 2471–82.

Gloor, P. (1997). *The Temporal Lobe and the Limbic System*. Oxford: Oxford University Press.

Goodale, M. A. & Milner, D. (1992). Separate visual pathways for perception and action. *Tins*, **15**, 20–5.

Gould, S. J. (1977). *Ontogeny and Phylogeny*. Cambridge, MA: Harvard University Press.

Gould, S. J. (2001). *The Book of Life*. New York: W. W. Norton & Co.

Gould, S. J. (2002). *The Structure of the Evolutionary Theory*. Cambridge,MA: The Belknap Press of the Harvard University Press.

Graña, F., Rocca, D. E. & Graña, L. (1954). *Las trepanaciones en el Perú de la época pre-hispánica*. Lima: Imprenta Santa Maria, pp. 15–7.
Gratiolet, L. P. (1854). *Mémoire sur les plis cérébraux de l'homme et des primates*. Paris: Bertrand apud Pearce, J. M. (2006). Luis Pierre Gratiolet (1815–1865): the cerebral lobes and fissures. *European Neurology*, **56**, 262–4.
Gross, C. G. (1973). Inferotemporal cortex and vision. *Progress in Physiological Psychology*, **5**, 77–123 apud Goodale, M. A. and Milner, D. (1992). Separate visual pathways for perception and action. *Tins*, **15**, 20–5.
Gusmão, S., Reis, C., Silveira, R. L. & Cabral, G. (2001). [Relationships between the coronal suture and the sulci of the lateral convexity of the frontal lobe: neurosurgical applications] [Portuguese]. *Arquivos de neuro-psiquiatria*, **59**, 570–6.
Gusmão, S., Silveira, R. L. & Cabral, G. (2000). [Broca and the birth of modern neurosurgery] [Portuguese]. *Arquivos de neuro-psiquiatria*, **58**, 1149–52.
Gwinn, R. (2015). *6th Annual SNI Brain Anatomy with Neurosurgical Applications Course*, Seattle, USA, March 20–21.
Haeger, K. (1988). *The Illustrated History of Surgery*. New York: Bell Publishing.
Haglund, M. M., Berger, M. S. & Hochman, D. W. (1996). Enhanced optical imaging of human gliomas and tumor margins. *Neurosurgery*, **38**, 308–17.
Hakuba, A., Liu, S. & Nishimura, S. (1986). The orbitozygomatic infratemporal approach: a new surgical technique. *Surgical Neurology*, **26**, 271–6.
Hamby, W. B. (1964). Pterional approaches to the orbits for decompression or tumor removal. *Journal of Neurosurgery*, **21**, 15–8 apud Altay, T. & Couldwell, W. T. (2012). The frontotemporal ("pterional") approach, and historical perspective. *Neurosurgery*, **71**, 481–91.
Hansebout, R. R. (1977). Surgery of epilepsy, current technique of cortical resection. In H. H. Schmidek, and W. H. Sweet, eds., *Current Techniques in Operative Neurosurgery*. New York: Grune and Stratton, ch. 9, pp. 101–17.
Hansebout, R. R. (1982). Surgery of epilepsy, current technique of cortical resection. In H. H. Schmidek and W. H. Sweet, eds., *Operative Neurosurgical Techniques*. New York: Grune and Stratton, pp. 963–79.
Harkey, H. L., Al-Mefty, O., Haines, D. E. & Smith, R. R. (1989). The surgical anatomy of the cerebral sulci. *Neurosurgery*, **24**, 651–4.
Heimer, L. (1995). *The Human Brain and Spinal Cord: Functional Neuroanatomy and Dissection Guide*, 2nd edn, New York: Springer Verlag.
Heimer, L. (2003). A new anatomical framework for neuropsychiatric disorders and drug abuse. *American Journal of Psychiatry*, **160**, 1726–39. [Erratum in: *American Journal of Psychiatry*, 160, 2258].
Heimer, L. & Van Hoesen, G. W. (2006). The limbic lobe and its output channels: implications for emotional functions and adaptive behavior. *Neuroscience and Biobehavioral Reviews*, **30**, 126–47.
Heimer, L., Harlan, R. E., Alheid, G. F., Garcia, M. M. & de Olms, J. (1997). Substantia innominata: a notion which impedes clinical-anatomical correlations in neuropsychiatric disorders. *Neuroscience*, **76**, 957–1006.
Heimer, L., Switzer, R. C. & Van Hoesen, G. V. (1982). Ventral striatum and ventral pallidum. *Trends in Neurosciences*, **5**, 83–7.
Heimer, L., Van Hoesen, G. W., Trimble, M. & Zahm, D. S. (2008). *Anatomy of Neuropsychiatry: The New Anatomy of the Basal Forebrain and its Implications for Neuropsychiatric Illness*. Amsterdam: Elsevier.
Held, L. I. (2009). *Quirks of Human Anatomy: an Evo-Devo Look at the Human Body*. Cambridge: Cambridge University Press.
Henneberg, R. (1910). Messung der Obergflachenausdehnung der Grosshirnrinde. *J Psychol Neurol*, **17**, 144–58 apud Catani,M. & Schotten, M. T. (2012).Surface neuroanatomy. In *Atlas of Human Brain Connections*. New York: Oxford University Press, ch. 2, pp. 7–20.
Hinck, V. C. & Clifton, G. L. (1981). A precise technique for craniotomy localization using computerized tomography. *Journal of Neurosurgery*, **54**, 416–8.
Hirsh, J. F., Zouaoui, A., Renien, D. & Pierre Kahn, A. (1979). A new surgical approaches to the third ventricle with interruption of the striothalamic vein. *Acta Neurochirurgica*, **47**, 135–47.
His, W. (1895). *Anatomishe Nomenklatur* (Nomina anatomica). Leipeiz: Verlag von Veit.
Horel, J. A. (1978). The neuroanatomy of amnesia: a critique of the hippocampal memory hypothesis. *Brain*, **103**, 403–45.
Horel, J. A. & Misantone L. J. (1974). The Klüver-Bucy syndrome produced by partial isolation of the temporal lobe. *Experimental Neurology*, **42**, 101–12.
Horel, J. A. & Misantone, L. J. (1976). Visual discrimination impaired by cutting temporal lobe connections. *Science*, **193**, 336–8.
Hori, T., Tabuchi, S., Kurosaki, M., *et al.* (1993). Subtemporal amygdalohippocampectomy for treating medically intractable temporal lobe epilepsy. *Neurosurgery*, **33**(1), 50–6.
Horsley, V. (1892). Cranio-cerebral topography. In C. J. Cunningham, ed., *Contribution to the Surface Anatomy of the Cerebral Hemispheres*. Dublin: Academy House apud Horwitz, N. H. (1995). Library historical perspective. *Neurosurgery*, **36**, 428–32.
Horsley, V. (1892). On the topographical relations of the cranium and the surface of the cerebrum. In C. J. Cunningham, ed., *Contribution to the Surface Anatomy of the Cerebral Hemispheres*. Dublin: Academy House, pp. 306–55 apud Ebeling, U., Rikli, D., Huber, P. & Reulen, H. J. (1987). The coronal suture, a useful landmark in neurosurgery? Craniocerebral topography between bony landmarks on the skull and the brain. *Acta Neurochirurgica*, **89**, 130–4.
Hugher, T. S., Abou-Khalil, B., Lavin, P. J. M., *et al.* (1999). Visual field defects after temporal lobe resection: a prospective quantitative analysis. *Neurology*, **53**(1), 167–72.
Jackson, J. H. (1863). Convulsive spasms of the right hand arm preceding epileptic seizures. *Medical Times and Gazetta*, **1**, 110–1 apud Finger, S. (1994). *Origins of Neuroscience*. New York: Oxford University Press.
Jane, J. A., Yashon, D., DeMyer, W. & Bucy, P. C. (1967). The contribution of the pre-central gyrus to the pyramidal tract of man. *Journal of Neurosurgery*, **26**, 244–8.
Johnston, J. B. (1923). Further contribution to the study of the evolution of the forebrain. *Journal of Comparative Neurology*, **35**, 337–481 apud de Olmos, J. S. and Heimer, L. (1999). The concept of ventral striatopallidal system and extended amygdala. *Annals of the New York Academy of Sciences*, **877**, 1–32.
Kaye, A. H. & Laws, E. R. Jr., eds. (2001). *Brain Tumors*, 2nd edn, London: Churchill Livingstone.
Kelly, P. J., Goerss, S. J. & Kall, B. A. (1988). Evolution of contemporary instrumentation for computed assisted stereotactic surgery. *Surgical Neurology*, **30**, 204–15.
Key, A. & Reteius, G. (1875). *Studien in der anatomy des nervensystems und des blindegewebes*. Stockholm, Norstad apud Yasargil, M. G. (1984). *Microneurosurgery*. Stuttgart: Georg Thieme, Vol. I.
Kier, A. L., Staib, L. H., Davis, L. M. &, Bronen, R. A. (2004). MR imaging of the temporal stem: anatomic dissection tractography of the uncinate fasciculus, inferior occipitofrontal fasciculus and Mayer's loop of the optic radiation. *AJNR American Journal of Neuroradiology*, **25**, 677–91.
King, J. S. & Walker J. (1980). Precise preoperative localization of intracranial mass lesions. *Neurosurgery*, **6**, 160–3.

Klinger, J. (1935). Erleichterung der makroskopischen Präparation des Gehirn durch den Gefrierprozess. *Schweiz Arch-Neurol Psychiat*, **36**, 247–56 apud Türe, U., Yasargil, M. G., Friedman, A. H. & Al-Mefty, O. (2000). Fiber dissection technique: lateral aspect of the brain. *Neurosurgery*, **47**, 417–27.

Kocher, E. T. (1907). *Chirurgishe operationslehre*, 5th edn, Jena: Gustav Fischer apud Krause, V. (1912). *Chirurgie du cerveau et de la moelle épinière*. Paris: Société D'Editions Scientifiques et Médicales.

Kocher, E. T. (1907). *Chirurgishe Operationslehre*, 5th edn, Jena: Gustav Fischer.

Koutsarnakis, C., Liakos, F., Kalyvas, A.V., Liouta, E., Emelifeonwu, J., Kalamatianos, T., Sakas, D. E., Johnson, E., Stranjalis, G., (2017). Approaching the atrium through the intraparietal sulcus: Mapping the sulcal morphology and correlating the surgical corridor to underlying fiber tracts. *Oper Neurosurg*. **13(4)**, 503–16.

Koutsarnakis, C., Liakos, F., Kalyvas, A.V., Skandalakis, G.P., Komaitis, S., Christidi, F., Karavasilis, E., Liouta, E., Stranjalis, G. (2017). The superior frontal transsulcal approach to the anterior ventricular system: Exploring the sulcal and subcortical anatomy using anatomic dissections and diffusion tensor imaging tractography. *World Neurosurgery*, **106**, 339–54.

Krause, F. (1912). *Chirurgie du cerveau et de la moelle épinière*. Paris: Société D'Editions Scientifiques et Médicales.

Krings, T., Reinges, M. H. T., Thiex, R., Gilsbach, J. M. & Thron, A. (2001). Functional and diffusion-weighted magnetic resonance images of space-occupying lesions affecting the motor system: imaging the motor cortex and pyramidal tracts. *Journal of Neurosurgery*, **95**, 816–24.

Krol, G., Galicich, J., Arbit, E., Sze, G. & Amster, J. (1988). Preoperative localization of intracranial lesions on MR. *AJNR American Journal of Neuroradiology*, **9**, 513–6.

Krönlein, R. U. (1898). *Topographie cranio cérébrale*. V. Bruns' Beiträge zur Keinishen Chirurgie, Vol. XXII, p. 364 apud Krause, V. (1912) *Chirurgie du cerveau et de la moelle épinière*. Paris: Société D'Editions Scientifiques et Médicales.

Kurze, T. & Doyle, S. B. (1962). Extradural intracranial (middle fossa) approach to the internal auditory canal. *Journal of Neurosurgery*, **19**, 1033–7.

Lang, J. (1985). *Mikroanatomischer Kurs für junge Neurochirurgen*. Anatomisches Institut der Universität Würzburg apud Ebeling, U., Rikli, D., Huber, P. & Reulen, H. J. (1987). The coronal suture, a useful landmark in neurosurgery? Craniocerebral topography between bony landmarks on the skull and the brain. *Acta Neurochirurgica*, **89**, 130–4.

Lavyne, M. H. & Patterson, R. H. (1983). Subchoroidal trans-velum interpositum approach to mid-third ventricular tumors. *Neurosurgery*, **12**(1), 86–94.

Lavyne, M. H. & Patterson, R. H. (1988). The subchoroidal trans-velum interpositum approach. In M. J. Apuzzo, ed., *Surgery of the Third Ventricle*, 2nd edn. Baltimore: Williams & Wilkins, pp. 453–70.

Lawton, M. T., Golfinhos, J. G. & Spetzler F. (1996). The contralateral transcallosal approach: experience with 32 patients. *Neurosurgery*, **39**(4), 729–35.

Lee, J. E., Bigler, E. D., Alexander, A. L., *et al.* (2007). Diffusion tensor imaging of white matter in the superior temporal gyrus and temporal stem in autism. *Neuroscience Letters*, **424**, 127–32.

Leuret, F. & Gratiolet, P. (1857–1959). *Anatomie comparée du système nerveux consideré dans ses rapports avec l'intelligence*. Paris: Baillière, Vol. II apud Türe, U., Yasargil, M. G., Friedman, A. H. & Al-Mefty, O. (2000). Fiber dissection technique: lateral aspect of the brain. *Neurosurgery*, **47**, 417–27.

Liu, C. N. & Chambers, W. W. (1964). An experimental study of the cortico-spinal system distribution of degenerating fibers following discrete lesions of the pre- and postcentral gyri and bulbar pyramid. *Journal of Comparative Neurology*, **123**, 257–84 apud Brodal, A. (1981). *Neurological Anatomy in Relation to Clinical Medicine*, 3rd edn, New York: Oxford University Press.

Livingstone, M. & Hubel, D. (1988). Segregation of form, color, movement, and depth: anatomy, physiology, and perception. *Science*, **240**, 740–9 apud Goodale, M. A. & Milner, D. (1992). Separate visual pathways for perception and action. *Tins*, **15**, 20–5.

Lobel, E., Kahane, P., Leonards, U., *et al.* (2001). Localization of human frontal eye fields: anatomical and functional findings of functional magnetic resonance imaging and intracerebral electrical stimulation. *Journal of Neurosurgery*, **95**, 804–15.

Lockard, I. (1977). *Desk Reference for Neuroanatomy. A Guide to Essential Terms*. New York: Springer.

Ludwig, E. & Klinger, J. (1956). *Atlas cerebri humani*. Basel: S. Karger.

Lyons, A. S. & Petrucelli, R. J. (1978). *Medicine, An Illustrated History*. New York: Abradale Press.

McArthur, L. L. (1912). An aseptic surgical access to the pituitary body and its neighborhood. *JAMA*, **58**, 2009–11 apud Altay, T. & Couldwell, W. T. (2012). The frontotemporal ("pterional") approach, and historical perspective. *Neurosurgery*, 71, 481–91.

McArthur, L. L. (1918). Tumor of the pituitary gland: technic of operative approach. *Surg Clin Chic*, **2**, 691–9 apud Altay, T. & Couldwell, W. T. (2012). The frontotemporal ("pterional") approach, and historical perspective. *Neurosurgery*, **71**, 481–91.

MacLean, P. D. (1973). *A Triune Concept of the Brain and Behavior*. Toronto: University of Toronto Press.

McClellan, G. (1896). *Regional Anatomy in its Relation to Medicine and Surgery*. Philadelphia: Published by the author.

McComb, J. G. (1988). Methods of cerebrospinal fluid diversion. In M. L. J. Apuzzo, ed., *Surgery of the Third Ventricle*, 2nd edn. Baltimore: Williams and Wilkins, ch. 27, pp. 607–34.

McComb, J. G. & Apuzzo, M. L. J. (1988). Posterior intrahemispheric retrocallosal and transcallosal approaches. In Apuzzo, M. L. J., ed., *Surgery of the Third Ventricle*, 2nd edn. Baltimore: Williams and Wilkins, ch. 25, pp. 611–40.

McGinty, J. F., ed. (1999). Advancing from the ventral striatum to the extended amygdala: implications for neuropsychiatry and drug abuse. *Annals of the New York Academy of Sciences*, **877**, XII–XV.

McKissock, W. (1951). The surgical treatment of colloid cyst of the third ventricle, a report based upon twenty-one personal cases. *Brain*, **74**, 1–9.

Mahaney, K. B. & Abdulrauf, S. I. (2008). Anatomic relationship of the optic radiations to the atrium of the lateral ventricle: description of a novel entry point to the trigone. *Neurosurgery*, **63**, ONS195–ONS202.

Makris, N., Kennedy, D. N., McInerney, S., *et al.* (2005). Segmentation of subcomponents within the superior longitudinal fascicle in humans: a quantitative, in vivo, DT-MRI study. *Cerebral Cortex*, **15**, 854–69.

Martino, J. & Brogna, C. (2011).Anatomy of the white-matter pathways. In H. Duffau, ed., *Brain Mapping: From Neural Basis of Cognition to Surgical Applications*. Vienna: Springer-Verlag, ch. 2, pp. 27–41.

Martino, J., Brogna, C., Gil Robles, S., Vergani, F. & Duffau, H. (2010). Anatomic dissection of the inferior fronto-occipital fasciculus revisited in the lights of brain stimulation data. *Cortex*, **46**, 691–9 apud Duffau, H. (2011). *Brain Mapping: From Neural Basis of Cognition to Surgical Applications*. Vienna: Springer-Verlag.

Martino, J., Vergani, F., Gil Robles, S. & Duffau, H. (2010). New insights into the anatomic dissection of the temporal stem with special emphasis on the inferior fronto-occipital fasciculus: implications in surgical approach to left mesiotemporal and temporoinsular structures. *Neurosurgery*, **66**, 4–12.

Matsuno, H., Rhoton, A. L. Jr. & Peace, D. A. (1988). Microsurgical anatomy of the posterior fossa cisterns. *Neurosurgery*, **23**(1), 58–80.

Maxwell, R. E. & Tummala, R. (2004) Standard temporal lobectomy and transsylvian amygdalohippocampectomy. In H. R. Winn, ed., *Youmans Neurological Surgery*. Philadelphia: WB Saunders, Vol. II, ch. 158, pp. 2605–13.

Mello, L. E. & Villares, J. (1997). Neuroanatomy of the basal ganglia. *Psychiatric Clinics of North America*, **20**, 691–704.

Meneses, M. S., ed. (1999). *Neuroanatomia aplicada*. Rio de Janeiro: Guanabara-Koogan.

Mesulam, M. M. (1987). Patterns in behavioral neuroanatomy: association areas, the limbic system, and hemispheric specialization. In *Principles of Behavioral Neurosurgery*. Philadelphia: F. A. Davis, pp. 1–70.

Mesulam, M. M. (1990). Large-scale neurocognitive networks and distributed processing for attention, language and memory. *Annals of Neurology*, **28**, 597–613.

Mesulam, M. M. (2011). Foreword. In H. Duffau, ed., *Brain Mapping: From Neural Basis of Cognition to Surgical Applications*. Vienna: Springer-Verlag, pp. v-vi.

Meynert, T. (1867–1868). Der Bau der Grosshirnrinde und seine ortlichen Verschiedenheiten, nebst einem pathologisch-anatomischen Corollarium. *Vierteljahresschrift für Psychiatrie*, **1**, 77–93; 198–217; **2**, 88–113 apud Catani, M. & Schotten, M. T. (2012). Surface neuroanatomy. In *Atlas of Human Brain Connections*. New York: Oxford University Press, pp. 7–20.

Meynert, T. (1885). *A Clinical Treatise on Diseases of the Fore-Brain Based upon a Study of its Structures, Functions, and Nutrition* (Translated by B. Sachs). New York: G. P. Putnam's Sons apud Catani, M. & Schotten, M. T. (2012). Surface neuroanatomy. In *Atlas of Human Brain Connections*. New York: Oxford University Press, pp. 7–20.

Meynert, T. H. (1872). Vom der Saugethiere. In Stricker, ed., *Handbbuck der Lehre von Geweben des Menschen und der Thiere*, Vol. II, pp. 694–808. Engelmann: Leipzig apud Türe, U., Yasargil, M. G., Friedman, A. H. & Al-Mefty, O. (2000). Fiber dissection technique: lateral aspect of the brain. *Neurosurgery*, **47**, 417–27.

Nagata, S., Rhoton, A. L. Jr. & Barry, M. (1988). Microsurgical anatomy of the choroidal fissure. *Surgical Neurology*, **30**, 3–59.

Naidich, T. P., Valavanis, A. G. & Kubik, S. (1995). Anatomic relationships along the low-middle convexity: Part I – normal specimens and magnetic resonance imaging. *Neurosurgery*, **36**, 517–32.

Neeley, E. S., Bigler, E. D., Krasny, L., *et al.* (2007). Quantitative temporal lobe differences: autism distinguished from controls using classification and regression tree analysis. *Brain Development*, **29**, 389–99.

Neolithic skull. Nogent-les-Vierges, Oise, France. Musée de l'Homme, Paris.

Niemeyer, P. (1958). The transventricular amygdalo-hippocampectomy in temporal lobe epilepsy. In N. Baldwin, and P. Bailey, eds., *Temporal Lobe Epilepsy*. Springfield, IL: Charles C. Thomas, pp. 461–82.

Nieuwenhuys, R., Voogt, J. & Van Huijzen, C. (1988). *The Human Central Nervous System*, 3rd edn, Berlin: Springer-Verlag.

Nishikuni, K. & Ribas, G. C. (2013). Study of the fetal and postnatal morphological development of the brain sulci. *Journal of Neurosurgery Pediatrics*, **11**(1), 1–11.

Nyberg-Hansen, R. & Brodal, A. (1963). Sites of termination of corticospinal fibers in the cat: an experimental study with silver impregnation methods. *Journal of Comparative Neurology*, **120**, 369–91 apud Brodal, A. (1981). *Neurological Anatomy in Relation to Clinical Medicine*, 3rd edn, New York: Oxford University Press.

O'Leary, D. H. & Lavyne, M. H. (1978). Localization of vertex lesions seen on CT scan. *Journal of Neurosurgery*, **49**, 71–4.

Ojemann, G., Ojemann, J., Lettich, E. & Berger M (1989). Cortical language localization in left, dominant hemisphere: an electrical stimulation mapping investigation in 117 patients. *Journal of Neurosurgery*, **71**, 316–26.

Oka, K., Rhoton, A. L. Jr., Barry, M. & Rodriguez, R. (1985). Microsurgical anatomy of the superficial veins of the cerebrum. *Neurosurgery*, **17**(5), 711–48.

Olivier, A. (1991). Relevance of removal of limbic structures in surgery for temporal lobe epilepsy. *Canadian Journal of Neurological Science*, **18**, 628–35.

Ono, M., Kubik, S. & Abernathey, C. D. (1990). *Atlas of Cerebral Sulci*. Stuttgart: Thieme.

Ono, M., Rhoton, A. L. Jr. & Barry, M. (1984). Microsurgical anatomy of the region of the tentorial incisura. *Journal of Neurosurgery*, **60**, 365–99.

Oró, J. J. (2004). Evolution of the brain: from behavior to consciousness in 3.4 billion years. *Neurosurgery*, **54**, 1287–97.

Papez, J. W. (1937). A proposed mechanism of emotion. *Archives of Neurology and Psychiatry*, **38**, 725–43.

Park, M. S., Nguyen, A. D., Aryan, H. E., *et al.* (2007). Evolution of the human brain: changing brain size and fossil record. *Neurosurgery*, **60**(3), 555–62.

Park, T. S., Bourgeois, B. F., Silbergeld, D. L. & Dodson, W. E. (1996). Subtemporal transparahippocampal amygdalohippocampectomy for surgical treatment of mesial temporal lobe epilepsy. Technical note. *Journal of Neurosurgery*, **85**(6), 1172–6.

Párraga, R. G., Ribas, G. C., Gómez Llata, S. & de Oliveira, E. (2011). Microsurgical anatomy of the posterior cerebral artery in three-dimensional images. *World Neurosurgery*, **75**, 245–69.

Párraga, R. G., Ribas, G. C., Welling, L. C., Alves, R. V. & de Oliveira, E. (2012). Microsurgical anatomy of the optic radiation and related fibers in 3-dimensional images. *Neurosurgery*, **71**(ONS Suppl 1), ONS160–ONS172.

Passet, J. (1882). Über einige Unterschiede des GroBhirns nach dem Geschlecht. *Archiv. für Anthropologie* (Braunschweig), **14 Band**, 89–141 apud Ebeling, U., Rikli, D., Huber, P. & Reulen, H. J. (1987). The coronal suture, a useful landmark in neurosurgery? Craniocerebral topography between bony landmarks on the skull and the brain. *Acta Neurochirurgica*, **89**, 130–4.

Pearce, J. M (2006). Luis Pierre Gratiolet (1815–1865): the cerebral lobes and fissures: *European Neurology*, **56**, 262–4.

Peltier, J., Travers, N., Destrieux, C. & Velut, S. (2006). Optic radiations: a microsurgical anatomical study. *Journal of Neurosurgery*, **105**, 294–300.

Peltier, J., Verclytte, S., Delmaire, C., *et al.* (2010). Microsurgical anatomy of the temporal stem: clinical relevance and correlations with diffusion tensor imaging fiber tracking. *Journal of Neurosurgery*, **112**, 1033–8.

Peltier, J., Verclytte, S., Delmaire, C., *et al.* (2011). Microsurgical anatomy of the anterior commissure: correlations with diffusion tensor imaging fiber tracking and clinical relevance. *Neurosurgery*, **69**, ONS241–ONS247.

Penfield, W. & Baldwin, M. (1952). Temporal lobe seizures and technique of subtotal temporal lobectomy. *Annals of Surgery*, **136**, 625–34 apud Hansebout, R. R. (1977) Surgery of epilepsy, current technique of cortical resection. In H. H. Schmidek and W. H. Sweet, eds., *Current Techniques in Operative Neurosurgery*. New York: Grune and Stratton, ch. 9, pp. 101–17.

Penfield, W. & Boldrey, E. (1937). Somatic motor and sensory representation in the cerebral cortex of man as studied by electrical stimulation. *Brain*, **60**,389–443 apud Brodal, A. (1981). *Neurological Anatomy in Relation to Clinical Medicine*, 3rd edn, New York: Oxford University Press.

Penfield, W. & Flanigin, H. (1950a). Surgical therapy of temporal lobe seizures. *Arch Neurol*, **64**, 491–500 apud Maxwell, R. E. and Tummala, R. (2004). Standard temporal lobectomy and transsylvian amygdalohippocampectomy. In H. R. Winn, ed., *Youmans Neurological Surgery*, Vol. II, Philadelphia: WB Saunders, pp. 2605–13.

Penfield, W. & Rasmussen, T. (1950b). *The Cerebral Cortex of Man*. New York: Macmillan.

Penning, L. (1987). CT localization of a convexity brain tumor on the scalp. *Journal of Neurosurgery*, **66**, 474–6.

Perlmutter, D. & Rhoton, A. L. Jr. (1978). Microsurgical anatomy of the distal ante cerebral artery. *Journal of Neurosurgery*, **49**, 204–28.

Pernkoff, E. (1980). *Atlas of Topographical and Applied Human Anatomy*. Baltimore: Urban & Schwarzenberg.

Petrides, M. (2012). *The Human Cerebral Cortex*. London: Elsevier.

Peuskens, D., van Loon, J., van Calenbergh, F., *et al.* (2004). Anatomy of the anterior temporal lobe the frontotemporal region demonstrated by fiber dissection. *Neurosurgery*, **55**, 1174–84.

Pia, H. W. (1986). Microsurgery of gliomas. *Acta Neurochirurgica*, **80**, 1–11.

Quesada, V. Q. (2015). *Abordaje supracerebeloso transtentorial suprameatal a la totalidade de la región mediobasal del lóbulo temporal* (doctoral thesis). Valencia: Universitat de València Facultat de Medicina i Odontologia Departament de Cirurgia.

Quiñones-Hinojosa, A., Ojemann, S. G., Sanai, N., Dillon, W. P. & Berger, M. S. (2003). Preoperative correlation of intraoperative cortical mapping with magnetic resonance imaging landmarks to predict localization of the Broca area. *Journal of Neurosurgery*, **99**, 311–8.

Rasmussen, A. T. (1943). The extent of recurrent genicukicakcarine fibers (loop of Archambault and Meyer) as demonstrated by gross brain dissection. *The Anatomical Record*, **85**, 277–82.

Rasmussen, T. (1979). Cortical resection for medically refractory focal epilepsy: results, lessons and questions. In T. Rasmussen and R. Marino Jr., eds., *Functional Neurosurgery*. New York: Raven Press, pp. 253–69.

Rasmussen, T. (1991a). Surgery for central, parietal and occipital epilepsy. *Canadian Journal of Neurological Science*, **18**, 611–6.

Rasmussen, T. (1991b). Tailoring of cortical excisions for frontal lobe epilepsy. *Canadian Journal of Neurological Science*, **18**, 606–10.

Rasmussen, T. B. (1975). Surgical treatment of patients with complex partial seizures. In J. K. Penry and D. D. Daly, eds., *Advances in Neurology*. New York: Raven Press, Vol. XI, pp. 440–60 apud Hansebout, R. R. (1977). Surgery of epilepsy, current technique of cortical resection. In H. H. Schmidek and W. H. Sweet, eds., *Current Techniques in Operative Neurosurgery*. New York: Grune and Stratton, Ch 9, pp. 101–17.

Rasmussen, T. B. & Milner, B. (1975). Clinical and surgical studies of the cerebral speech areas in man. In K. J. Zulch, O. Creutzfeldt and G. C. Galbraith, eds., *Cerebral Localization*. New York: Springer-Verlag, pp. 238–57 apud Hansebout, R. R. (1982). Surgery of epilepsy, current technique of cortical resection. In H. H. Schmidek and W. H. Sweet, eds., *Operative Neurosurgical Techniques*. New York: Grune and Stratton, Vol. II, ch. 65, pp. 963–79.

Rasmussen, T. B. & Jasper, H. (1958). Temporal lobe epilepsy: indication for operation and surgical technique. In M. Baldwin and P. Beiley, eds., *Temporal Lobe Epilepsy*. Springfield, IL: Charles C. Thomas, pp. 440–60 apud Hansebout, R. R. (1977). Surgery of epilepsy, current technique of cortical resection. In H. H. Schmidek and W. H. Sweet, eds., *Current Techniques in Operative Neurosurgery*. New York: Grune and Stratton, ch. 9, pp. 101–17.

Régis, J., Mangin, J. F., Ochiai, T., *et al.* (2005). "Sulcal Root" generic model: a hypothesis to overcome the variability of the human cortex folding patterns. *Neurol Med Chir* (Tokyo), **45**, 1–17.

Reil, J. C. (1812). Nachträge zur anatomie des groβen und kleinen Gehirns. *Arch Physiol*, **11**, 345–76 apud Catani, M. & Schotten, M. T. (2012). Surface neuroanatomy. In *Atlas of Human Brain Connections*. New York: Oxford University Press, ch. 2, pp. 7–20.

Rhoton, A. L. Jr. (1999). General and micro-operative techniques. In J. R. Youmans, ed. *Neurological Surgery*, 4th edn. Philadelphia: WB Saunders, pp. 724–66.

Rhoton, A. L. Jr. (2003). Cranial anatomy and surgical approaches. *Neurosurgery*, **53**, 1–746.

Rhoton, A. L. Jr., Fujii, K. & Fradd, B. (1979). Microsurgical anatomy of the ante choroidal artery. *Surgical Neurology*, **12**, 171–87.

Ribas, G. C. (1991). Study of the anatomic relationships of the lambdoid, occipitomastoid and parietomastoid sutures with the transverse and sigmoid sinuses, and of regional burrholes sites [Portuguese] Doctoral thesis. São Paulo: University of São Paulo Medical School.

Ribas, G. C. (2005a). Comment of: Siwanuwatn, R., Deshmukh, P., Zabramski, J. M., Preul, M. C., Spetzler, R. F. Microsurgical anatomy and quantitative analysis of the transtemporal-transchoroidal fissure approach to the ambient cistern. *Neurosurgery*, **57**, ONS233–ONS234.

Ribas, G. C. (2005b). Surgical anatomy of microneurosurgical sulcal key-points [Portuguese] (thesis). São Paulo: University of São Paulo Medical School.

Ribas, G. C. (2006). Considerations about the nervous system phylogenetic evolution, behavior, and the emergence of consciousness [Portuguese]. *Revista Brasileira de Psiquiatria*, **28**, 326–38.

Ribas, G. C. (2007a). Neuroanatomical basis of behavior: history and recent contributions [Portuguese]. *Revista Brasileira de Psiquiatria*, **29**, 63–71.

Ribas, G. C. (2007b). The suprapetrosal craniotomy. *Journal of Neurosurgery*, **106**, 449–54.

Ribas, G. C. (2010). The cerebral sulci and gyri. *Neurosurgical Focus*, **28**(2), E2.

Ribas, G. C. (2015). Cerebral hemispheres. In S. Standring, ed., *Gray's Anatomy: The Anatomical Basis of Clinical Practice*, 41st edn. United Kingdom: Elsevier, ch. **25**, pp. 373–98.

Ribas, G. C. & Rodrigues, A. J. (2007). The suprapetrosalcraniotomy. *Journal of Neurosurgery*, **106**(3), 449–54.

Ribas, G. C., Rhoton A. L. Jr., Cruz, O. R. & Peace, D. (2005b). Suboccipital burr holes and craniotomies. *Neurosurgical Focus*, **19**, E1.

Ribas, G. C., Ribas, E. C. & Rodrigues, C. J. (2005a). The anterior Sylvian point and the suprasylvian operculum. *Neurosurgical Focus*, **18**(6), E1–E6.

Ribas, G. C., Yasuda, A., Ribas, E. C., Nishikuni, K. & Rodrigues Jr., A. J. (2006). Surgical anatomy of microneurosurgicalsulcal key points. *Neurosurgery*, **59**(4 Suppl 2), ONS177–ONS210.

Roberts, D. W., Hartov, A., Kennedy, F. E., Miga, M. I. & Aulsen, K. D. (1998). Intraoperative brain shift and deformation: a quantitative analysis of cortical displacement in 28 cases. *Neurosurgery*, **43**, 749–60.

Rolando, L. (1829.). *Della struttura degli emisferi cerebrali*. Turin: Memorie de Regia Accademia delle Scienze di Torino apud Türe, U., Yasargil, M. G., Friedman, A. H. & Al-Mefty, O. (2000). Fiber dissection technique: lateral aspect of the brain. *Neurosurgery*, **47**, 417–27.

Romer, A. S. (1970). *The Vertebrate Body*, 4th edn, Philadelphia: WB Saunders apud Sarnat, H. B. and Netsky, M. G. (1981). *Evolution of the Nervous System*, 2nd edn, New York: Oxford University Press.

Rowland, L. P. & Mettler, F. A. (1948). Relation between the coronal suture and cerebrum. *Journal of Comparative Neurology*, **89**, 21–40.

Rutten, G. J. M., Ramsey, N. F., Van Rijen, P. C., Noordmans, H. J. & Van Veelen, C. W. M. (2002). Development of a functional magnetic resonance imaging protocol for intraoperative localization of critical temporoparietal language areas. *Annals of Neurology*, **51**, 350–60.

Sachs, E. (1952) *The History and Development of Neurological Surgery*. New York: Paul B. Hoeber.

Sarnat, H. B. & Netsky, M. G. (1981). *Evolution of the Nervous System*, 2nd edn, New York: Oxford University Press.

Sarton, G. (1954). *Galen of Pergamon*. Lawrence: The University of Kansas Press.

Sartor, K. M. R. (1992). *Imaging of the Skull and Brain*. Berlin: Springer-Verlag.

Saunders, J. B. C. M. & O'Malley, C. D. (1950). *The Illustrations from the Works of Andreas Vesalius of Brussels*. Cleveland: World Publishing.

Schiffbauer, H., Berger, M. S., Ferrari, P., *et al.* (2002). Preoperative magnetic source imaging for brain tumor surgery: a quantitative comparison with intraoperative sensory and motor mapping. *Journal of Neurosurgery*, **97**, 1333–42.

Schiller, F. (1992). *Paul Broca, Explorer of the Brain*. New York: Oxford University Press.

Schneider, G. E. (1969). Two visual systems. *Science*, **163**, 895–902 apud Goodale, M. A. and Milner, D. (1992). Separate visual pathways for perception and action. *Tins*, **15**, 20–5.

Seeger, W. (1978). *Atlas of Topographical Anatomy of the Brain and Surrounding Structures*. Vienna: Springer.

Seeger, W. (1995). *Microsurgery of Intracranial Tumors*. Vienna: Springer-Verlag.

Shimizu, S., Tanriover, N., Rhoton, A. L. Jr., Yoshioka, N. & Fujii, K. (2005). MacCarty keyhole and inferior orbital fissure in orbitozygomatic craniotomy. *Neurosurgery*, **57**, 152–9.

Shucart, W. (1988). The anterior transcallosal and transcortical approaches. In M. J. Apuzzo, ed., *Surgery of the Third Ventricle*, 2nd edn. Baltimore: Williams & Wilkins, pp. 369–90.

Simos, P. G., Papanicolaou, A. C., Breier, J. I., *et al.* (1999). Localization of language-specific cortex by using magnetic source imaging and electrical stimulation mapping. *Journal of Neurosurgery*, **91**, 787–96.

Sincoff, E. H., Tan, Y. & Abdulrauf, S. I. (2004). White matter fiber dissection of the optic radiations of the temporal lobe and implications for surgical approaches to the temporal horn. *Journal of Neurosurgery*, **101**, 739–46.

Singer, C. (1952). *Vesalius on the Human Brain*. London: Oxford University Press.

Spencer, D. D., Spencer, S. S., Mattson, R. H., Williamson, P. D. & Novelly, R. A. (1984). Access to the posterior medial temporal lobe structures in the surgical treatment of temporal lobe epilepsy. *Neurosurgery*, **15**(5), 667–71.

Squire, L. R., Bloom, F. E., McConnell, S. K., *et al.* (2003). *Fundamental Neuroscience*, 2nd edn, Amsterdam: Academic Press.

Standring, S., ed., (2008). *Gray's Anatomy*, 40th edn, Spain: Churchill Livingstone Elsevier.

Steinmetz, H., Ebeling, U., Huang, Y. X. & Kahn, T. (1990). Sulcus topography of the parietal opercular region: an anatomic and MR study. *Brain & Language*, **38**(4), 515–33.

Steno, N. (1669). *Discours de Monsieur Stenon sur l'anatomie du cerveau* [Translated in Clarke, E. and O'Malley, C. D., eds. (1996). *The Human Brain and Spinal Cord: A Historical Study. Illustrated by Writings from Antiquity to the Twentieth Century*. San Francisco: Norman Publishing.]

Stone, J. L. (1991). Paul Broca and the first craniotomy based on cerebral localization. *Journal of Neurosurgery*, **75**, 154–9.

Sure, U., Alberti, O., Petermeyer, M., Becker, R. & Bertalanffy, H. (2000). Advanced image guided skull base surgery. *Surgical Neurology*, **53**, 563–72.

Sylvius, F. (1663). *Disputationes medicarum pars prima, primarias corporis humani functiones naturales ex anatomicis, praticis et chymicis experimentiis deductas complectens*. Amsterdam: J. Van den Berg apud Catani, M. & Schotten, M. T. (2012). Surface neuroanatomy. In *Atlas of Human Brain Connections*. New York: Oxford University Press, pp. 7–20.

Talairach, J. & Tornoux, P. (1993). *Referentially Oriented Cerebral MRI Anatomy*. New York: Thieme apud Yousry, T. A., Schmid, U. D., Alkadhi, H., *et al.* (1997). Localization of the motor hand area to a knob on the precentral gyrus a new landmark. *Brain*, **120**, 141–57.

Tamraz, J. C. & Comair, Y. G. (2000). *Atlas of Regional Anatomy of the Brain Using MRI: With Functional Correlations*. New York: Springer.

Taveras, J. M. & Wood, E. H. (1976). *Diagnostic Neuroradiology*, 2nd edn, Baltimore: Williams and Wilkins, Vol. 1.

Taylor, E. H. & Haughton, W. S. (1900). Some recent researches on the topography of the convolutions and fissures of the brain. *Transactions of the Royal Academy (Ireland)*, **18**, 511–9 apud Uematsu, S., Lesser, R., Fisher, R. S., *et al.* (1992). Motor and sensory cortex in humans: topography studied with chronic subdural stimulation. *Neurosurgery*, **31**, 59–72.

Testut, L. & Jacob, O. (1932). *Text of Topographic Anatomy* [in Spanish], 5th edn. Barcelona: Salvat.

Timurkaynak, E., Rhoton, A. L. Jr. & Barry, M. (1986). Microsurgical anatomy and operative approaches to the lateral ventricles. *Neurosurgery*, **19**, 685–723.

Tubbs, R. S., Loukas, M., Shoja, M. M. & Cohen-Gadol, A. A. (2010). Refined and simplified surgical landmarks for the MacCarty keyhole and orbitozygomatic craniotomy. *Neurosurgery*, **66**, 230–3.

Türe, U., Harput, M. V., Kaya, A. H., *et al.* (2012). The paramedian supracerebellar-transtentorial approach to the entire length of the mediobasal temporal region: an anatomical and clinical study. Laboratory investigation. *Journal of Neurosurgery*, **116**(4), 773–91.

Türe, U., Yasargil, D. C. H., Al-Mefty, O. & Yasargil, M. G. (1999). Topographic anatomy of the insular region. *Journal of Neurosurgery*, **90**, 730–3.

Türe, U., Yasargil, M. G., Friedman, A. H. & Al-Mefty, O. (2000). Fiber dissection technique: lateral aspect of the brain. *Neurosurgery*, **47**, 417–27.

Turner, W. (1866). *The Convolutions of the Human Cerebrum Topographically Considered*. Edinburgh: Maclachlan & Stewart apud Catani, M. & Schotten, M. T. (2012). Surface neuroanatomy. In *Atlas of Human Brain Connections*. New York: Oxford University Press, pp. 7–20.

Turner, W. (1873). Relations of the convolutions to the skull. In D. Ferrier, ed. (1876). *The Functions of the Brain*. London: Smith, Elder, p. 311 apud Greenblatt, S. H. (1997) Cerebral localization: from theory to practice. In S. H. Greenblatt, ed., *A History of Neurosurgery*. Park Ridge: American Association of Neurological Surgeons, pp. 137–52.

Uematsu, S., Lesser, R., Fisher, R. S., *et al.* (1992). Motor and sensory cortex in humans: topography studied with chronic subdural stimulation. *Neurosurgery*, **31**, 59–72.

Ungerleider, L. G. & Mishkin, M. (1982). Two cortical visual systems. In D. J. Ingle, M. A. Goodale, & R. J. W. Mansfield, eds., *Analysis of Visual Behaviour*. Cambridge, MA: MIT Press, 549–86 apud Goodale, M. A. and Milner, D. (1992). Separate visual pathways for perception and action. *Tins*, **15**, 20–5.

Unsgaard, G., Ommedal, S., Muller, T., Gronningsaeter, A. & Nagethus Hermes, T. A. (2002). Neuronavigation by intraoperative three-dimensional ultrasound: initial experience during brain tumor resection. *Neurosurgery*, **50**, 804–12.

Vajkoczy, P., Krakow, K., Stodieck, S., Pohlmann-Eden, B. & Schmiedek, P. (1998). Modified approach for the selective treatment of temporal lobe epilepsy: transsylvian-transcisternal mesial en bloc resection. *Journal of Neurosurgery*, **88**(5), 855–62.

Varolio, C. (1573). *De nervis opticis nonnullisque aliis, praeter communem opinionem in human capite observatis, epistolae*. Padua: Meitti. [Translated in Clarke, E. and O'Malley, C. D., eds. (1996). *The Human Brain and Spinal Cord: A Historical Study. Illustrated by Writings from Antiquity to the Twentieth Century*. San Francisco: Norman Publishing.]

Vesalius, A. (1543). *De humani corporis fabrica libri septem*. Basel: Oporinus apud Catani, M. & Schotten, M. T. (2012). Surface neuroanatomy. In *Atlas of Human Brain Connections*. New York: Oxford University Press, pp. 7–20.

Viale, G. L. & Turtas, S. (1980). The subchoroidal approaches to the third ventricle. *Surgery*, **14**, 71–6.

Vicq d'Azyr, F. (1786). *Traité d'anatomie et de physiologie*. Paris: Didot l'Aine [Translated in Clarke, E. and O'Malley, C. D., eds. (1996). *The Human Brain and Spinal Cord: A Historical Study. Illustrated by Writings from Antiquity to the Twentieth Century*. San Francisco: Norman Publishing.]

Vieussens, R. (1690). *Nevrographia universalis*. Frankfurt: Georgium Wilmelmum Künnium.

Vogt, C. & Vogt, O. (1926). Die vergleichend-architektonische und vergleichend-reizphysiologische Felderung der Grosshirnrinde unter besonderer Berücksichtigung der menschlichen. *Naturwissenschaften*, **14**, 119–94 apud Catani, M. & Schotten, M. T. (2012). Surface neuroanatomy. In *Atlas of Human Brain Connections*. New York: Oxford University Press, pp. 7–20.

Voigt, K. & Yasargil, M. G. (1976). Cerebral cavernous haemangiomas or cavernomas. Incidence, pathology, localization, diagnosis, clinical features and treatment. Review of the literature and report of an unusual case. *Neurochirurgia (Stuttg)*, **19**(2), 59–68.

von Economo, C. (1987). *Encephalitis Lethargica: Its Sequelae and Treatment*.Tucson, AZ: Books on Demand UMI.

von Economo, C. (2009). *Cellular Structure of the Human Cerebral Cortex* (Translated by L. C. Triarhou). Basel: Karger.

von Economo, C. & Koskinas, G. N. (1925). *Die Cytoarchitektonik der Hirnrinde des erwachsenen Menschen* apud Tamraz, J. C. and Comair, Y. G. (2000). *Atlas of Regional Anatomy of the Brain Using MRI: With Functional Correlations*. New York: Springer.

von Economo, C. & Koskinas, G. N. (1925). *Die Cytoarchitektonik der Hirnrinde des erwachsenen Menschen. Atlas mit 112 mikrophotographischen Tafeln*. Vienna: J. Springer apud Williams, P. L. and Warwick, R., eds. (1980). *Gray's Anatomy*. 36th edn, Philadelphia: WB Saunders.

Waldron, J. S. & Lawton, M. T. (2009). The supracarotid-infrafrontal approach: surgical technique and clinical application to cavernous malformations in the anteroinferior basal ganglia. *Neurosurgery*, **64**, 86–95.

Walsh, F. B. & Hoy, W. F. (1969). *Clinical Neuro-Ophthalmology*, 3rd edn, Baltimore: Williams & Wilkins, pp. 43–60.

Wang, F., Sun, T., Li, X. G. & Liu, N. J. (2008). Diffusion tensor tractography of the temporal stem on the inferior limiting sulcus. *Journal of Neurosurgery*, **108**, 775–81.

Watanabe, E., Watanabe, T., Manaka, S., Mayanagi, Y. & Takakura, K. (1987) Three-dimensional digitizer (neuronavigator): new equipment for computed tomography-guided stereotatic surgery. *Surgical Neurology*, **6**, 543–7.

Wen, H. T., Rhoton, A. L. Jr. & Marino, R. Jr. (2006). Gray matter overlying anterior basal temporal sulci as an intraoperative landmark for locating the temporal horn in amygdalohippocampectomies. *Neurosurgery*, **59**(4 Suppl 2), ONS221–ONS227.

Wen, H. T., Rhoton, A. L. Jr. & Oliveira, E. (1998). Transchoroidal approach to the third ventricle: an anatomic study of the choroidal fissure and its clinical application. *Neurosurgery*, **42**(6), 1205–17.

Wen, H. T., Rhoton, A. L. Jr., de Oliveira, E., *et al.* (1999). Microsurgical anatomy of the temporal lobe: Part 1: mesial temporal lobe anatomy and its vascular relationships as applied to amygdalohippocampectomy. *Neurosurgery*, **45**, 549–92.

Wernicke, C. (1874). *Der aphasische Symptomencomplex. Ein psychologische Studie auf anatomischer Basis*. Breslau: Cohn e Wigert apud Catani, M. & Schotten, M. T. (2012). Surface neuroanatomy. In *Atlas of Human Brain Connections*. New York: Oxford University Press, pp. 7–20.

Wiebe, S., Blume, W. T., Girvin, J. P. & Eliasziw, M. (2001). A randomized, controlled trial of surgery for temporal-lobe epilepsy. *New England Journal of Medicine*, **345**, 311–8.

Wieser, H. G. & Yasargil, M. G. (1982). Selective amygdalohippocampectomy as a surgical treatment of mesiobasal limbic epilepsy. *Surgical Neurology*, **17**(6), 445–57.

Williams, P. L. & Warwick, R., eds. (1980). *Gray's Anatomy*, 36th edn, Philadelphia: WB Saunders.

Wirtz, C. R., Bonsanto, M. M., Knauth, M., *et al.* (1997). Intraoperative MRI to update interactive navigation in neurosurgery: method and preliminary experience. *Computer Aided Surgery*, **2**, 172–9.

Witmer, B. P., Moftakhar, R., Hasan, K. M., *et al.* (2002). Diffusion-tensor imaging of white matter tracts in patients with cerebral neoplasm. *Journal of Neurosurgery*, **97**, 568–75.

Yamamoto, I., Rhoton, A. L. Jr. & Peace, D. (1981). Microsurgery of the third ventricle, microsurgical anatomy. *Neurosurgery*, **8**, 334–56.

Yasargil, M. G. (1984a). *Microneurosurgery*. Stuttgart: Georg Thieme, Vol. I.

Yasargil, M. G. (1984b). *Microneurosurgery*. Stuttgart: Georg Thieme, Vol. II.

Yasargil, M. G. (1987). *Microneurosurgery*. Stuttgart: Georg Thieme, Vol. IIIa.

Yasargil, M. G. (1988). *Microneurosurgery*. Stuttgart: Georg Thieme, Vol. IIIb.

Yasargil, M. G. (1994). *Microneurosurgery*. Stuttgart: Georg Thieme, Vol. IVa.

Yasargil, M. G. (1996). *Microneurosurgery*. Stuttgart: Georg Thieme, Vol. IVb.

Yasargil, M. G. (1999). Legacy of microneurosurgery: memoirs, lessons, and axioms. *Neurosurgery*, **45**, 1025–91.

Yasargil, M. G. (2005). Experiences and reflections about selective amygdalohippocampectomy. *Epileptologie*, **22**, 74–80.

Yasargil, M. G. & Abdulrauf, S. I. (2003). Comment of: Tirakotai, W., Sure, U., Benes, L., Krishek, B., Bien, S. & Bertalanffy, H Image-guided transsylvian, transinsular approach for insular cavernous angiomas. *Neurosurgery*, **53**, 1299–305.

Yasargil, M. G., Cravens, G. F. & Roth, P. (1988a). Surgical approaches to "inaccessible" brain tumors. *Clinical Neurosurgery*, **34**, 42–110.

Yasargil, M. G., Fox, J. L. & Ray, M. W. (1975). The operative approach to aneurysms of the anterior communicating artery. In H. Krayenbül, ed., *Advances and Technical Standards in Neurosurgery*. Vienna: Springer-Verlag, pp. 114–70.

Yasargil, M. G., Kasdaglis, K., Jain, K. K. & Weber, H. P. (1976). Anatomical observations of the subarachnoid cisterns of the brain during surgery. *Journal of Neurosurgery*, **44**, 298–302.

Yasargil, M. G., Krisht, A. F., Türe, U., Al-Mefty, O. & Yasargil, D. C. H. (2002c). Microsurgery of insular gliomas: Part VI: surgical treatment and outcome. *Contemporary Neurosurgery*, **24**, 1–8.

Yasargil, M. G., Krisht, A. F., Türe, U., Al-Mefty, O. & Yasargil, D. C. H. (2002a). Microsurgery of insular gliomas: Part I: surgical anatomy of the Sylvian cistern. *Contemporary Neurosurgery*, **24** (11), 1–8.

Yasargil, M. G., Krisht, A. F., Türe, U., Al-Mefty, O. & Yasargil, D. C. H. (2002b). Microsurgery of insular gliomas: Part II: opening of the Sylvian fissure. *Contemporary Neurosurgery*, **24**(12), 1–5.

Yasargil, M. G., Teddy, P. J. & Roth, P. (1985). Selective amygdalohippocampectomy. Operative anatomy and surgical technique. *Advances and Technical Standards in Neurosurgery*, **12**, 93–123.

Yasargil, M. G., Türe, U. & Roth, P. (1988b). A combined approach. In M. J. Apuzzo, ed., *Surgery of the Third Ventricle*, 2nd edn. Baltimore: Williams and Wilkins, pp. 541–52.

Yasargil, M. G., Türe, U. & Yasargil, D. H. C. (2004). Impact of temporal lobe surgery. *Journal of Neurosurgery*, **101**, 725–38.

Yonekawa, Y., Imhof, H. G., Taub, E., *et al.* (2001). Supracerebellartranstentorial approach to posterior temporomedial structures. *Journal of Neurosurgery*, **94**(2), 339–45.

Yousry, T. A., Schmid, U. D., Alkadhi, H., *et al.* (1997). Localization of the motor hand area to a knob on the precentral gyrus: a new landmark. *Brain*, **120**, 141–57.

Yousry, T. A., Schmid, U. D., Jassoy, A. G., *et al.* (1995). Topography of the cortical motor hand area: prospective study with functional MR imaging and direct motor mapping at surgery. *Radiology*, **195**, 23–9.

Index

Please note that page references to Figures will be in *italics*; those representing Tables will be in **bold**

Printed by Integrated Books International,
United States of America